What Physicians and Authors Are Saying about *Miracle Moms* and the Wurn Technique^{SM}

Your work is a Godsend. Thank you for providing women all over the world with such a safe, natural, and effective therapy to enhance fertility and pelvic health.

– Dr. Christiane Northrup, MD, Ob/Gyn physician,
NYTimes best selling author of "Women's Bodies, Women's Wisdom", "Mother-Daughter Wisdom" and "The Wisdom of Menopause"

Miracle Moms reads like a novel, rich in information about how the body works, and why the therapy may benefit some people. This informative book is well documented and illustrated. The use of patient narratives makes the therapy more understandable for health professionals and potential patients.

– Dr. Lisa Conboy, Doctor of Science,
Instructor in Medicine, Harvard Medical School

Women who suffer from chronic pelvic pain will benefit greatly by reading this book, not only from the hope it exudes, but from the therapy it describes.

- Dr. Howard T. Sharp, Ob/Gyn physician,
President, International Pelvic Pain Society,
Director, University of Utah Pelvic Pain Center,
Vice Chair, Department of Obstetrics and Gynecology,
University of Utah School of Medicine

What a much-needed, useful and safe way to deal with the common, yet mystifying problem of adhesions. I am excited to see that you have studied and perfected a technique to treat adhesions, with years of experience, scientific 'backup' and case studies to prove it.

This technique makes sense: to put 'hands on' the problem and nurture the body's innate desire to heal from pelvic pain, hormonal imbalance, endometriosis, infertility, and related dysfunction. Read this book if you suffer from pelvic or digestive disorders, or if you are a doctor who sees patients with these problems.

- Dr. Leslie Mendoza Temple, Family Practice and Integrative Medicine MD, Medical Director, Integrative Medicine NorthShore Univ. Health System , Asst. Professor, Northwestern University, Feinberg School of Medicine

With clear explanations, research studies and patient narratives, this book brings a formerly "taboo" topic front and center, opening the door for greater healing and quality of life. *Miracle Moms, Better Sex, Less Pain* will bring awareness and hope to legions of women suffering from pelvic pain and infertility disorders. I recommend this to both patients and women's health specialists alike.

–Dr. Melinda Ring, Internal Medicine and Integrative Medicine Physician, Medical Director, Center for Integrative Medicine and Wellness, Northwestern Memorial Physicians Group, Asst. Professor, Northwestern University, Feinberg School of Medicine

After reading *Miracle Moms, Better Sex, Less Pain:The Clear Passage Story,* I have been instructed by Belinda and Larry Wurn. Their work in women's health is exciting, exhilarating, ground breaking, and amazing.

The 'Wurn Technique' in my professional opinion, is a blockbuster breakthrough both for physicians and women who have known for so long that there was something better out there for treatment of infertility, painful intercourse, sexual dysfunction, endometriosis, and chronic pelvic pain. Their approach highlights that which ought to be basic to medical care and treatment; believing and listening to the patient, and applying "hands on healing" with compassion and genuine concern.

The Wurns have published their work showing significant improvement in areas of infertility caused by endometriosis, fallopian tube occlusion, and hydrosalpinx. Their studies also document improvement in all areas of sexual function including desire, arousal/lubrication, orgasm/satisfaction and pain. I know of no other single therapy reported to increase all areas of sexual function. I am truly excited to learn about (this) therapy.

–Dr. Scott Miles, Gynecology and Sexology Physician, Medical Director, Miles Ahead Health and Wellness, Indianapolis, IN

As a gynecological surgeon I have seen first hand what happens after I operate on patients. As much as I try to prevent adhesions, I know that most patients after surgery are going to develop some form of adhesive disease. In the past treatment for adhesions has been even more surgery which caused even more adhesions. Now with the amazing "Clear Passage" technique patients have a safe and effective alternative to surgery. .. I know it does work and recommend it to all my patients with adhesive disease.

– Dr. Jacques Moritz, Ob/Gyn physician, Director of Endoscopy Section and Division of Gynecology St. Luke's-Roosevelt Hospital Center,
Asst. Professor of Obstetrics and Gynecology
Columbia University College of Physicians and Surgeons

It's about time! I've been waiting so long for Larry and Belinda Wurn to bring their magnificent healing modality to print. Over the many years I have known Larry, we have shared many patients who had previously been told that they would never conceive naturally, had complete tubal obstruction, scarring or intractable pelvic pain. I have seen their work help all of these conditions, and more.

Their therapy is beyond surgical intervention; it taps right into the body's inherent healing capacity.

The Wurns are revolutionizing women's health. Tried and proven, documented and studied again and again – the proof is in the results. There are children alive today who wouldn't be here without Clear Passage Therapies. I support and applaud this work.

– Dr. Randine Lewis, L.Ac. Ph. D. in Alternative Medicine
Founder, The Fertile Soul,
Author of "The Infertility Cure" and "The Way of the Fertile Soul"

The love story of Belinda and Larry Wurn, and the birth of the stunning Wurn Technique reveals beyond any doubt, that when we approach the body with reverence, intelligence and a desire to reduce suffering, we can repair what the most sophisticated technologies fail to fix. Read it and learn what a pair of skilled, listening hands can do.

– Julia Indichova, Director, Fertile Heart Studio,
Author of "Inconceivable" and "The Fertile Female"

What a remarkable book! It is so wonderful that this natural therapy has been so effective treating female infertility, without surgery or drugs.

I don't know which is more amazing: the adventure of discovering the treatment, the published medical studies, or the dozens of *Miracle Moms* who shared their stories of success with this 100% natural therapy.

– *Gilli Moorhawk Author of "Miracle Babies,"* and *"Meditations and Positive Thoughts for Pregnancy & Birth"*

Clear Passage Therapy is remarkable because it is the only therapy empirically shown to improve all four classical phases of female sexual function --- arousal, lubrication, orgasm, and satisfaction, as well as the current gremlins, "low desire" and "pain on intercourse".

And it does this, amazingly, without the negative side effects and multiple risks of treatments like surgery or drugs.

Unique among "hands-on" therapies, the Wurns have a solid understanding of, and they evidence experience with, "The G-Spot." Too many other hands-on therapists are, sadly, still looking for it! This is no place for the timid or faint of heart. This book shows how they do it.

– *Dr. John D. Perry, Ph. D. Psychologist, Author of "The G Spot"*

As a Fertility and IVF specialist, I am always looking for new options to improve success. Any therapy that helps restore natural pelvic organ function will help increase and preserve fertility. The "Wurn Technique" seems to do just that, as I have seen patients benefit from this treatment. This natural adjunct to traditional medicine and surgery makes sense.

– *Dr. Mark Kan, Ob/Gyn, IVF and Reproductive Medicine Physician, Newport Beach, CA*

Adhesions are a major problem for women with endometriosis, causing pain which can continue for decades, sexual and bowel function problems, difficulty with exercise and other movement. Previously, only surgery was available, which in itself could lead to more adhesions. This book will bring new hope to many women now suffering."

– *Dr. Mary Lou Ballweg, Ph.D., Co-founder, President, Executive Director, Endometriosis Association*

Patients Speak

After all the drugs, the painful, unnecessary surgeries and treatments, it was a natural, drug-free treatment that finally enabled me to become a mother.

– Madison, mother of two after multiple unsuccessful surgeries and IVF

By the end of the week, intercourse pain was completely gone – it was amazing.

– Katrina, who experienced severe pain after numerous surgeries

I became pregnant again naturally, six years after therapy! I am amazed that the positive results of the therapy lasted all that time.

– Roxanne, mother of two after two blocked fallopian tubes

In the months following therapy, I discovered I had an entire new body, which was flexible, strong, and ready to get back to work!

– Kelly, who experienced chronic pain after sexual abuse

Their therapy gave me hope and that's something I have not had in a long time.

– Autumn whose blocked tubes opened naturally after treatment

The headaches I have had daily for over three years are completely gone now!

– Michael, who experienced chronic pain and headaches after a severe work injury

I am so happy I decided to return to CPT. I could have gone through years of invasive treatment. Instead, I went to them and because of their hands, I got pregnant almost instantly!

– Jacqueline, mother of one after only remaining fallopian tube was blocked with hydrosalpinx

After CPT, I experienced a great reduction in intercourse pain. I had always thought the pain I experienced with intercourse was normal.

– Sydney, mother of two who struggled with infertility and chronic pain

I believe anyone with pregnancy issues should consider this therapy prior to trying to conceive.
– Savannah, mother of one after ectopic pregnancy

Before long, I stopped experiencing pain in my bowels, neck, and back. Things in life that most people take for granted, but that had been denied to me for so long slowly began to return.
– Ginny, who experienced chronic pain and bowel obstructions

I became pregnant naturally! After years of emotionally and physically taxing treatments – it was a natural, non-invasive treatment that enabled me to get pregnant. If we had known about CPT prior to everything we did, we would have saved ourselves a lot of time, money, and emotionally taxing years.
–Andie, mother of one after fourteen unsuccessful IUIs

I made more progress healing my body in five days at CPT than I had experienced in the past 12 years!
– Marcella, who experienced severe pelvic pain

I know they helped improve my hormones because after just a few days of their therapy, my period has returned!
– Chloe, mother of one at age 42 after being denied IVF due to hormonal levels

My last day of therapy was the first day of my period. Immediately, I felt a difference. All of my abdominal pain was gone without a trace! The therapy was totally worth doing to relieve my pain.
– Neveah, currently expecting after struggling with endometriosis pain and infertility

It is amazing to both of us that after all the drugs, all the surgeries, all the failed medical attempts, these two beautiful children came to us without surgery or drugs.
–Tamás and Bianka, parents of two after 3 unsuccessful IVFs and PCOS

It's been over six months since treatment now, and my libido and desire are still increasing. My husband and I have been having sex more often and I am still amazed at the difference. Another amazing outcome was that I no longer experienced pain from my endometriosis.

– Emily, currently expecting after struggling with intercourse pain, endometriosis, and infertility

We are convinced totally that miracles can happen and that Clear Passage was the open door to help it along – especially now because I just gave birth to a second baby girl!

– Dana, mother of two after two prior miscarriages

I wish I had known a treatment like this existed long before I had so many surgeries.

– Teena, who experienced relief after years of bowel obstructions and surgeries

They not only helped me conceive my daughter, but also conceive again naturally – I'm eleven weeks pregnant! They truly changed my life!

– Jennifer, mother of one and currently expecting after seven years of unexplained infertility

My pain decreased precipitously during my menstrual cycle. In fact, I didn't even know I had started my period until I saw it!

– Danielle, mother of one after struggling with endometriosis pain and infertility

They rejuvenated my body and prepared it for the greatest natural miracle.

– Nicole, mother of one after multiple unsuccessful IVFs

The first thing that happened following therapy is that the endometriosis pain I had lived with for over ten years completely disappeared.

– Ava, mother of one after struggling with endometriosis pain and infertility

This manual physical therapy does much more than just massage . . . it gives us hope, and in my case, a beautiful daughter despite years of infertility.

– Paulina, mother of one after unsuccessful IUIs and IVF

Miracle Moms, Better Sex, Less Pain

A remarkable journey in "hands-on" healing from infertility, pain, sexual dysfunction and adhesions

Authors:

Belinda Wurn, PT

Larry Wurn, LMT

Richard King, MD

Editors:

Jackie Schuld

Amy Parker

Mary L Dennis

Printed in the United States of America

Med-Arts Press
PO Box 358692
Gainesville, FL 32635

www.medartpress.com

ISBN-13: 978-0-9811868-0-1

Library of Congress control number:

2009921589

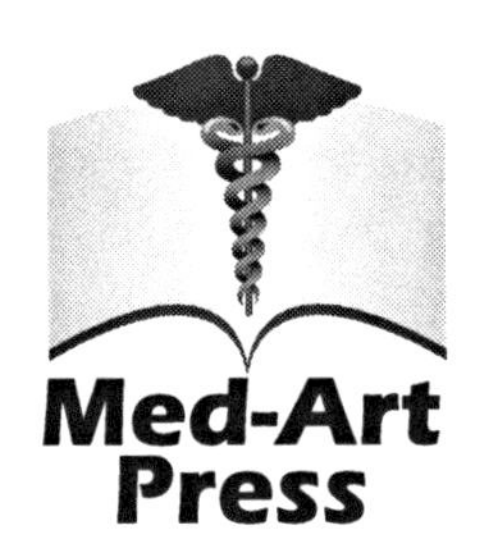

Miracle Moms Better Sex Less Pain

A remarkable journey in "hands-on" healing from infertility, pain, sexual dysfunction and adhesions

The Clear Passage Story

Eighty individual patient narratives

Belinda Wurn, PT
Larry Wurn, LMT
with Richard King, MD

Foreword by *NY Times* bestselling author Christiane Northrup, MD

Dedication

This book is dedicated to the patients, physicians, and co-workers who encouraged our ongoing clinical and scientific inquiry. You have helped make the last two decades of our lives a remarkable adventure.

The seeds we planted together have grown into fields of returned function and fufilled dreams. Many of the results that developed from our efforts are new to this world. We know that more discoveries will likely develop from our work, and will continue to unfold with each passing year.

Acknowledgments

Many talented hands went into the creation of this book. The authors are thankful that so many talented women chose to participate. We wish to especially thank the following for their contributions which went above and beyond in their assistance to us. They were all professionals, team players, and lovely people with whom to work.

Editors

Our Principal Editor was Jackie Schuld (www.focusonfoundations.com). Jackie believes that a great non-fiction literary work must begin with a strong foundation, built on truth, substance and structure. Point in fact, Jackie is not only a fine writer, she is an extraordinary organizer. Jackie interviewed most of the patients whose stories appear in this book, then distilled and edited many heartbreaking and heartwarming stories into manageable prose, including both the hard facts and the often strong emotional elements the patients wanted to convey. She then worked tirelessly with Larry to coordinate the 80 patient stories, published studies, artwork, and medical and theoretical text to create what we hope is a whole entity. The entire team is greatly indebted to Jackie's powerful mind, focus and efforts.

Mary L. Dennis (www.maryldennis.com) provided valuable assistance with the text. She was timely, professional and incredibly picky in making sure the text, case and syntax were always grammatically correct – not an easy task with this complex manuscript. In addition, the authors would like to thank Amy Parker, Jacqueline Wurn and Eugenia Scharf, PhD, for their editorial and conceptual design assistance.

Illustrators and Graphic Artists

Several illustrators and graphic artists provided valuable skills to help create this book. The two main illustrators for this book were Florida artist Lisa Ibarra-Rivera, who created the detailed medical drawings of adhesions and organs, and British illustrator Joanna Culley (www.medical-artist.com) who created about 60 specific illustrations of adhesions, techniques, and a variety of other drawings we asked her to create. Joanna and Lisa are both extraordinary artists who worked well in the team setting we required. Maria Rachwal created the lovely drawing of the ancient Egyptian method of determining fertility, along with several others that will likely appear in another book we plan to produce. Gainesville, Florida artist Leslie Vega (leslievegadesign.com) did a wonderful job creating the front cover.

Book Designer

When the text and illustrations were finally ready to prepare for press, we chose Canadian graphics artist Gisele Malenfant (www.timelessdigital.org). We could not have been more pleased. Gisele's artistry, timeliness, sensitivity and attention to detail are reflected in every page of this book. The lovely page layouts, spine and back cover are all Gisele's handiwork.

Table of Contents

Foreword

Christiane Northrup, MD

Like all conventionally trained physicians, I was taught to use drugs and surgery as the primary approaches to women's health problems such as infertility, pelvic pain, bleeding, menstrual cramps, and so on. And though these treatments have their place, all too often there are untoward side effects to common procedures such as episiotomy, hysterectomy, ovarian cyst removal, and Cesarean section that leave women with pelvic pain, infertility, digestive problems, and sexual dysfunction. Synthetic hormones such as birth control pills or even antidepressant medications are then prescribed to help women cope with these symptoms. But these too often have their own side effects. The end result is that countless women end up with chronic pain and dysfunction following common pelvic surgeries and procedures of all kinds.

Having spent many years on the frontlines of women's health, I have always known that there had to be better ways to treat women's bodies than simply drugs and surgery. This is why I have spent the majority of my career searching for non-toxic, safe, and natural ways to help women maintain or restore their pelvic and sexual health. Most of these methods, such as nutrition, meditation, and acupuncture, were considered heresy when I began my career back in the 1970's. Now holistic medicine has become much more mainstream, much to my surprise and delight.

One of the truly revolutionary and effective modalities that I discovered along the way is the manual therapy developed by Belinda and Larry Wurn known as "Clear Passage." Clear Passage is the term they use for the refinements in manual therapy they developed as physical and massage therapists who have helped thousands of people resolve chronic pain, infertility, and sexual dysfunction. Most of these symptoms are caused by adhesions—scar tissue that results from infection or simply from the process of surgical healing. Clear Passage helps break up these adhesions to restore normal function to nerves and organs.

Of course hands-on healing is nothing new. From the ancient time of Hippocrates, manual therapy in the form of treatments such as massage has been a standard part of the healing arts. Massage therapy and other manual therapies such as classical osteopathy have very well-documented benefits such as decreased pain, enhanced relaxation, and better immunity. But the Clear Passage therapy developed by the Wurns is more than just massage. It is a very systematic approach that not only decreases pain, but has also been shown to open up scarred fallopian tubes, improve pregnancy rates in women undergoing assisted reproductive technologies, enhance sexual function, and even reverse small bowel obstructions. Not bad for a perfectly safe, non-invasive technique!

I am always interested in the origins of a particular therapy because the history of something says a great deal about the healing intent behind it. Clear Passage grew out of Belinda Wurn's personal experience with the aftermath of cervical cancer surgery and radiation treatment—both of which left her with chronic pelvic pain and sexual dysfunction—conditions I've seen repeatedly in my own practice. After exhausting all the usual allopathic approaches, the Wurns turned to manual therapy, researching and working with various modalities and practitioners from all over the world. Belinda's health was restored with this approach—and it wasn't long before this husband and wife team began bringing their newfound manual therapy skills to others in their practice—with the amazing and heartening results you will read about in these pages.

But the Wurns have also provided another invaluable service. They have documented and published their work in a series of peer-reviewed scientific articles, thus building a bridge between more conventional approach es and the ancient but updated manual therapies. Moreover, they have trained many others in the Clear Passage techniques so that more people can benefit from their pioneering approach.

I thank the Wurns from the bottom of my heart for the gift of healing that their work represents. It is my sincere hope that, through the information in this book, people all over the world will realize that manual therapy is a proven healing modality that can help on so many levels—with no side effects whatsoever. More importantly, I dream of a time when treatments such as Clear Passage will be the standard of care for restoring and maintaining health, long before drugs and surgery are ever required.

Christiane Northrup, M.D. FACOG

Author of: *Women's Bodies, Women's Wisdom (Bantam 2006)*
The Wisdom of Menopause (Bantam 2006)
Mother Daughter -Wisdom (Bantam 2005)

How to Read this Book

There are several ways to read this book. If you read it from beginning to end, you can trace the discovery of a manual physical therapy that is very effective in treating adhesions and chronic pain in men and in women, and its subsequent development into an effective treatment for female infertility and sexual dysfunction.

If you prefer to go directly to your area of specific interest, we suggest you first read Section One. That portion of the book will provide the foundation for how a hands-on therapy can help repair tissues and return the body to a state of pain-free function despite decades of pain or dysfunction – including several types of female infertility. There you will read about the mechanics of the body, its mobility, and its function. You will also read about adhesions, why they exist in virtually all people, and the role they play in so many cases of unexplained pain and dysfunction.

Should you encounter unfamiliar words, concepts, or procedures, you may find help in the glossary at the end of the book.

Authors' Note

Patient Stories

When we compiled the patient stories in this book, it was very important to us to provide first-hand accounts. We are honored that so many of our patients wanted to share their stories with our readers.

Most patient stories were written in the first person by patients who wanted to pen their own stories. Others wanted to share their stories, but asked us to write them. Editor Jackie Schuld wrote these stories after interviewing patients or reviewing patient histories and charts. Then we had each patient check them for accuracy before including them in the book.

In a few (very old) stories, we recreated patient histories based on patients' charts and interviews with the treating therapists. All patients were assigned a pseudonym unless they specifically requested we use their real name.

Medical Disclaimer

This book is designed to support, not replace, the relationship that exists between a patient and his/her physician, and the information herein is not intended to replace the services of a physician. Information contained herein is provided for informational purposes only and is not a substitute for professional medical advice. This book contains fact, theory, and professional and personal assumptions and conclusions. You should not use the information in this book for diagnosing or treating a medical or health condition. You should consult a physician in all matters regarding your health, and particularly with respect to any symptoms that may require diagnosis or medical attention.

Non-invasive Therapy and The Hippocratic Oath

In the 5th century BC, the Greek philosopher Hippocrates began to create the principles for modern medicine. Even today, all US physicians are required to take and abide by the Hippocratic Oath before they are granted a license to treat patients. The guiding principal of the Hippocratic Oath is "Above all, do no harm." This principle is meant to guide and direct all phases of medicine and all diagnoses, from a broken bone to the most complex medical condition.

In essence, the Hippocratic Oath directs all physicians and healthcare professionals to first take the most conservative, risk-free course in treating any medical condition. In general practice, this translates to using a conservative therapy before drugs, and using drugs before surgery. After 2,500 years, it remains a guiding principle for the sequence of care that physicians and patients should choose.

Seeking Treatment via Manual Therapy

We encourage anyone who is seeking manual therapy for any condition to first obtain a referral from her/his physician, clearing her/him for any contraindication to therapy. Manual therapy to abdominal and pelvic organs can contain significant risks for certain conditions.

Before seeking treatment, make sure your therapist has advanced training and knowledge of anatomy, pathology, and contraindications to treating the areas where s/he will treat. At a minimum, you should obtain from your practitioner

- Contraindications to her/his therapy, and
- Proof of certification or advanced training if the therapist will be treating in the pelvis or abdomen.

Preface

Belinda Wurn, PT

> People who say "it cannot be done" should not interrupt those who are doing it.
>
> *- George Bernard Shaw*

> The body has the ability to adapt to minor stresses, but as you increase the number, the body has less room to adapt until you reach a point where the body cannot adapt any further.
>
> *- Gerald H. Smith, DDS.*

> The magic is not in the medicine but in the patient's body — in the recuperative or self-corrective energy of nature. What the treatment does is to stimulate natural functions or to remove what hinders them.
>
> *- Miracles, C. S. Lewis, 1940*

> ... primum no nocere (first do no harm) ...
>
> *- from the Hippocratic Oath*

It has been 35 years since I entered the pre-medical program at the University of Florida. As I began to better understand how my life would be as a physician, I began to feel that there might be a better opportunity for me to help the people I wanted to serve in the health care arena. Simply said, my heart was telling me that I wanted to be more "hands-on" with patients, helping relieve pain, and getting people back to active, functional lives after they had undergone a trauma or other debilitating incident.

My advisor was shocked that I would leave pre-med (I was top of my class and made the President's and Dean's List every semester), but I transferred into the Physical Therapy program. In the 35 years since that time, I have never regretted that decision.

While I never lost my love for medicine and my faith in physicians, I was to find that faith tested personally in ways I could never have imagined.

Nine years after becoming a physical therapist, I was diagnosed with cervical cancer. It was scary to have physicians cut away part of my delicate vaginal tissues and cervix to stop me from hemorrhaging. I attended the University of Florida's Medical Center for 40 external radiation treatments over a period of eight weeks. Physicians then inserted radioactive implants the full depth of my uterus and beside the tumor in my cervix. Then they asked me to lie in one position without moving for 72 hours in a lead-lined room. I had to do this twice, two weeks apart. That's when I understood first-hand that modern medicine could sometimes be brutal. No visitor was allowed to stay in my room for more than five minutes for fear of exposing them to the radiation that was placed deep inside of me — yet I was confined in that leaden sarcophagus for three solid days, twice. At that point, I experienced modern medicine at its most barbaric, insensitive, and draconian.

Before long, I was unable to work or even move without pain.

Six months after the treatment, I began experiencing debilitating pain in my pelvis, low back, and coccyx. Before long, I was unable to work or even move without pain. I had to quit my job. Eventually, my life became a quest and search for relief from constant pelvic, back, and coccyx pain.

My husband, Larry, and I first sought effective treatment in our home town, Gainesville, Florida — the site of the University of Florida's highly respected medical school. Gainesville is a small city with several thousand physicians and a dozen physical therapy groups. In this lofty setting, we expected to find relief from the pain I was experiencing and an answer to our prayers, but relief was not to be found.

We then began searching for relief in other settings. After attending many manual therapy courses taught by other respected physical therapists and osteopathic physicians, and also being treated by them, I slowly began to experience relief from my back and pelvic pain for the first time in years. Larry began studying with the same therapists and osteopaths as I had. He used and refined techniques we had learned, and we developed new ones to resolve the pain in my pelvis, back, and tailbone, as well as neck pain from a disc herniation and a failed cervical fusion. As we developed a therapy protocol that was to become our life work, the relief from debilitating chronic pain I experienced was like finding an oasis in the desert.

After two years of therapy, I was finally able to consider going back to work, but my life had changed. I told Larry, "I would like to open a clinic for people who have problems like I had. I'd like to treat people with chronic, complex pain symptoms in an atmosphere that is relaxed, friendly, and healing, as well as professional. I'd like it to be beautiful, warm, and nurturing to the soul, and effective for the body."

Larry and I developed the Wurn Technique® as a compassionate but effective way to address the adhesions that formed as my body's response to the trauma I endured from my medical cure.

Now, 20 years after the traumatic event that started us on this road, we have come a long way, but we feel we have only opened the door. My life turned dramatically and indelibly the day that I learned that I had cervical cancer in 1984, and I feel there was a reason that God or fate placed that obstacle in my path.

As I look back at the incredible journey we have taken, I remember the patients who put their faith in us when they had no more reason to hope that there would be an answer to their prayers. I am pleased that most of them left us with decreased pain and increased function, but also having known that they were loved, nurtured, listened to, cared for deeply, and assisted and supported in reaching their own physical and spiritual goals. Larry and I have found that it is only by studying intensely, listening deeply, and treating others with compassion and faith (as we ourselves would like to be treated) that we can help them achieve their goals.

The purpose of this book is to provide a theoretical foundation, an awareness and understanding of the underlying principles and context of our therapy, and a level of confidence in this new therapy. Through real-life stories, this book provides the rationale for the manual techniques we have learned, synthesized, refined, and developed over the past 20 years. We will share with you individual stories and clinical experiences of many of our patients. The techniques are very effective in treating chronic and adhesion-based pain, female sexual dysfunction, and many cases of female infertility. In fact, they appear to help many heretofore unexplained or confusing conditions.

The Wurn Technique® practiced at Clear Passage Therapies® clinics is a unique and eclectic soft tissue therapy focused on restoring balance and mobility to the entire body, with a special focus on abdominopelvic and neighboring structures and tissues. We developed it after extensive study with some of the finest, most dedicated osteopathic and physical therapy clinicians in the world. Their teachings and treatment philosophies started us on a path, a journey that has led us through more than 50,000 treatment hours to date (2009). We have published several studies and citations in highly respected peer-reviewed medical journals. Over the years we developed and refined our treatment protocol, we were granted US patent protection for the Wurn Technique®.

We would like to acknowledge some of the outstanding clinicians who went before us. Their pioneering discoveries in the field of musculoskeletal mechanics and soft tissue therapy guided us to develop a treatment protocol focused on the needs of our unique patient population.

We would especially like to acknowledge John Barnes, PT, for his development of Myofascial Release. John introduced the concept of sustained release to address dysfunctions in the fascial system that is basic to much of our therapy. We would also like to acknowledge Jean-Pierre Barral, DO, for developing Visceral and Urogenital Manipulation, showing the interrelationship of structure and function among the organs in the pelvic and abdominal cavities. Frank Lowen, LMT, and Gail Wetzler, PT, refined Dr. Barral's Visceral Manipulation techniques; Sharon Weiselfish, PhD, PT, refined Fred Mitchell, DO's muscle energy techniques for the pelvis, sacrum and extremities. Janet Travel, MD, physician to John F. Kennedy, was formative in exploring and researching myofascial trigger points and their significance in myofascial pain syndromes (MPS). John Upledger, DO, developed Craniosacral Therapy to treat the dura mater, the environment of the central nervous system. Paul Chauffour, DO, developed the Mechanical Link approach to reduce structural tensions within the fascial system. There were many others, too numerous to mention here.

We took knowledge, thoughts, and ideas from each of these pioneers, and then modified, refined, refocused, and added to them techniques we developed to serve the needs of patients with infertility and abdominopelvic pain and dysfunction. This is a population who has heretofore not been addressed in any systematic manner by non-surgical or non-pharmaceutical techniques.

Our approach is unique in its effectiveness with this patient population. We apply our techniques to treat numerous diagnoses including abdominopelvic adhesions, endometriosis pain, female infertility, sexual dysfunction, and many other disorders. Most of our patients and therapists find it is effective for treating pain and mechanical dysfunction anywhere in the body. We feel very honored that we have become a part of returning true healing to modern healthcare.

We wish you the best on your own journey. Our suggestion to you is:

> **Create your vision, and step into it, with clarity and assurance that you will achieve your goal, one step at a time.**
> *- Belinda Wurn, PT*

Introduction

Richard King, MD

In the early 1990s I was working as the Chief of Staff at North Florida Regional Hospital in Gainesville, Florida. During this time, Belinda Wurn, a local physical therapist, and her husband, Larry, a massage therapist, approached me with preliminary results of their success treating tubal infertility cases. They told me that they had opened totally occluded (blocked) fallopian tubes with a manual physical therapy they were developing, and that women were achieving pregnancy.

I was initially quite skeptical when they came to me with their results. As a gynecologist and surgeon with more than twenty-five years of experience at the time, I knew that surgery to open occluded tubes had low success rates; it was hard for me to imagine that a nonsurgical procedure could have any effect at all.

My first question to the Wurns was, "How are you accessing the tubes?" On average, fallopian tubes are less than a centimeter in diameter near the ovaries, as small as one millimeter in diameter as they enter the uterus, and only about 10 centimeters (four inches) in length. They lie deep within the pelvis, between the endometrial and peritoneal cavities. Surgery on the fallopian tubes requires delicate micro techniques under magnification.

The Wurns first expressed to me how all of their cases shared a common history of confirmed or suspected abdominopelvic adhesions. Then they described how they palpated bi-manually (internally and externally) the soft tissues (viscera and fascia) in the abdominopelvic regions for restricted mobility. When they located any area with adhered or restricted mobility, they would use their manual techniques to apply specific forces to the adhered tissues until the cross-links (which are the building blocks of adhesions) dissipated. Instead of cutting or burning an adhesion as a surgeon might do, they peeled it apart like opening the run in a sweater.

They told me that they had originally discovered this could open blocked fallopian tubes by accident while working on a patient who developed severe abdominal and pelvic adhesions after a slip and fall. They had used the same techniques that they were creating to resolve Belinda's chronic pain and dysfunction after surgery and radiation therapy for cervical cancer. Yet, this patient later called to say that she was pregnant. She was very shocked because her physician had diagnosed her with blocked tubes seven years earlier and she had never been pregnant — that is, until she received the Wurns' therapy.

Before coming to me, the Wurns had paired with another local gynecologist/surgeon. They used their therapy to treat a difficult case of "frozen pelvis" and total bilateral occlusion (total blockage of both fallopian tubes) which the surgeon diagnosed by both laparoscopy and open surgery. The adhesions were so bad that the surgeon was unable to open either tube; HSG dye tests after surgery confirmed surgical findings that total occlusion remained in both tubes after surgery.

Then the Wurns treated her. After the patient received their therapy, the diagnostic physician's HSG showed "copious free spillage" of the dye from one tube, and further advancement of the dye in the other tube. The Wurns had opened one tube and improved the other. They had proven their point, and my curiosity piqued.

As they continued treating patients, I began reviewing patient charts and talking to the patients. Upon further study, I not only became a believer but an advocate. Frankly, I was amazed, but the data was there.

The Wurns confessed that, being neither gynecologists nor researchers, they felt a bit overwhelmed with the data they were witnessing. They asked for my help as a physician and a researcher. I offered to guide the Wurns, offer medical feedback, and provide research oversight as they continued their journey to scientifically explore, test, and measure their results.

Together we have seen their manual physical therapy help women with pain, infertility, and sexual dysfunction in areas generally reserved to physicians. The unique approach they have developed has helped women in areas that were previously underserved (or unserved) by other areas of women's medical health. I have seen many full-term natural pregnancies in women who arrived at their clinic diagnosed infertile due to blocked fallopian tubes, endometriosis, or hormonal factors. We have also seen many natural successes with secondary infertility, and unexplained infertility in women who were treated with the Wurn Technique®.

In their study on treating women with blocked fallopian tubes, nearly two-thirds of the participants achieved patency in one or both tubes, and many of the women became pregnant naturally. This is a phenomenal statistic, better than surgical results. And the results appear to last — some of those women conceived and then went on to have subsequent natural pregnancies and births.

We have also seen therapy increase the chances of pregnancy via IVF. In women who underwent the Wurns' treatment before an IVF transfer, their pregnancy success rate increased from 41% in the control group (no therapy) to 67% in the group that received therapy.[1]

Side effects of therapy have generally been beneficial, including significant increases in sexual function (e.g. desire, orgasm, and lubrication) and dramatic decreases in intercourse pain. Over the course of nearly 20 years, we have been able to document and measure these changes scientifically, and publish the results in several respected medical journals.

Patients have been very receptive and thankful that this dedicated couple developed a natural adjunct to gynecologic medicine that has been shown to be effective, and appears to have lasting results. This treatment is a wonderful opportunity for women to achieve their goals without the side effects of pharmaceuticals or the risks and costs of surgery. The techniques they have developed now offer women options that have never existed before.

For Belinda, Larry, and me, our discoveries evolved from Belinda's pain. Her cancer, surgeries, radiation therapy, and the adhesions that grew within her from those experiences created a background of pain and dysfunction that was intolerable to the Wurns. When they came to me, I was deeply moved by their story, their quest, and their determination to find relief for Belinda, and for others with chronic pain and dysfunction.

Our professional lives together have been an adventure that continues to unfold and benefit patients from across the country, and around the world. Through nearly four decades of medicine, I have seen and heard many stories of pain, dysfunction, and unrealized goals. During the past decade and a half, it has been my pleasure to work with the Wurns as an unpaid medical and research advisor, and to watch their fascinating story become public. I am pleased to offer medical insights and guidance, and to help them tell their story in a way that is scientific, accurate, and medically appropriate. My hopes are that some of the truths revealed herein will help others to find the pain-free, functional life that they seek.

Introduction

Larry Wurn, LMT

Basically I am a pretty simple guy with a few core values. I love my wife, I cherish my friends, and I believe in the dignity and goodness of humankind.

I was not born into healthcare. In fact, I really knew very little about it except that "the doctor is always right," as my parents would say. Early on, they imbued me with a deep respect for physicians.

My father, a hard-working but very philanthropic businessman taught me tenacity; he inspired me to an attitude which he called "stick-to-it-ive-ness." My mother, a remarkably strong woman, was a romantic at heart. She taught me to embrace the fairy tale dream that says, "The Prince and the Princess reunited, and lived happily ever after."

They both encouraged me to relentlessly seek out the truth in all situations, because uncovering the truth gives us knowledge and insight. I have found that to be the case. Whenever I persisted in my quest for answers, I found that the truth revealed itself — for better or for worse. Together, all of these lessons from my parents became guiding principles in my life.

The real problem came for me when my fairy tale perspective on life conflicted with my belief that "the doctor is always right." A few years after marrying my childhood sweetheart, Belinda, she was diagnosed with cancer of the cervix. It was in an advanced stage and apparently spreading quickly, so she had to undergo surgery and intensive radiation therapy. Thankfully the treatments saved her life; yet, she was left in terrible pain, often doubling over from the adhesions that formed in the wake of her cure.

A year after my dear wife finished her cancer treatments, the doctors said, "Nothing more can be done to give Belinda back the pain-free life she had a year ago; she will only stay the same, or get worse." This presented some serious problems for me: first of course, was that I was losing my wife to increasingly debilitating pain. But I also had a difficult time coming to grips with the fact that their dire predictions were a direct contradiction to my inner voice telling me that the Prince and Princess live happily ever after. I knew where our life was supposed to be going — but the doctors and the facts before us were telling an entirely different story.

Not knowing how I would do it, I was determined to resolve the quandary so Belinda and I could get back to the life I knew was supposed to be ours. I felt the most reasonable thing to change was the part that predicted "Nothing more can be done." Knowing that truth always won out, Belinda and I began a tenacious search to resolve her condition and get back to our fairy tale ending — the "happily ever after" that I knew was there for us.

I am pleased this decision not only helped Belinda, but also set us on a path of discovery that continues to unfold and reap benefits for other people. In truth, the principles in this book and the inquiries we have begun by this quest have opened more doors, and will ultimately lead to more adventures of discovery in healthcare than all three of your authors could investigate in a lifetime.

Along the way, we discovered that tiny adhesions, the first step in the healing process, are responsible for many of the "mystery ailments" we hear about from our patients. The idea that adhesions can form in virtually all systems of the body is simply fact. It is also a fact that Western medicine's ability to deal with these tiny but powerful collagenous cross-links (the building blocks of adhesions) is very limited. The main response in medicine is surgery, but that process often adds to the problem since (in more cases than not) more adhesions form as the body heals from the surgical process. For example, surgery has been implicated as the main cause of bowel obstruction.

Initially in our search, we found that some techniques (e.g., John Barnes's wonderful invention: Myofascial Release) appeared to improve mobility in muscles and joints, relieving pain and returning function for many people. As we went on to develop our own work, we were stunned to find that women with blocked fallopian tubes were becoming pregnant with techniques we developed to treat adhesions between organs, in the visceral and reproductive tracts. It was both exciting and a little scary. No one had ever thought — or even suggested — that something like this could happen.

When we unexpectedly found that we could open blocked fallopian tubes, tiny structures at the deepest area in the pelvis, it seemed almost unbelievable. And yet, there it was. We tested it over and over again with independent diagnostic radiologists and gynecologists, and it kept happening, over and over again. When the Chief of Staff of our local hospital encouraged us to prepare a scientific report on this phenomenon for a major medical journal, we felt good. When that was completed, we were sure we had reached the zenith of what we could accomplish with our hands alone.

But fate was not done with us yet; our patients led us on into other uncharted (and sometimes unintended) areas of discovery. Apparently, there was more truth left in the bottom of the barrel. From opening blocked fallopian tubes, we moved on to reversing smalll bowel obstructions in the larger "tubes"— the intestines.

We started seeing dramatic positive changes in endocrine hormone levels and in reproductive function in women who had been diagnosed with hormone-related infertility. These were patients whom we had initially refused to treat, because we didn't think we could help them. We didn't want to waste their time or money. And yet again, there it was. Truth was staring us in the face as women diagnosed hormonally infertile or menopausal were having one, then (in some cases) two natural full-term pregnancies after therapy. Again, this seemed beyond the realm of possibilities — but there it was.

When we conducted clinical trials and treated woman after woman with aberrant hormone levels, the results kept coming back with overwhelmingly positive changes. It is almost as if God or fate was drawing us along to where we were supposed to go.

We are not sure what is on the horizon next. Certainly we want to further investigate our effect on hormones in a large controlled clinical study. The possibility that our treatment for faulty biomechanics and adhesive processes could change endocrine levels for glands that lie deep within the cranium is something that opens doors and minds to many wonderful possibilities for humanity.

A physician member of our team reviewed our results treating the pituitary gland (which you will read in this book) with a group of neurosurgeons who were curious about our work in this area. These physicians asked us, "If you can improve hormonal secretions from the pituitary deep within the brain, why wouldn't you be able to improve function and dopamine levels in the nearby *substantia nigra* — the area responsible for Parkinson's disease?"

My heart skipped a beat. While this was something we had considered in private, not one of us had dared to breathe it to anyone outside the team. And yet, the slow squeezing of that part of the brain by microscopic collagenous cross-links could certainly cause the kind of slow cell death and decreasing function that accompanies Parkinson's disease — much as it causes slowly decreasing function on other body parts and systems.

Over the years, we have begun to wonder if the biomechanical effects of collagen formation associated with healing may be a factor in other unexplained conditions. For example, is there a relationship between the collagen cross-links that form in the body wherever we heal, and the colloid "plaques and tangles" that are so often found in the brains of Alzheimer's victims?

Western medicine has become highly specialized with remarkable diagnostic instruments, surgeries, and pharmaceuticals. So many of these inventions and developments are wonderful, and many great milestones have been discovered. But nearly all diagnostic tools bypass the tiny but powerful cross-links that form like glue wherever we heal. Of these developments, surgery alone addresses adhesions, but surgeons are stymied by adhesion reformation as a natural by-product of surgical recovery.

I hope that this book will become an inspiration to physicians to broaden their vision when it comes to the possibility that tiny, sometimes microscopic adhesions may be at work in some of their unexplained cases. I encourage them to team with allied professionals to try some risk-free soft tissue therapy techniques in cases where they suspect an etiology of adhesions — and in cases where surgery is not a viable option.

This book is also a call to body workers to investigate diligently and to not make unwarranted claims. Only tedious and vigorous scientific testing can bring us the truths we seek in this area.

Finally, it is an invitation to patients and their loved ones to know that there is a reason for their pain and dysfunction, and that reason can be found – often in the most logical and simple way. Following our hearts and intuitions, with one step slowly leading the other, let us move forward to help find the way for most people to live happily ever after.

Section One

The Big Picture

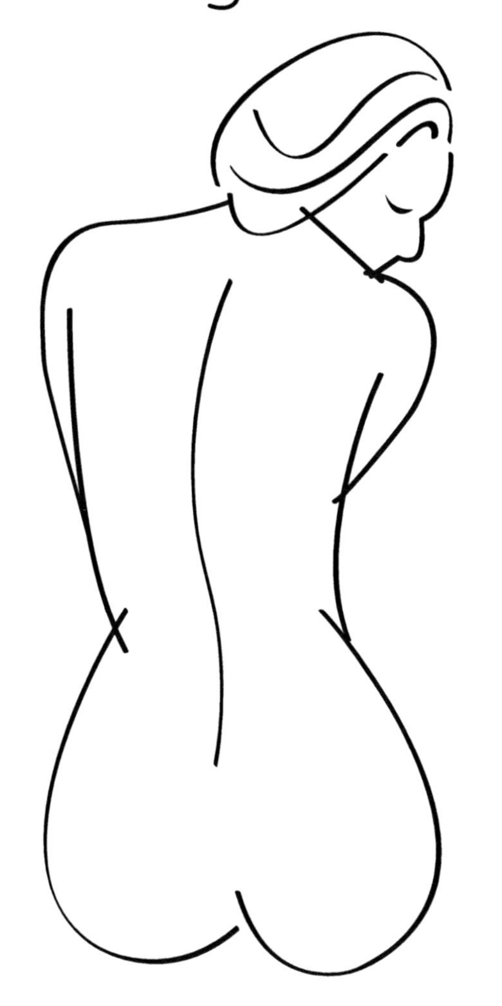

"Life is what happens when you're making other plans"
– John Lennon

Chapter One
Humble Beginnings

(Chapter by Larry Wurn)

"She's so radiant," I thought. In the years since Belinda and I grew up together as kids, the scrawny girl I had played with had become a brilliant and lovely woman at 30. Leaving her pre-medical program for a career she felt would give her more quality time with her patients, Belinda graduated top of her class from the physical therapy school at the University of Florida. Now, I was meeting my childhood friend again as an adult: bright, mature, radiant – and fun! How lucky could I be? A professional artist in my 30s, and back in Florida to help my aging parents, I ran into Belinda as an adult and we fell in love all over again. We happily married but were soon shocked and then devastated to learn that Belinda had developed cancer of the cervix. In her case, it was a potentially life-threatening condition that her doctors feared had begun to spread rapidly.

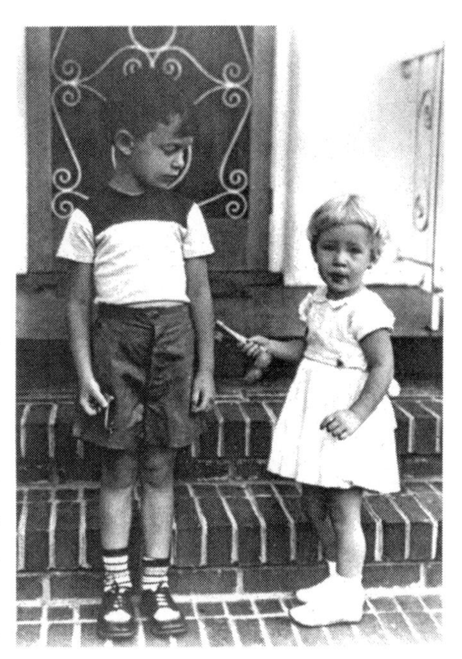

Authors Larry and Belinda Wurn during an earlier time.

Physicians at the nearby University of Florida Medical School suggested immediate, aggressive action to stem the progress of her disease. They started with surgery to cut the diseased tissues from the most sensitive structures of my dear wife's body. Then, they used radiation therapy to stop the growth of any cancer cells that escaped the surgeon's scalpel. They never warned us about the potential for adhesion formation, with its deleterious effects, but it probably would not have mattered to us at the time. We just wanted her cured, alive, and cancer free.

Searching for Relief from Debilitating Pain

In the end, Belinda was pronounced healed, but that healing came at a great price. A few months after her treatments, Belinda began to notice an uncomfortable pulling sensation in her pelvis. As time went on, the pull developed into a more persistent pain. Raised on traditional medicine, we consulted the best physicians and specialists we could find, trying to resolve her pain. They offered no solution except more surgery, with guarded prospects for success.

Unfortunately, the pain now came with more and more frequency, and the severity seemed to be worsening. But our experiences with surgery had been a two-sided road. While the surgery likely saved her life, it had also left her with increasingly debilitating pain. In the end, we decided that further surgery would lead us into even worse problems.

We started researching less invasive, more natural approaches to heal her pain. Belinda had taken many continuing education courses in physical therapy after her graduation. Most of these involved exercises or new electrical modalities that were being researched, some of which were being billed as "state of the art" physical therapy, such as ultrasound and cold laser stimulation. We tried both the new and the traditional techniques, but they did not help resolve her pain. In fact, much to our distress, her pain was getting worse.

Belinda had read stories about manual physical therapy — a controversial compendium of various types of hands-on manipulations to the body. Most of her colleagues had little good to say about it — after all, there was just no proof that it did anything. Despite the fact that manual therapy has been practiced in virtually all cultures throughout history, many professionals still consider it unproven, or simply a sham. Notwithstanding, most doctors felt it would do us no harm.

As Belinda's pain increased, we became more determined to find an answer and we decided to take a few courses in different hands-on manipulative physical therapy techniques. We were drawn to physical therapy because of its strong foundation in medicine and its acceptance by physicians, scientists and insurers throughout the US.

After each course we took, we adapted, refined, and modified new techniques we learned in order to address Belinda's pelvic pain. Slowly, her pain and dysfunction (poor digestion, fatigue, painful intercourse, etc.) began to resolve. Two long years after we started our research, she was finally able to return to work full-time. She was regaining her life and her capabilities.

The more we studied various methods and techniques, the more fascinated we became. Our curiosity turned into passion. Over the next several years, Belinda and I continued to take many manual therapy courses from wonderful physicians and physical therapists in the US and Europe. Far from being the charlatans our doctors had warned us about, the teachers we encountered were educated, well-grounded healthcare professionals who generally appreciated the advances of Western medicine, but were frustrated with its failures and myopic views of treating certain conditions. Like us, they had found that many of Western medicine's biggest failures were in the treatment of chronic pain and unexplained dysfunction, both of which plagued Belinda. Allopathic medicine seemed limited to drugs and surgery, which were not appropriate treatments for Belinda.

The experiences and knowledge we had gained through our ordeals and the results we achieved in Belinda were inspiring. During courses and seminars, we heard other people's stories. As we did, we began to realize that others with chronic pain or dysfunction might benefit from our investigation and the synthesis of techniques. In 1989, I became a massage therapist, and Belinda and I opened a small manual physical therapy clinic with three treatment rooms. We specialized in treating men and women with chronic pain who did not want surgery and patients with persistent unresolved pain, despite all attempts by their physicians to resolve their symptoms.

As we used the techniques we had learned, developed, and synthesized, our patients began to report relief from years and even decades of pain. Physicians responded by sending more complicated chronic pain patients to our door. As we continued to witness dramatic turnarounds, we began to develop an organized system of treatment protocols to address longstanding pain issues for various areas of the body. We were becoming extremely busy treating very complicated cases. It was incredibly gratifying to be able to return a pain-free lifestyle to so many people.

Our tiny physical therapy clinic grew with our referral base, until we had five clinics that covered much of the geography of our state. Doctors were happy to send us their most challenging pain patients – what one physician called his "chronic pain hall of fame."

Most of our patients were physician-referred, and we were enjoying an excellent reputation among the roughly 700 orthopedic surgeons, neurologists, internal and family practice doctors, and pain specialists who referred patients to us.

Over time, we found that we were helping pain and dysfunctions beyond our original intent and out of the usual scope of practice for physical therapy. Many of these "discoveries" were uncovered by chance. Patients who came for treatment of chronic pain would often report that they also seemed to have dramatic improvement in seemingly unrelated areas, such as digestion, elimination, or sexual function. Through feedback and encouragement from our patients and referring physicians, we documented many of these unexpected turnarounds.

Then the impossible happened. Nothing in our professional lives would ever be the same again. In fact, our world was about to turn upside down.

In 1989, Belinda and I treated a patient, Andrea, at our clinic. Andrea reported chronic pelvic pain and dysfunction following an invasive surgery and a fall. She and her physician had been unable to find relief for her via the conventional physical therapy, exercise, and electrical modalities that had been prescribed for her. In fact, like Belinda, her condition seemed to be worsening. As her pain became more chronic and severe, her doctor sent her to us as a "last resort."

When we treated Andrea, she and her doctor were pleased to find that her longstanding pain went away. Five months after therapy, she was surprised that she had unexpectedly become pregnant.

Andrea told us that her pregnancy was remarkable because both of her fallopian tubes had been diagnosed blocked during medical testing, seven years earlier. Fallopian tubes typically block due to adhesions, and once closed they are not known to open again naturally. "I've been sexually active with the same partner for seven years; I never used any form of birth control — we knew for a fact that both of my tubes were blocked. How could this happen?" she asked.

Dr. Falk, the physician who referred Andrea to our manual physical therapy clinic, learned of Andrea's pregnancy. He became curious and asked us if we felt we had anything to do with opening her tubes. While we had similar thoughts, we did not know. The idea that we had opened her tubes seemed at once far-fetched and intriguing.

Andrea had her child and then Dr. Falk referred a woman with three years of "unexplained" infertility to us. He said, "Let's see if you can do that again." After a few hours of treatment, she became pregnant naturally and had an easy, successful birth — of twins! This was exciting. Belinda and I were very happy with the results, as were the physician and of course, the new moms.

Then Dr. Falk revealed to us that his wife, Shannon, had been infertile for twelve years. Her infertility history was incredibly complex. He explained, "She only has one fallopian tube and it is totally blocked. Her other tube and ovary were removed years ago. Her history includes Stage IV endometriosis (the most severe form) and massive surgical adhesions. Over the years, she has had several surgeries for the endometriosis and to remove ovarian cysts, and another surgery to remove her ovary, remove one tube, ease her pain, and help her conceive. Each of these surgeries left its own internal scars. Due to her only tube being blocked and her extensive scarring, her doctors gave up on her fertility years ago."

"Oh, and she is now 41, so she is fast approaching menopause," Dr. Falk said. "Do you think you can help her?"

With a deep inhale, Belinda and I resolved to give it our best shot. A few weeks after therapy, Shannon came to see Belinda. She stood in the doorway, just staring. "I don't know if I should hug you or hit you," Shannon said with a broad grin. "I'm turning 42 years old — and now I'm pregnant — naturally!"

Dr. Falk was amazed that through the therapy we were developing, his wife was pregnant naturally, despite all the procedures medical science had attempted over 12 years of infertility. Shannon gave birth to a beautiful little girl who is now 17 years old — and an accomplished equestrian and rising tennis star at her school.

By now, our curiosity was piqued. As healthcare professionals, we felt a strong obligation to investigate this phenomenon, which appeared to be having positive effects on seemingly unrelated bodily systems. We had seen it dramatically increase reproductive function in women who were considered medically beyond hope. At the same time, it was significantly decreasing pain in most of our chronic pain sufferers despite years of debilitating pain, and improving digestion for most patients with abdominopelvic complaints.

Excited and looking for answers, we approached the Chief of Staff of our local hospital. Richard King, MD, was a highly respected physician, scientist, and research gynecologist. While Dr. King was initially quite skeptical, he agreed to review the charts of the three unexpected mothers. The more he read, the more fascinated he became. Before long, he was telling Belinda and me that these were important findings and that we needed to start conducting some serious scientific research. Our curiosity and passion combined with Dr. King's, and we began a journey that would help many women and men, and lead to over 15 years together (thus far) researching new phenomena and discoveries in non-surgical treatment of pain, infertility, and several unexplained dysfunctions.

We never dreamed that our quest to relieve Belinda's pain would lead us on a path to discover and develop a natural treatment, not just for patients with chronic pain, but for women with endometriosis, menstrual or intercourse pain, sexual dysfunction, and other, often unexplained conditions – including unexplained infertility. Nor did we ever expect to conduct clinical research or to publish studies and abstracts in some of the most respected medical journals in the world.

Belinda and I learned how drastically fate could turn our lives in an instant. Just as we were starting our life together as newlyweds and looking forward to great careers treating patients (for Belinda) and creating art (for me), a few tiny cancer cells deep within Belinda's body changed everything for both of us, immediately and indelibly.

Now, 20 years after her diagnosis, our lives have come full circle. Belinda is still practicing physical therapy, but she is largely teaching patients and their partners the reasons for their unexplained pain and dysfunction, and what to do about it. She is also teaching select therapists around the country how to treat these complex patients with our new therapy, the Wurn Technique®. We also conduct, publish, and share our scientific research and findings with doctors and other healthcare providers when we are invited to speak at professional conferences.

As for me, I am once again creating art, but that too is very different from anything I had ever imagined. I no longer sit in front of a blank canvas with brushes and paints. Instead, my canvases are patients who arrive at the clinic every day in search of help.

These canvases have very complex histories: a lifetime of experiences, traumas, and the emotions associated with them. My art now, like Belinda's and that of all of our therapists, is to help uncover the trail of adhesions left by the healing processes deep within the bodies of our patients over time. As we peel apart these adhesions strand by strand, we return patients to an earlier state of pain-free function and mobility.

Chapter Two

Structure and the Body

"Structure governs function . . .
abnormal structure governs dysfunction"
David J. Martinke, D.O.[54]

The body begins as a single cell. One egg, the largest cell in the human body, and one sperm, the smallest, unite to create a fertilized egg. Life is born.

The human body begins to grow. Each cell is intimately connected to its neighbor in the ever-evolving symphony which becomes our body. Cells split and generate new cells. Eventually, muscles, organs, nerves, and connective tissue begin to differentiate from each other. Various parts of the body continue to relate to each other, both as neighbors and as intricate, interrelated parts of the whole.

As the body grows, a sweater-like structure begins to form. This sweater wraps around cells, organs, muscles, and bodily structures, holding them together. It also separates each of them from its neighbor. This three-dimensional sweater is called fascia.

Just as the white of an orange surrounds and separates every section of an orange all the way down to the pulp, fascia surrounds and separates every structure and every cell in our body with strong collagenous fibers, all the way down to the cellular level.

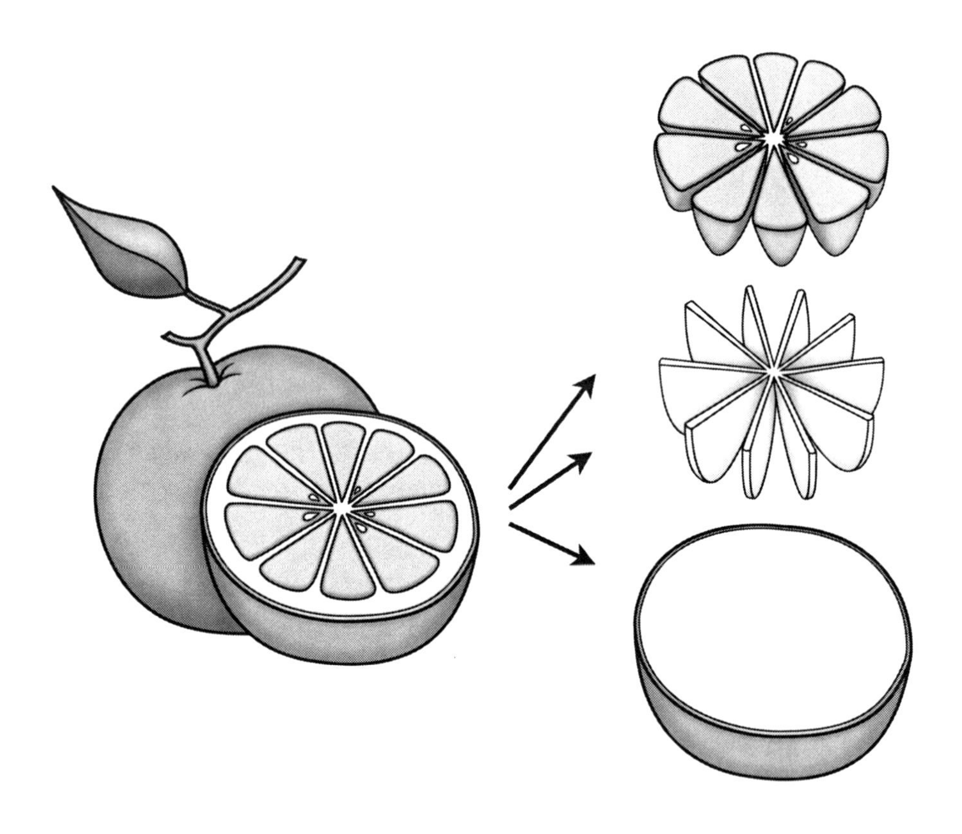

As the white of an orange separates individual wedges of fruit, a woven sweater of fascia surrounds and separates all the body's structures

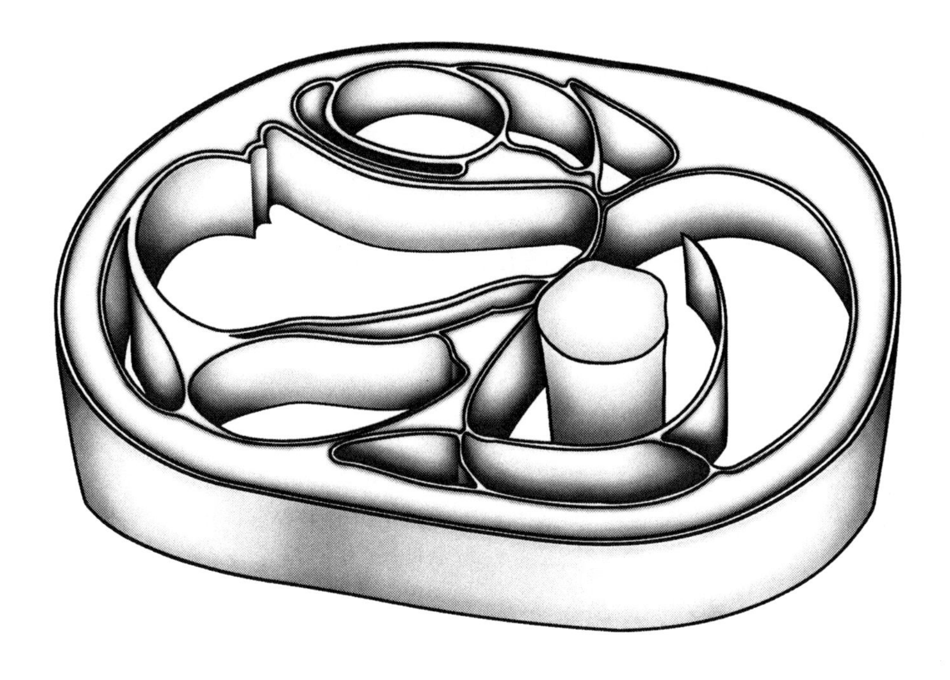

A cross-section of a leg with the muscle and bone removed reveals the layers of fascia that surround and separate all the structures of the leg.

The Body as a Whole: An Interconnected Puzzle

Adhesions (which we examine in detail in Chapter Three) can form anywhere in the body, wherever we heal. When they attach to the fascia, they can (and often do) create powerful bonds between structures within this fascial web. Like boats bound together side to side by ropes, movement in one area will cause a pull in another. Said another way, adhesions act like a run in the sweater of our fascia. Any bond or pull on that sweater will cause a concurrent pull further up or down the line.

Because of this whole body nature of fascia, we have found that the area of pain or dysfunction in a patient is not always the geographic center of the problem. In many cases, a distant area or site may be the primary cause of the pain or dysfunction in another location. While our patients may seek our treatment for pain or symptoms in one specific area, such as the uterus for pelvic pain or the head for headaches, we generally look at that area in relation to the entire body in order to see the full picture as to what may be causing problems for our patient.

For example, as the psoas muscle passes through the pelvis, it connects the vertebrae of the low back to the front of the leg. While the delicate ovaries have little functional relationship to the large psoas muscle, the ovaries and psoas muscle share an intimate space. Any trauma to the psoas or low back may indirectly cause damage and inflammation to the delicate tissues where life begins, in the ovaries.

As we will see through examples later in this book, if we do not regard the patient's problem area in relation to the many neighboring structures and the entire body joined by the fascial sweater, we may miss some of the most valuable information available to address and resolve our patient's complaints.

This "whole body" approach to our patients' goals is something that we have found to be missing as Western medicine has progressed into greater and greater specialization.

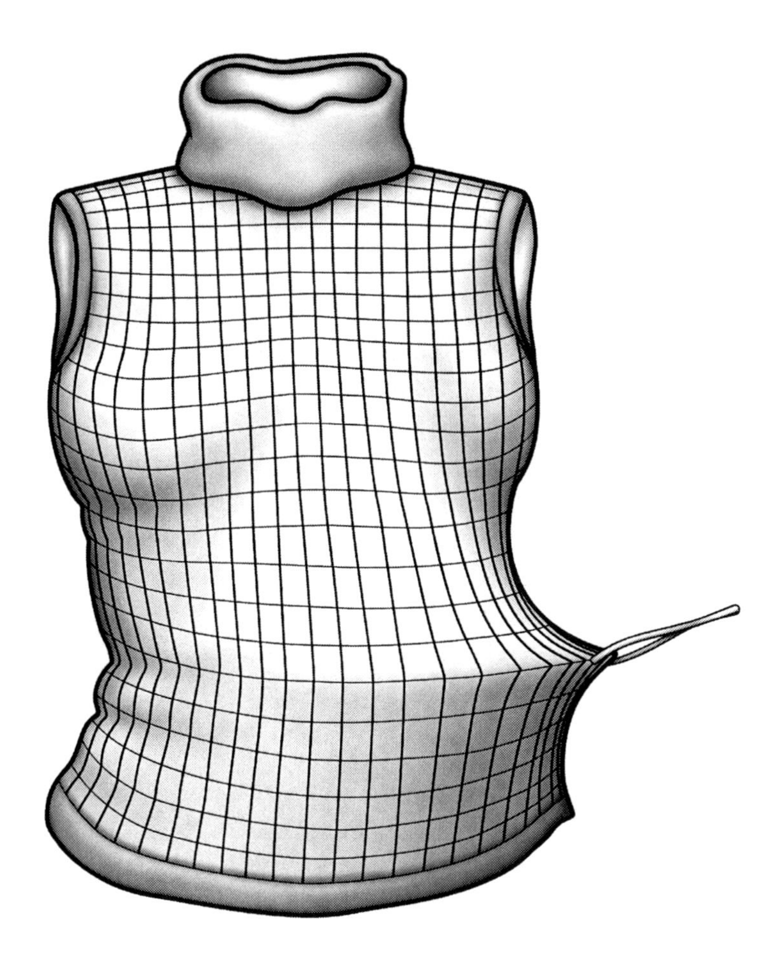

Fascia acts like a three-dimensional sweater, connecting all our body parts into a whole structure. Thus, when one area tightens, the pull can manifest itself in distant tissues and structures, sometimes far from the site of the original injury.

The Body as Parts: The Myth of Specialization in Modern Medicine

As western medicine has evolved, healthcare providers have become more and more knowledgeable about the various bodily systems. With this increased knowledge, physicians and medical professionals have become more and more specialized.

Specialists are highly trained, well versed experts in their fields. While they realize that a physical relationship exists with nearby structures, they are not necessarily trained to think in a "whole body" manner. Thus, a reproductive endocrinologist may concentrate on hormonal response and the function of the ovaries, but s/he may overlook an earlier hip injury that traumatized tissues just a half-inch away. If microscopic fascial adhesions formed within the hip after the trauma, they may have easily created a physical pull through adhesions or the fascial sweater, affecting the ovary and delicate finger-like fimbriae at the end of the fallopian tube on the other side of the pelvic bone.

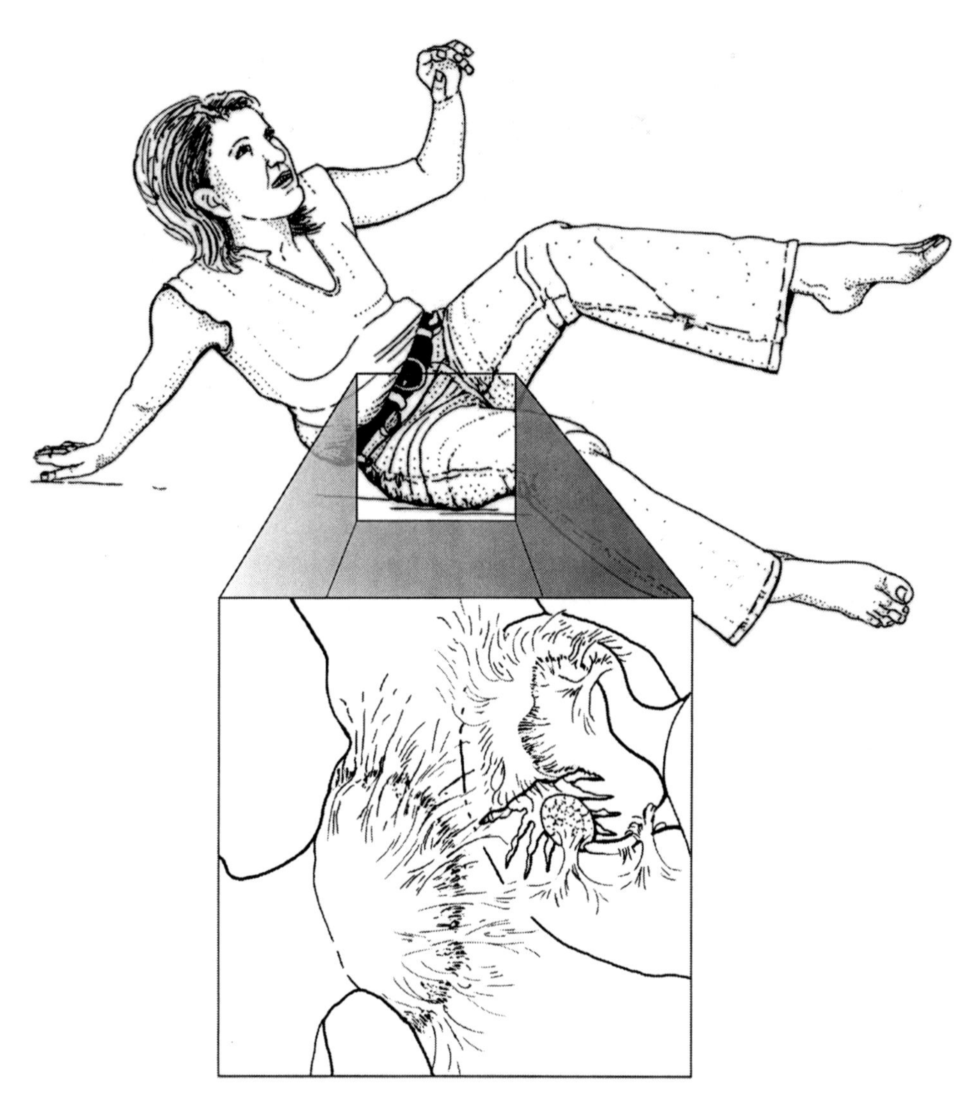

A fall onto the hip can cause glue-like adhesions to form in delicate reproductive structures, just a half-inch away.

Unexplained Infertility after Motor Vehicle Accident

- Stacy's Story

Stacy, one of our former patients, came to us with just this problem. She sought our treatment to help resolve her unexplained infertility. Stacy had been treated for two years by the head of reproductive endocrinology at a large medical school. Her physician was a highly respected infertility specialist, but despite his skills, she remained childless. In fact, she never had a single pregnancy during that time.

When we conducted her onsite evaluation, we learned that Stacy had sustained injuries to her hips and pelvis in a motor vehicle accident several years before. The more we spoke, the more this trauma stood out to us as a possible source of her infertility problems.

When we treated her, we addressed all of her reproductive structures, but also paid special attention to her hips, which are the joints where her legs join her pelvis. Anatomically, we noted that the inside of this joint was very close to the ovaries, at the ends of her fallopian tubes. We thought it was reasonable that adhesions which formed here after her accident may have spread over time, and now involved her nearby tube and ovary.

As it happens, Stacy became pregnant naturally two months after therapy and delivered a baby boy. She has since reported another natural pregnancy and live birth, so her infertility is a thing of the past.

We often find that patients never discuss seemingly unrelated injuries or traumas with their specialists. This is unfortunate for patients like Stacy whose infertility was apparently initiated by trauma to neighboring structures, rather than directly to the reproductive organs. As holistic practitioners, we review our patient's specific focus and goals, and then step back to regard, examine, and palpate their body as a whole. Even if a person comes to us for treatment as specific as opening blocked fallopian tubes, we find it is important to examine all of the soft tissues of the body and resolve any mechanical mobility problems we find. This is critical in our minds, due to the interconnectivity of fascia and the interrelated structure of the body.

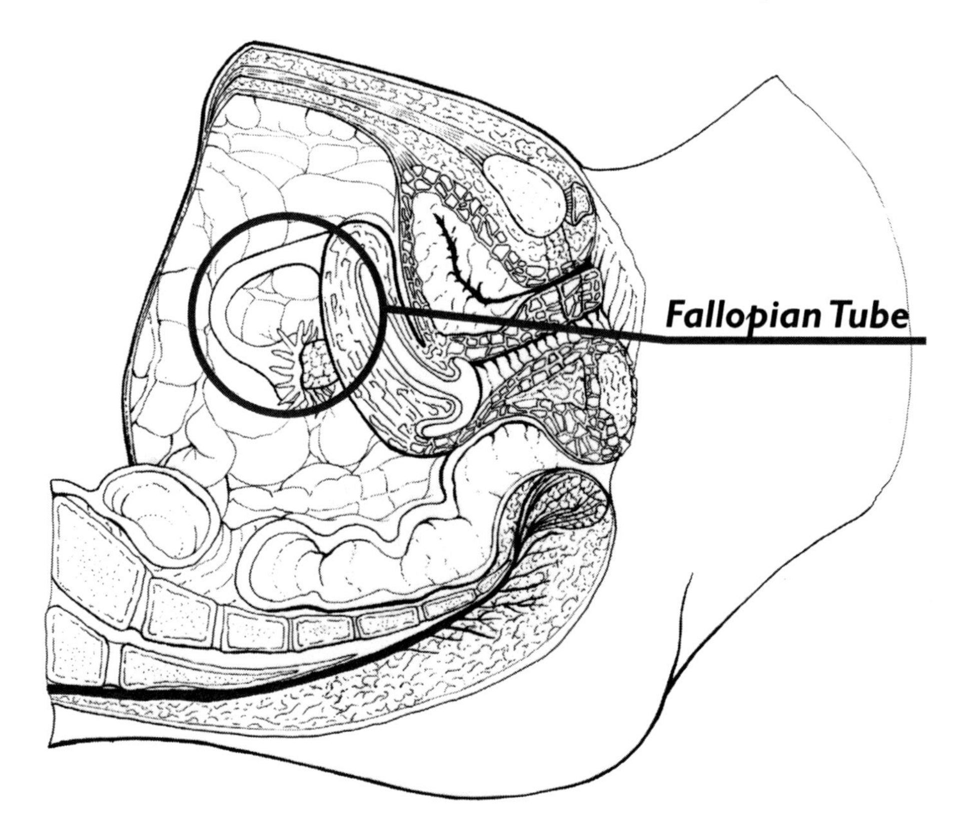

The fallopian tubes lie much deeper in the body than we can palpate. We access them indirectly through the fascia that joins all structures.

The fallopian tubes lie very deep within the body. In order to access them, we have to palpate through multiple layers of tissues, and around other body structures. If there are restrictions in surrounding layers or neighboring tissues or structures, we have to clear those if we expect to achieve success and lasting function of the tubes. Thus, we take the treatment layer by layer. Once we have cleared adhesive cross-links and spasm in surrounding tissues and structures, we can access and treat the actual organs that are the focus of our patient's goals.

We know that this therapy opens fallopian tubes, and we understand that adhesions are the most common cause of fallopian tube blockage. We use the interconnected sweater of fascia to indirectly access and treat these tiny, deep organs, and help restore their function.

The Patient is an Expert

We have found that relying on the patient's intuition and opinions often helps tremendously in this process. For example, we ask our patients to tell us specifically what they are feeling in their bodies while we are treating them. After all, it is their body we are treating. In our view, who can better tell us what is going on within our patient's body than our patient? Each patient has extensive, intimate knowledge of his/her body — from traumas, falls, inflammations, and surgeries to thoughts, hypotheses, and physical and emotional responses to these experiences.

In essence, the sum of patients' lifetime experiences and their thoughts and feelings about them comprise their present physical and emotional state. For this reason, we regard each patient as an expert on her case. Part of our job is to help patients tap into their "inner knowledge" of themselves. This helps us discover, then unravel the physical barriers that stand in the way of their goals.

As we are taking an extensive history, our initial evaluation requires that we listen deeply to each patient's personal experiences and feelings. As we palpate the body, we feel the adhered tissues and structures with our hands. As we do, we note body tension patterns to determine which areas can move properly and which structures are adhered, inflamed, irritated, or less mobile. We also regard our patients' reactions and emotional responses as we palpate their various tissues and structures to get a sense of any guarding or history about which we may inquire.

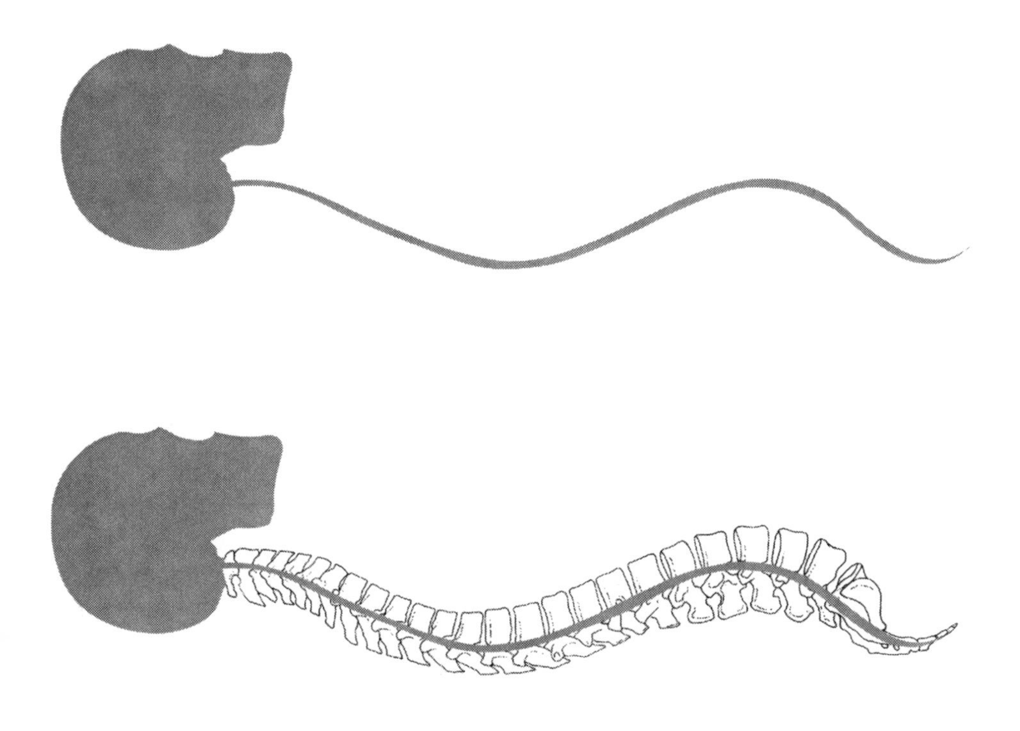

The dura (shown above) is a dramatic example of the interconnected nature of the body. This strong sheath of fascia starts at the coccyx (tailbone) and sacrum at the base of the spine. From there, it travels up the body, surrounding the spinal cord and central nervous system. It has strong attachments at the top of the neck and the base of the skull. From there, it enters the cranium, then spreads like a sweater to totally surround the brain, and all of its internal structures.

Shouldn't Patients be Involved in Their Treatment?

The approach of treating the body as a whole and listening to our patients' personal experiences is not only necessary in our view, it is also exciting for us. In fact, many patients find therapy becomes a marvelous journey as we unravel together the layers of pain, adhesions, and dysfunctions to help free the symmetrical, functional, and pain-free individual from adhesive straight-jackets. Therapy is like uncovering an unfolding mystery with every patient.

In the following chapters of this book, we discuss some of the specific conditions and dysfunctions we have seen resolved through this approach. No matter what our final focus, we do not find it helpful to treat our patients in parts. When patients come to our office, our goal is to improve the overall function and mobility of their organs, muscles, joints, glands, and support structures. Thus, we not only treat their main complaint, but work with a view to restore proper structure, function, and mobility to the entire body.

Chapter Three

Structural Changes Throughout Life

Adhesions form as we heal — it's as simple as that. For this reason, virtually all of us have adhesions.

In fact, by the time we reach puberty, literally everyone who has ever had a fall, infection, inflammation, or surgery has developed adhesions. They are part of the natural process of healing and aging. Adhesions become an intimate part of the geography of our body and of our fascial sweater. Let's look at an example.

Healing and Adhesions

Think back to a time you were very young, four or five years old. While playing with friends you fell off your tricycle or slipped while running, landing on your hip. The trauma of the fall set in motion a series of events in your body.

First, you suffered tissue damage from the fall. Small blood vessels ruptured, and cells in the area were crushed or injured. Within minutes, the healing mechanisms of your body started sending out tiny, but very strong strands of collagen. These tiny collagen threads are called cross-links.

As they attached to the injured tissue and to each other, the cross-links created an adhesive blanket to protect and isolate the injured area from the rest of the body. In the beginning, this blanket was small. It helped stop any bleeding, and it helped prevent bacteria that may have entered your body during the trauma from spreading beyond the injury site. Thus, it prepared the tissues in that area to heal.

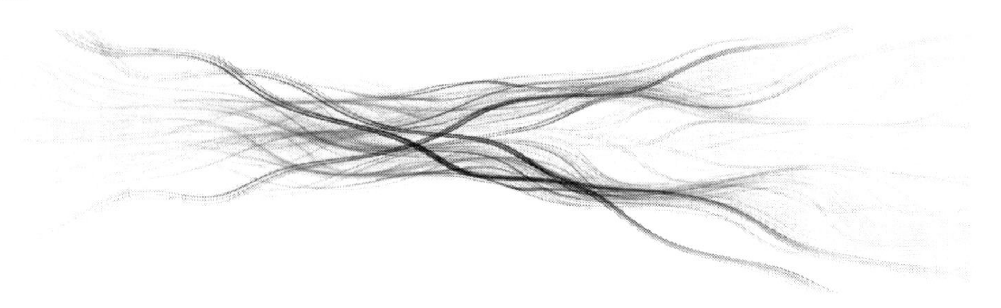

Adhesions may initially form as microscopic ropes, curtains or blankets.

If you were lucky, your body reabsorbed some or all of the cross-links, lessening their glue-like affect. But if the inflammation in the area persisted, the number of cross-links increased. Thus, the micro-adhesions grew into adhesions – or a scar. Cross-links, micro-adhesions, adhesions, and scars refer to the same adherent tissue, the main difference being the size and appearance. Whether large or small, these collagen threads represent the first step in the process of healing.

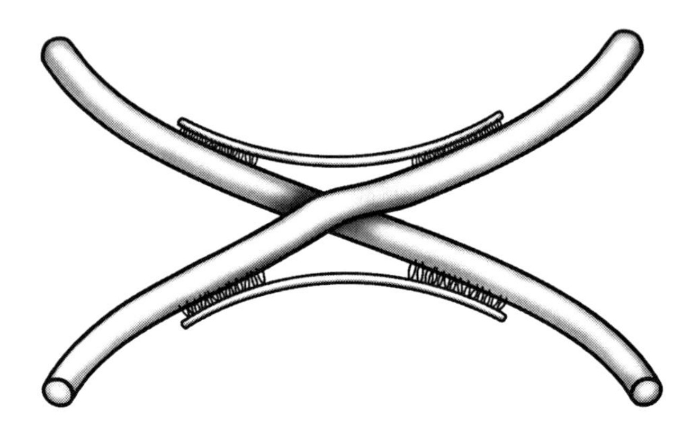

As the body heals, small but powerful cross-links form between individual fibers of the fascial sweater, permanently restricting movement and sometimes causing pain or dysfunction.

Over the next several weeks, your skin may have undergone some interesting color changes. The trauma may have turned the injured area "black and blue" as your body progressed through the various stages of healing. After several weeks (or months with a bad injury), you noticed that you finally felt little or no pain when that area brushed up against a wall or a piece of furniture. To all your senses, you were healed, and you went about your prior activities.

However, inside of the body, the tissues underwent a significant change. In fact, the adhesive tissues that originally formed to help the body heal after the injury remain in the body. There, they could continue to affect your bodily structures for decades, even for your entire life.

Collagen fibers or cross-links are the "building blocks" of adhesions. Collagen fibers have been measured as having a tensile strength of nearly 2,000 pounds per square inch in the body. Because of its tremendous strength, collagen is ideally suited to be the main structural element of tendons and ligaments, as well as adhesions.

Collagen is one of the main structural elements in fascia. In fact, collagen is so prevalent in the body that it surrounds and separates virtually all of the body's structures, giving them strength and stability, from the largest muscle to the most delicate gland.

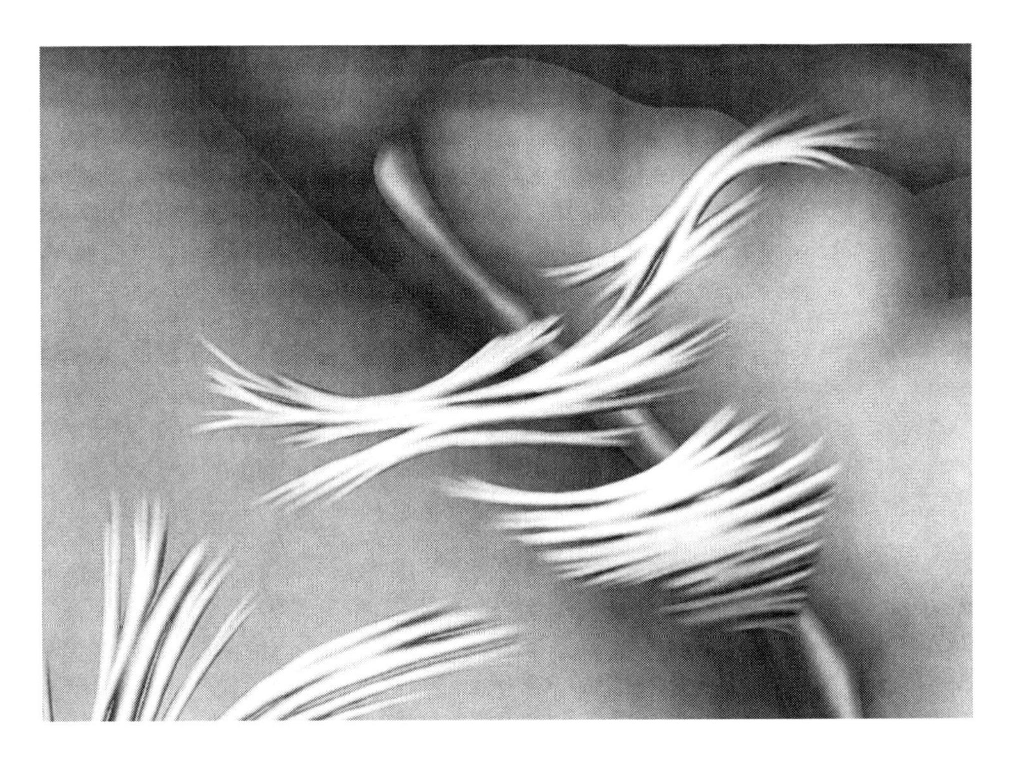

Collagenous cross-links can join to form adhesions which glue bodily structures to their neighbors.

But collagen's strength and prevalence in the body can also be a drawback. Collagenous cross-links, adhesions, and scars form within the fascial sweater, or attach to bodily structures after trauma or inflammation. Once formed, these adhesive structures often remain in place long after the original healing process has completed. Since collagen occurs throughout the body, the body produces no solvent to dissolve adhesions or scars. In fact, while you have "healed" from your injury, the tiny adhesions which formed during those first days of the healing process remain in your body — and stay there for the rest of your life!

What Causes Adhesions to Form?

Many people think that because they have not had any major surgery, injury, or accidents, their body is free from adhesions. However, adhesions can form from a variety of causes, including simple infections or inflammations. The next section examines some of the causes we see frequently.

Infection

Infections affect nearly everyone at some time during their life. During the course of an infection, inflammation often forms in the affected area, as the body attempts to contain the infection and fight it off. With luck, the adhesions that form due to infection or the associated inflammatory response will be localized and will not cause great harm. In most cases, they go unnoticed. However, inflammation and the resulting cross-link formation can adversely affect the more delicate tissues of the body.

SIX COMMON CAUSES OF ADHESION FORMATION

- Infection
- Inflammation
- Surgery
- Trauma
- Radiation therapy
- Chronic poor posture

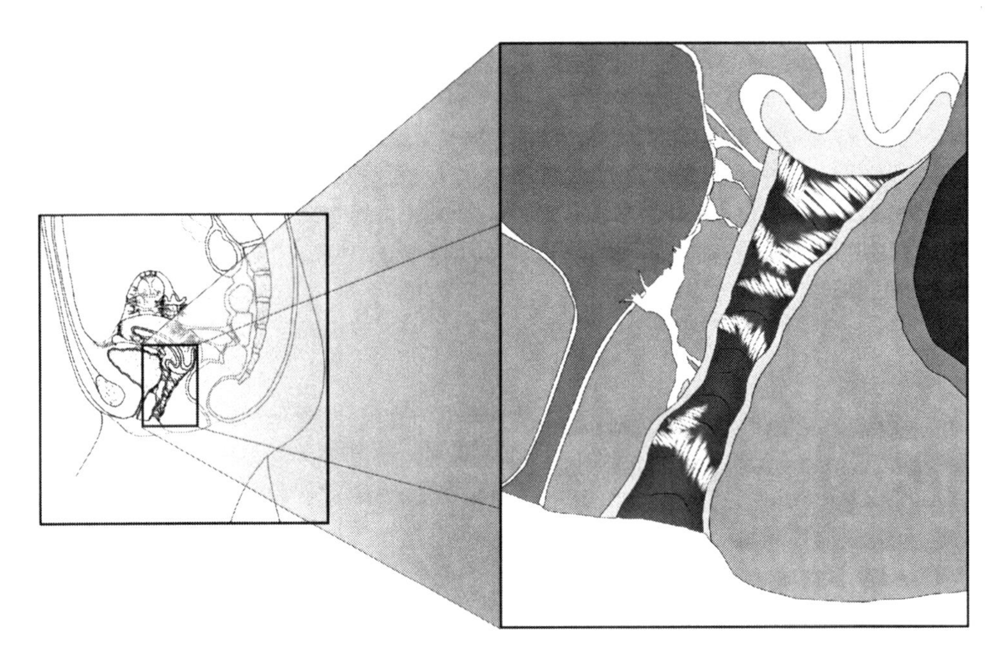

Adhesions may form on the warm, moist walls of the vagina due to bacterial infection, trauma, or abuse.

The female reproductive tract is one of the most common areas of infection in the body. The warm, moist tissues of the vaginal walls are designed to promote life, as are the nearby tissues and structures of the cervix and uterus. Thus, they form a near-perfect environment for bacterial infection. Besides trauma to the coccyx (tailbone) which is the closest neighbor to the cervix, the vagina itself is a frequent site of infection and cross-link formation.

Items that enter the vagina may not always be as clean as we hope. Through tampons, a partner, or even self-exploration, items enter the semi-closed tissues of the vagina from the outside environment, exposing those delicate tissues to bacteria from the world outside.

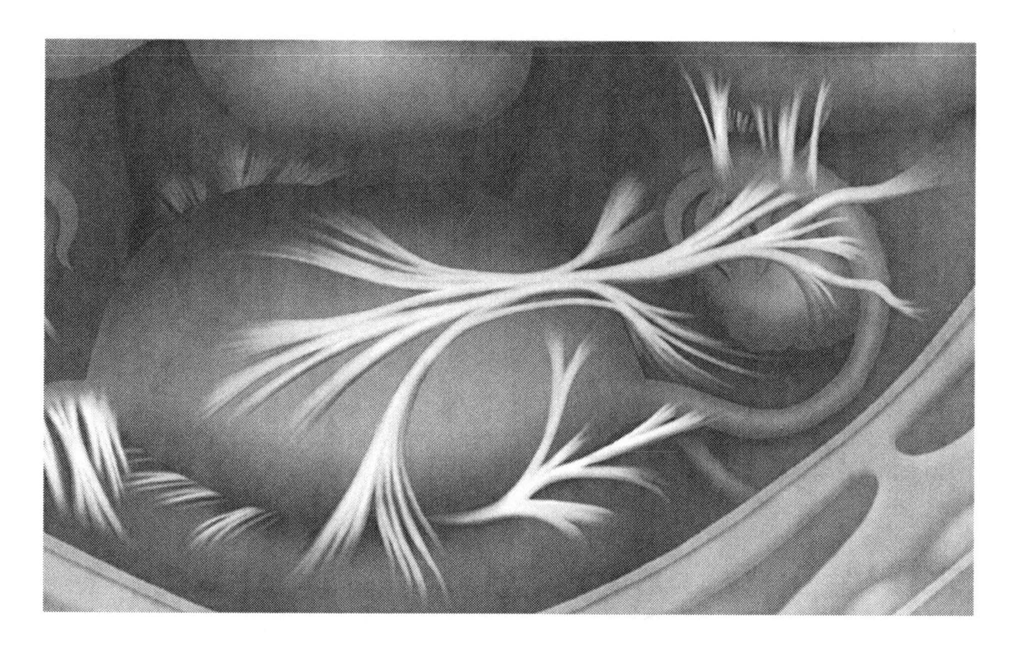

Adhesions from vaginal or bladder infections can spread into the uterus, fallopian tubes or ovaries.

Vaginal and bladder infections are considered by many to be a normal part of life. Unfortunately, even minor bacterial infections may create tiny adhesions as the body responds to the bacterial invasion. These infections can cause inflammation deep within the vagina that can later produce adhesions. These vaginal adhesions may later cause pain with intercourse, or create an adhesive pull into nearby structures such as the cervix, bladder or rectum, causing pain or decreased function of the organs responsible for reproduction or elimination. Chronic constipation or infertility are common complaints of women we treat with histories of vaginal or bladder infections.

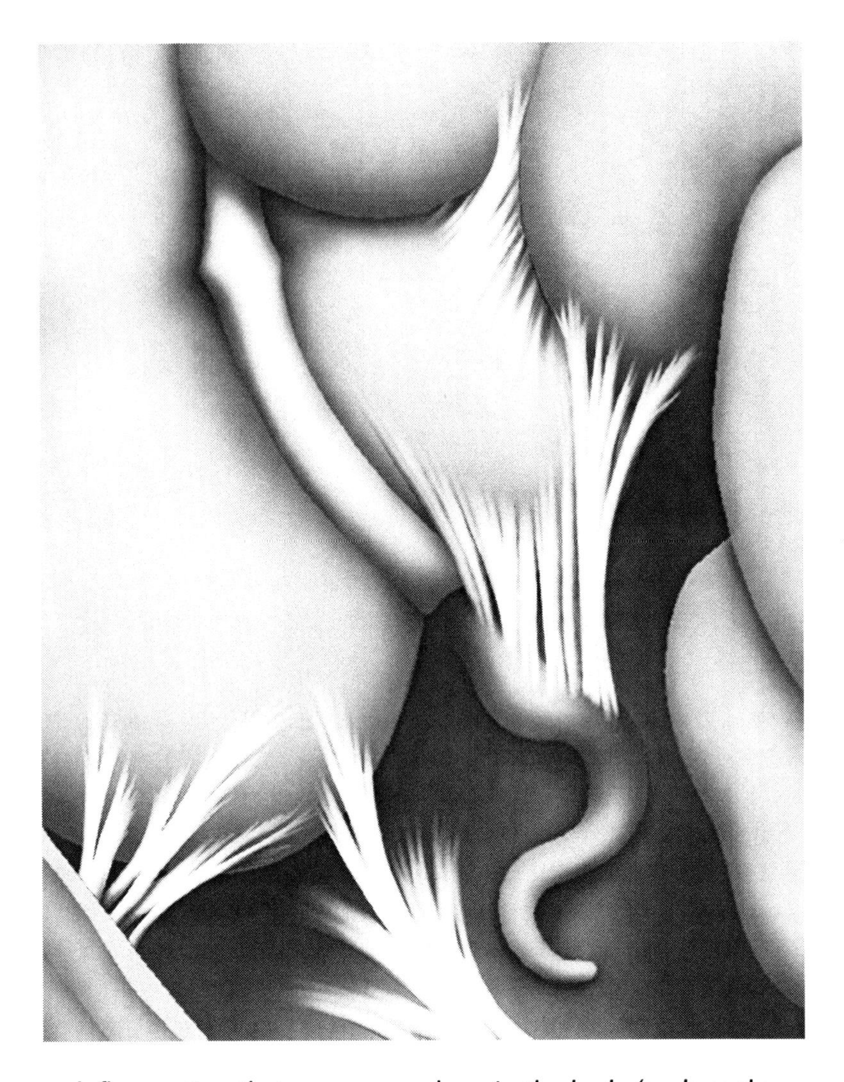

Inflammation that occurs anywhere in the body (such as the intestines shown here) can cause adhesions to form, binding structures that must move freely, for proper function.

Inflammation

Inflammatory conditions such as endometriosis, pelvic inflammatory disease (PID), cystitis, and vaginitis are often intimately associated with adhesion formation. As with physical injury, the body's response to inflammation is to lay down collagenous cross-links, the building blocks of adhesions. As noted earlier, these cross-links are designed to create a blanket which covers and isolates the inflamed tissue, but in doing so, they can glue structures together with a tensile strength of nearly 2,000 pounds per square inch.

Even when the body is fully able to recover from the inflammation, the adhesive blanket that formed to contain the original inflamed tissues remains in the body for life. When this happens, these tiny but strong straight-jackets become part of the intricate network of the structure of the body, a permanent record of the times that the body healed.

Once glue-like adhesions form, they may pull on structures as we walk, breathe, or perform other daily activities. This pull can itself cause inflammation. Thus the process of inflammation and adhesions may continue as a process of ongoing adhesion growth, binding more tissues and structures over time.

A few examples of inflammatory disorders that can create adhesions in the abdomen and pelvis are listed below:

- Colitis
- Irritable bowel syndrome
- Diverticulitis
- Bowel obstruction
- Gastritis gastroenteritis
- Cholecystitis
- Perforated ulcer
- Pelvic inflammatory disease (PID)

- Endometriosis
- Cystitis or vaginitis
- Perforated diverticulum, small or large bowel
- Appendicitis, ruptured appendix
- Hepatitis
- Ruptured ovarian cyst

Chronic poor postures

Over the years, we have noted that adhesions appear to form in patients along tension vectors due to chronic, poor, or compensatory postures. Scientists have documented adhesion formation in areas that receive less movement than normal, such as when a joint is placed in a cast. In fact, scientists took a dog that was perfectly healthy and put his knee in a cast so he could not bend it. When they observed the knee joint six weeks later (arthroscopically), adhesions had already begun to form, presumably due to the lack of movement in that joint.

The same process appears to happen in humans when we are forced to maintain chronic poor postures for extended periods of time. Clinically, we often note significant thickening and hardening in the muscles that support these chronic postures — such as in the neck and shoulders of dentists, therapists, hairdressers, gynecologists, students, and office workers who must work with their head and arms in front of them or in asymmetrical positions for hours at a time, day after day.

It is an unfortunate fact of modern life that people who sit in front of computers for many uninterrupted hours tend to develop spasms due to the constant strain on muscles in the neck and upper back, muscles that are working overtime to hold the head in place. Over time, this spasm creates chronic inflammation. The body's response to this inflammation is to form adhesions in the necks, shoulders and upper backs of office workers and other people who adopt chronic forward head postures.

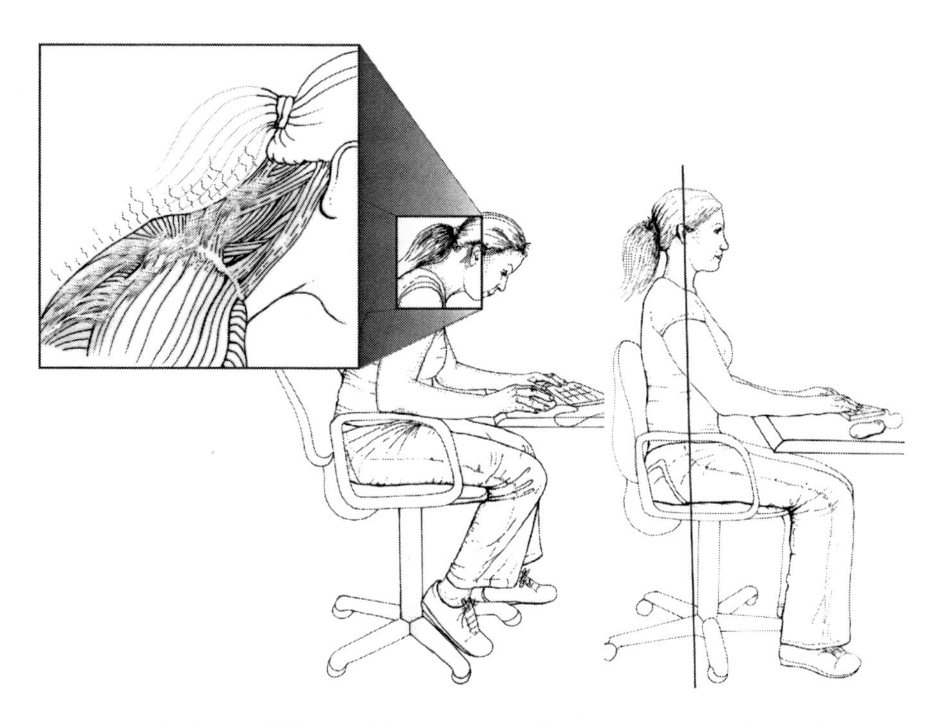

Prolonged "forward head posture" can cause muscles to fire continuously. The resulting spasm and inflammation can create adhesions that cause pain and tightness.

Good seated posture happens when the head is balanced upright over the shoulders, letting the muscles of the neck relax. When sitting or standing properly, a vertical line can be drawn from the ear though the shoulder and hip joints. This posture occurs naturally in most young children. But later in life, when people sit for hours at a time at desks at school and work, their bodies tend to change that posture into a "forward head position." In that position, the muscles in the back of the neck, shoulders, and upper back need to tighten for hours at a time, just to keep the head from falling forward onto the chest.

While the muscles in the back of the neck are strong, they are not designed to hold static positions (such as at a desk or computer) for hours at a time. As hours, months, and years go by, recurrent poor posture causes the muscles to become inflamed, and cross-links begin to form within the muscles in the back or sides of the neck. When the head lifts up to look at a computer screen, stiffness or pain in the neck or at the base of the skull often occurs, sometimes accompanied by headaches. Uncorrected over time, the pain and stiffness can migrate into the shoulders, mid-back, and finally into the low back as all the muscles of the back struggle to correct the poor posture. Thus, a "stiff neck" or a "stiff back" results, and may grow worse over time if not corrected.

Surgery

Surgeries save lives every day. The very idea that during laparoscopic surgery, a physician can enter the body via a viewing scope or scalpel, repair damaged structures, and exit again, leaving the body in better shape than before, is an incredible testament to the wonders of modern medicine. The advances in surgery over the last 50 years have been remarkable, and surgeons develop more effective and less traumatic surgical techniques with each passing year.

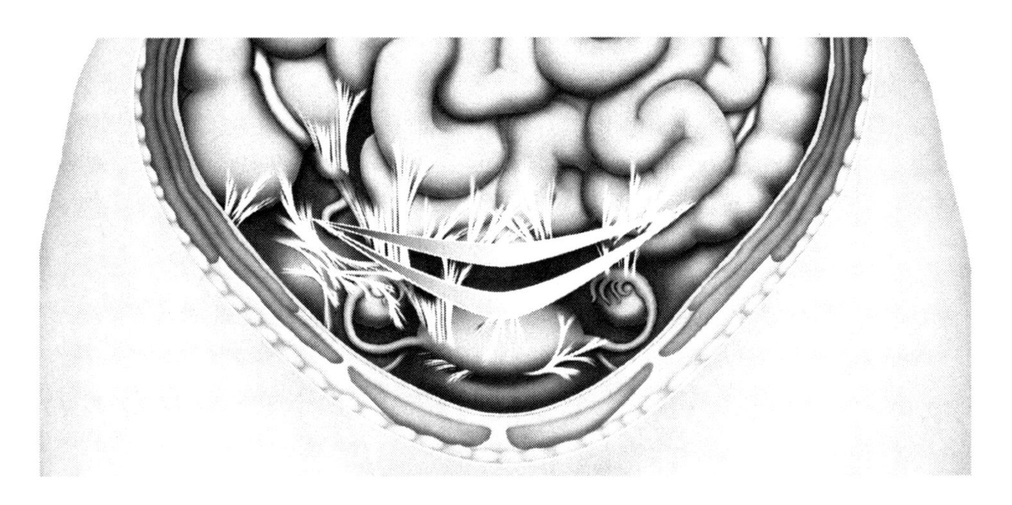

Surgery is a major cause of adhesion formation

Unfortunately, surgery is also a major cause of adhesion formation; adhesions are one of the most common side effects of surgery. No matter how skilled a surgeon, the body lays down adhesive cross-links to help the body heal from the surgery, just as it would from any other trauma.

Numerous methods and devices have been developed to slow or lessen the adverse affects of post-surgical adhesions. But despite surgeons' best efforts and the advances of modern medicine, post-surgical adhesions are a vexing problem that continue to complicate the lives of patients who undergo surgeries. We discuss post-surgical adhesion formation and pain extensively in Chapter Sixteen.

Radiation therapy

Designed to kill cancer cells, radiation therapy also kills some surrounding healthy living tissue. Like surgery, radiation therapy can be a valuable, life-saving technique. But the process of irradiating a tumor can create severe tissue damage and massive adhesion formation at the site of the tumor, and in nearby, previously healthy tissue. Adhesions can bind organs together, severely restrict mobility and function, and cause pain, digestive conditions, or other problems.

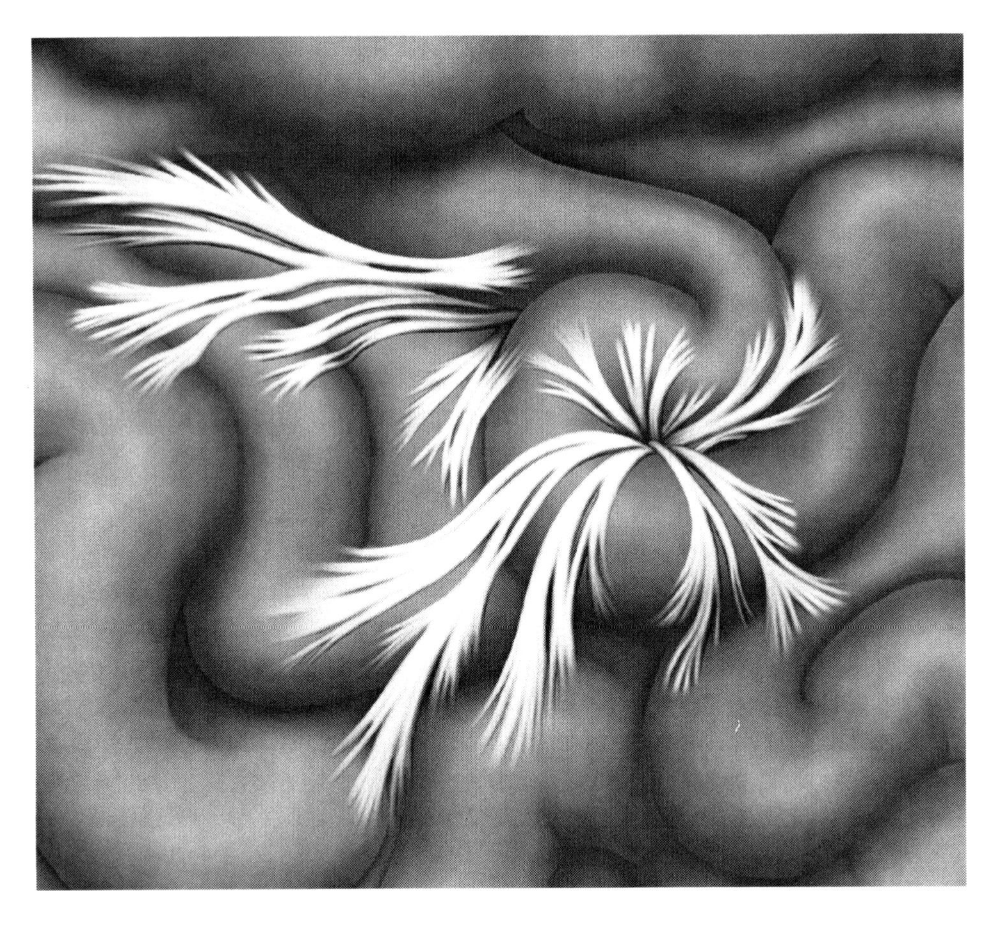

Used to treat cancer, radiation therapy can cause massive adhesion formation, depicted here in the intestines.

Adhesions from radiation therapy to the abdomen or pelvis can become life-threatening when they obstruct the bowel, causing the delicate tissues of the intestines to become restricted, twisted, or closed due to adhesive straight-jackets. While oncologists and radiologists continue to develop ways to shield and protect healthy tissues from its deleterious effects, radiation therapy remains a major cause of adhesions, with resulting pain or dysfunction.

Trauma

As seen in the example at the beginning of this chapter, a fall at a young age can cause adhesions with long-term deleterious effects later in life. Early life traumas such as falls onto the hip, tailbone, chest, or head can create strong glue-like adhesions at the site of tissue injury.

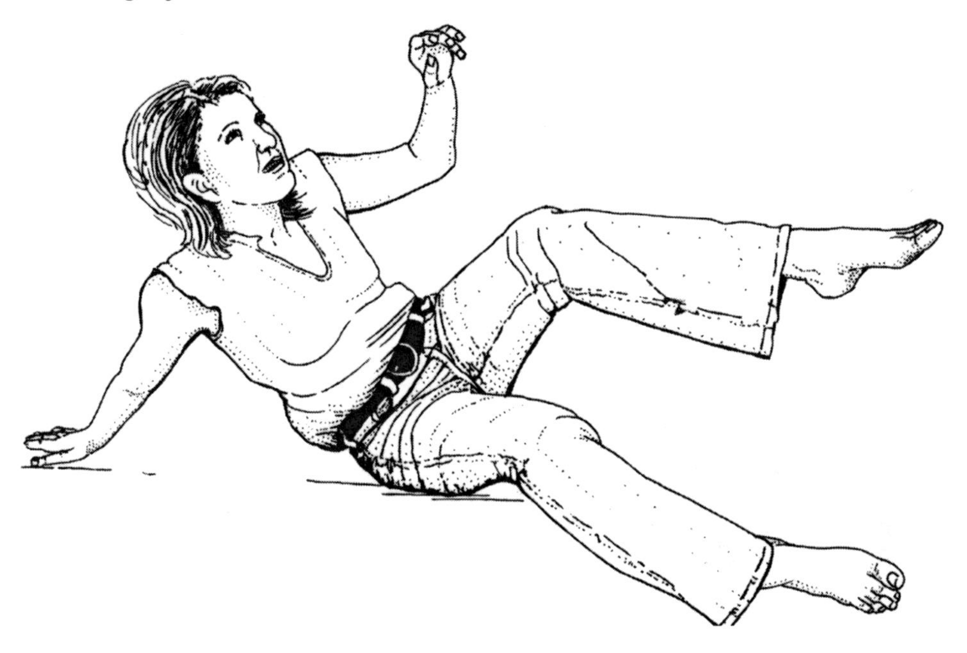

Falls and traumas cause adhesions to form at the site of tissue impact. These adhesions may spread to other areas over time.

As the body grows, adhesions do not always stretch along with the nearby growing structures. Thus, the adhesions can create a pull into muscles, nerves, organs, and support structures during youth and into adulthood. This pull can continue through life, creating internal bonds from which some tissues never escape.

During the school years, athletic injuries from falls or sporting events can create more adhesions. And so it goes through life, as trauma (whether minor or severe) often adds to the adhesive straight-jackets that grow wherever the body heals.

Abuse

Physical and sexual abuse are too prevalent in the world. The trauma of abuse can tear or chafe delicate tissues at the entrance, or deep within the vagina, rectum, face, or elsewhere in the body. Trauma leads to inflammation, and the body responds by laying down adhesive cross-links to contain, protect, and isolate the injured area. The affected tissues can remain adhered thereafter for life, unless treated by a knowledgeable soft-tissue therapist, or removed by a surgeon.

The body's emotional response to sexual or physical abuse is often as tangible as the physical response. The body's compensatory postures of guarding against an imminent threat can create recurrent spasm, eventually leading to inflammation and adhered tissues in the affected areas. The consequent decreases in mobility and function can last for years or decades beyond the original abuse.

We have witnessed the effects of physical and sexual abuse, not just in the areas that were directly traumatized, but also in areas such as the neck, shoulders, low back, hips, and legs as the survivor's body reacted to a terrible situation by creating a pattern of guarding and muscle spasm in areas that were physically, mentally, or emotionally affected by the abuse.

Auto accidents

Motor vehicle accidents (especially sudden acceleration from or deceleration to a total stop) are significant causes of adhesion formation in the body. Since the body may brace for a sudden, oncoming change, the muscles are often tense when the trauma occurs, increasing the shock and degree of injury from the impact.

As the force of the impact travels through the car into the driver or passenger, the various soft tissues of the body absorb the trauma or whiplash. Solid organs like the kidneys, liver, brain, and spleen lack pliability, so they tend to absorb the trauma of the impact immediately. Stretched beyond their normal anatomy, the ligaments and support attachments experience micro-tears as they attempt to contain organs that have been violently jarred from their normal anatomical positions.

Following trauma, injured areas become inflamed. Tiny cross-links form at the areas of trauma to contain the damage and start the healing process. Depending on the extent of the inflammation, cross-links may spread to neighboring structures, increasing the geographic impact of the trauma within the body. Wherever they develop, adhesive straight-jackets begin to form as a response to the injury.

How Adhesions Impact the Body

Many people notice the pull of adhesions as decreased range of motion, or pulls in specific areas of the body. Initially this may feel like a dull pain or ache in these areas that continues or increases over time.

Adhesions create problems when they:

- Put pressure on pain-sensitive tissues or other structures
- Pull on nerves causing pain
- Glue structures that should be mobile, causing dysfunction.

Depending on where and how adhesions form, people experience the pull of adhesions in different ways. Some people are totally asymptomatic – there is virtually no sensation of pain or pulling in the body. These people may never know they have adhesions until they note decreased function (such as infertility or digestive problems) or undergo a diagnostic test such as a laparoscopy or HSG dye test that shows problems.

In fact, we have examined people with severe tightness, adhesions, and spasm in their necks, upper shoulders, or back with no complaint of pain or discomfort in those areas.

For some people, this tightness may manifest itself further up or down the line with TMJ pain or other problems in the head, face, and jaw. Some have difficulty turning their head and shoulders to full range – for example to look out the rear window when backing up a car. Because a physician cannot diagnose adhesions without surgery, many people do not realize they have developed them, nor understand the impact that adhesions may be creating on their comfort or quality of life.

When nerves or pain-sensitive structures become bound by adhesions, the result is pain. Adhered organs and muscles become inefficient, ineffective, or unable to properly do the job for which they were designed when their normal ability to move over and around each other becomes restricted. Eventually, they can stop working altogether, as the adhesive glue slowly shuts down their ability to function. As tissues become adhered, they can exert significant force or pull on other structures, creating pain and dysfunction in remote areas.

Chapter Four

The Wurn Technique®

The numerous successes and life-changing experiences shared in this book are a direct result of the Wurn Technique®. Our treatment is a 100% individualized treatment; it addresses each patient's pain or dysfunction and goals individually. We began to develop the Wurn Technique® in the 1980s when we used manual soft tissue therapy techniques to address pain and adhesions in Belinda's pelvis which physicians called "untreatable." When the therapy returned Belinda to pain-free function, we modified the technique to help others with conditions that were labeled "difficult" or "untreatable."

Finding and Treating the Cause

While we developed this system of therapy, we cannot take total credit for all of the procedures used in it. Like all eclectic systems, we created our work from a foundation of knowledge that we gained from several sources, including continuing education, personal investigation, and experimentation on each other. We expanded our protocols by treating over a thousand patients with diverse and complex diagnoses in the decade after opening our first private physical therapy clinic in 1989.

At that time, we told doctors, "When you see patients no one else has been able to help, send them to us." As we treated patients with complex, chronic pain, we realized that the therapy we were using to decrease adhesions was proving extremely beneficial — sometimes in areas we never expected. We continued to develop and expand our skills, eventually creating a program that included several hundred manual techniques which collectively became known as the Wurn Technique®.

When we discovered this therapy could return function to structures that had been bound, impaired, or closed by adhesions, we founded Clear Passage Therapies® — or CPT. Over the many years since CPT opened its first tiny clinic, CPT-certified therapists have used the work we developed to help many patients whose goals were not met at other facilities.

While the Wurn Technique® defines the manual treatment at CPT, our approach to patient care can be broken into four successive steps. The way we perform these steps appears to set us apart from most other physical therapists and healthcare providers:

1) Extensive Patient History Review

2) Patient Participation, Team Goal Setting

3) Thorough Palpatory Evaluation

4) Manual Treatment (Wurn Technique®)

How Past Events Affect the Body's Present Condition

Our work starts before we ever meet our patient, as we examine each patient's medical and life history. All applicants for therapy must complete an extensive questionnaire before treatment. This document helps us to determine if our treatment may help them meet their goals, or if there are any contraindications to our therapy.

We then encourage prospective patients to review their cases with one of our physical therapists during a pre-therapy telephone consultation. The therapist will answer all of the applicant's questions, and help them determine whether treatment would be appropriate for them. Based on that interview and the patient's history and goals, the therapist can generally advise the patient of the results she may expect to achieve from therapy.

After we accept a patient into our program, our review of patient history continues during the initial physical evaluation and throughout treatment. Many patients do not note past events or experiences on their initial questionnaires because they do not see them as important or relevant to their present situation. During the course of therapy, patients begin to understand how a past trauma, surgery, inflammation, or infection can have a lasting impact on the body. During treatment, they may recall an event from the past that sheds light on their present condition – and finally mention that incident to the therapist.

When speaking of the past, patients often state, "I don't know if this is important but...," or "This may sound silly but...." In many cases, whatever words come next are important clues to help us understand the cause of the patient's pain or dysfunction. We have lost track of the number of times this information has helped our therapists access an adhered area we needed to treat to reach that patient's goal. Over the years, all CPT therapists have become attentive to these phrases, and the words that follow those innocent openings.

The Patient and Therapist: Working as a Team

Whether due to specialization or the busy atmosphere of modern medicine, many patients feel somewhat detached from the evaluation, treatment, and decision-making process involved in their healthcare today. Patients take their bodies to a doctor for repair, just as they would take their car to a mechanic. Physicians make informed decisions or suggestions based on their training and specialty schooling, but often will not ask the patient if s/he has a sense of what his or her body needs. We feel this approach prevents providers from learning valuable clues and information that can help achieve patients' goals.

When we enroll each patient as a valued member of the treatment team, we find that success comes much more easily. At CPT, we do not invite patients into the team out of mere courtesy, but because it significantly enhances their final results.

We have learned to regard each patient as an expert of her body. Over the course of life, a patient experiences and understands her body in ways no health professional ever will. Only the patient has lived through every trauma, surgery, injury or pain affecting her body. This history helped the patient develop a pretty good understanding of her body's processes – how much sleep she needs, what meals agree and disagree with the digestive system, what movements elicit pain, and what activities she loves – or can no longer do, because of tightness or pain.

Discovering Intuition

The lifetime of knowledge a patient develops about her/his body is often overlooked by allopathic medicine. If your body or mind led you to this book, you likely have unresolved questions or complaints that Western medicine has been unable to answer.

When you started seeking help for your pain, dysfunction, or unfulfilled goals, you may have undergone diagnostic tests and then heard the results. Some of the information you were given made good sense, and perhaps some did not ring true for you.

Some patients have consulted several specialists to get a diagnosis, and were given a drug to treat the symptoms — but nothing to address the cause. If that happened to you, did you feel something might be missing that could help you achieve resolution? Perhaps you even have an "inner sense" of what might need to happen in your body for you to reach your goal...but no one has ever asked.

Throughout your life, a small voice called "intuition" has always been in the back of your mind, speaking to you. Some people dismiss intuition as a whim, while others trust it implicitly; many struggle with it, especially when it appears to be in conflict with professional advice.

After observing hundreds of patients and their struggles to choose the right paths for themselves, we have come to believe that intuition is extremely important. The small voice which speaks to you is the result of all you have experienced in your life, coupled with a vision of where you want your life to go from here.

We realize that this attitude is not scientific and is controversial itself. Yet over time, we have noticed that the patients who make decisions based on a combination of medical advice and their own intuition have been more successful and reached their goals faster than those who lived by empirical scientific advice alone.

We encourage you to develop your intuition and ask questions like, "Where do I want to take my life?" and "What do I need to get there?" If these questions prove too daunting, start with questions that may be more manageable, such as "What feels like a good first step?" Our clinical experience shows that you may need to give yourself permission to take that step. While you may make a mistake or "mis-step" from time to time, we have found that this process generally takes our patients to the fulfillment of their goals.

After you take that first step, the next question becomes, "What seems like the next step?" As this system becomes second nature, the mantra becomes "I envision where I am taking my life — and simply step into my vision, one step at a time."

One experiment we suggest is easy and fun. Mentally ask yourself an important question as you are drifting off to sleep. Then notice what answer pops into your head when you first wake up. So often, that answer is coming from the intuitive right brain, giving you the correct answer — directly from your subconscious.

During therapy, we invite you to employ your "inner wisdom" as part of your physical treatment. We may ask you questions like, "Do you have a sense of what is going on in this area of your body?" If something comes up for you, we think of that as a possible clue. We listen to your intuition and file it away as potentially valuable information toward achieving your success.

We also use your inner knowledge of your body in simple, straightforward ways that increase results significantly. When we are treating in one area, we ask if you are feeling a "pull" somewhere else in your body. If you do, this tells us exactly where the adhesive "run" is pulling in your fascial sweater. Similarly, if we are ever treating and you feel your therapist is close to something significant, we ask you to let us know. It's so easy to say, "It feels like there is something significant right there" or "about an inch to the right." We encourage (but do not require) your focus, input, and intuition to increase treatment results.

In essence, we'd like you to consider giving some credence to your inner voice. We also encourage you to share with us and with all of your healthcare providers your intuition about what you feel is happening in your body.

Evaluating the Body

On the first day of therapy, we conduct an extensive physical therapy evaluation of the patient. Our measurement of structure and function of the body is very thorough, due to the complexity of the conditions we treat and our whole-body view. Our assessment includes all the elements associated with a traditional physical therapy evaluation (such as evaluating symptomatic areas), but we also evaluate each patient based on his or her individual history and goals. This evaluation generally takes about an hour.

The physical evaluation starts with a thorough postural assessment while the patient stands. We assess each patient from the front, back, and sides, noting any unusual asymmetries or tensions. At that time, we start to get a sense of which internal areas and structures may be pulling our patient out of alignment, symmetry, or balance. We examine the head and shoulders, noting if they are pulled forward or down, or if one shoulder is lower than the other. As therapists, we are always asking ourselves, "How might the tensions we are noting in the body affect this patient's pain, function, fertility, or ability to meet his or her goals?"

We may ask the patient questions about what we are seeing, such as, "Do you notice a pull into your low back, pelvis, or legs? Is there any achiness in your neck, shoulders or head? What is the frequency, intensity, and duration of your pain?"

Since the adhesive process which helped the patient heal from an earlier lifetime event may indicate a cause or precipitating factor for the present symptoms, we often review history in greater depth. "When did you first notice that ache? What was going on in your life at that time, and during the year before? Did you have a fall, infection, inflammation, surgery, or life transition a while (up to two years) before you started noticing that?" This time element gives us a sense of whether adhesions may have formed in the tightened area(s).

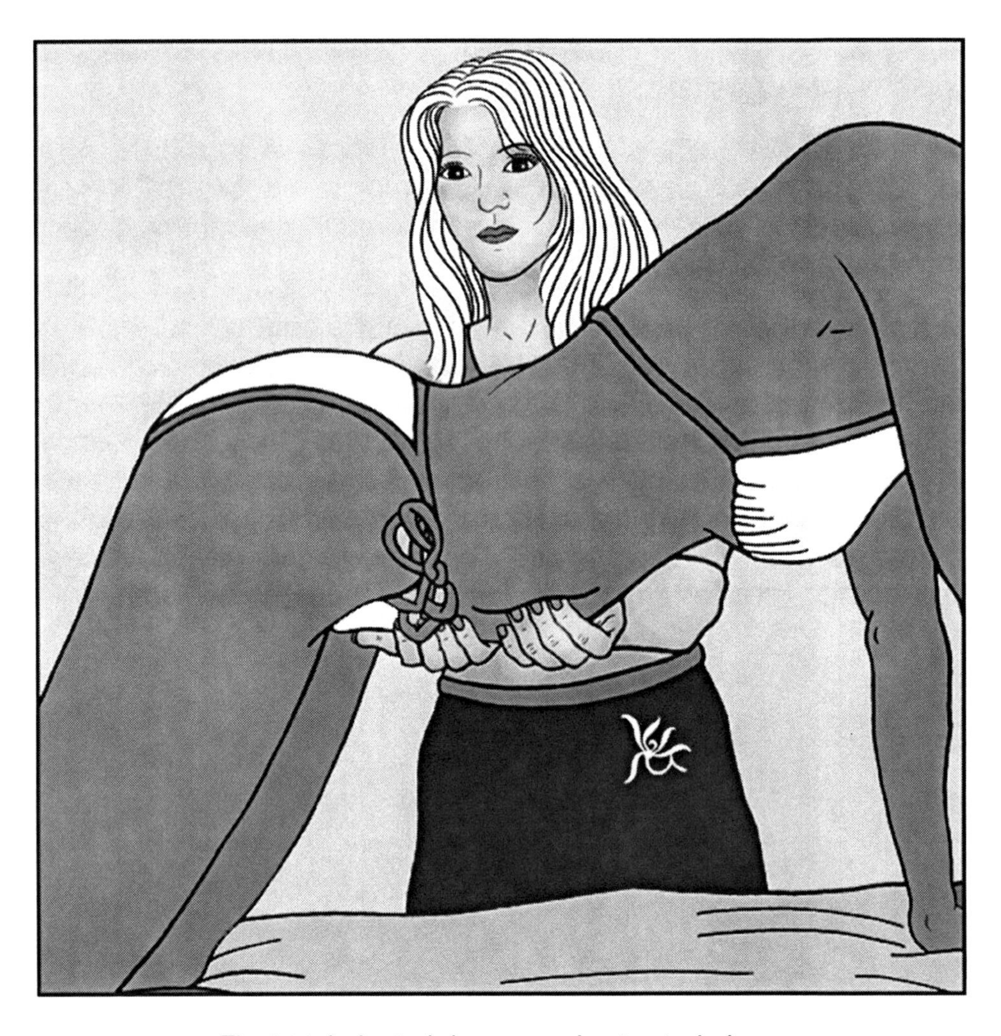

The initial physical therapy evaluation includes a thorough palpation of the body's organs and soft tissues

We then assess the patient's mobility and range of motion. How easily do the major joints move? Does s/he have unrestricted, pain-free range of motion in all areas, or is there restriction or pain with any movement?

After assessing the structure and mobility of the musculoskeletal system, we begin to palpate the organs and connective tissues of the abdomen, pelvis, and the rest of the body. We use various manual tests we developed or learned to help us zero in on restricted areas. We test for restricted mobility and motility within virtually every body system, e.g., digestive, urogenital, reproductive, musculoskeletal, endocrine, and nervous. We assess for free vs. restricted mobility front to back, side to side, top to bottom, diagonally, externally and if indicated (with patient permission) internally.

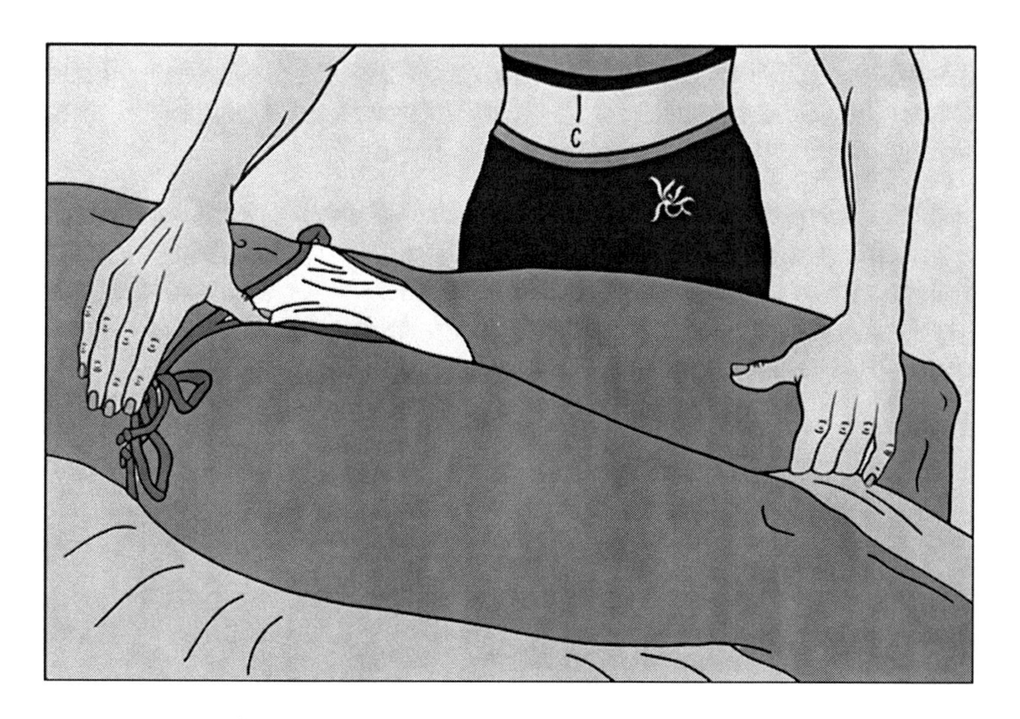

Joint and organ range of motion is measured in relation to the attachments at neighboring structures.

We palpate the structures and connections of all three layers of the fascia from the superficial fascia of the skin, through the deep fascia of the muscles, joints and organs, and then into the deepest layer of fascia, the dura which surrounds and protects the spinal cord, from the tailbone up into the structures of the brain.

After twenty years of experience palpating the viscera of the body, we can ascertain which organs or structures can move normally and which have restricted mobility or motility (the inner movement inherent within each organ).

Treating Adhesions

The principle intent of the Wurn Technique® is to find adhered tissues and structures wherever they exist in the body. As noted earlier, adhesive cross-links act like the thousand tiny fibers of a nylon rope. When they bind together, they can create persistent pain or dysfunction, gluing together structures within the body.

While a surgeon might cut or burn the adhered tissues, our therapy uses a different mechanism. Our focus is to detach the chemical bonds that attach the tiny cross-links to each other. Our work is analogous to peeling apart a nylon rope strand by strand. We use more than 200 specific manual techniques to treat our patients.

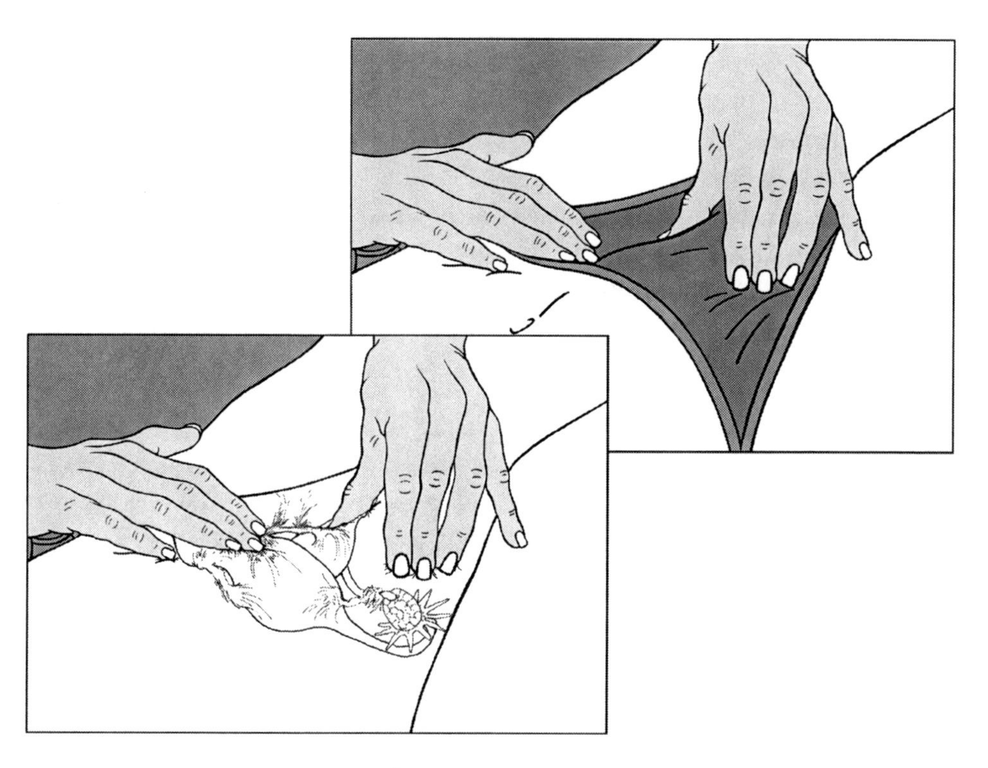

The Wurn Technique® is much less traumatic than surgery. We use more that 200 different techniques to achieve results.

Our patients, physician-advisers, and published study results indicate that this process tends to return the patient's body to a more functional, pain-free state, like the one they had before these areas became adhered. It is almost like going back in time for the areas we treat. When this happens, we give our patients a better chance to achieve their life goals.

Training, Testing, and Certifying Great Therapists

To be accepted for training and certification as a CPT therapist, an applicant must be professionally licensed to practice physical therapy in his/her state and must demonstrate several years of background in manual therapy. Each applicant must take specific physical therapy courses we require before being considered for training. In addition, applicants must demonstrate their skills by treating one of us personally.

Once a therapist has passed these requirements, we send him/her a 650 page *Therapist Training Manual* that we wrote. Each manual contains theory and information on how to treat various conditions not generally addressed by most physical therapists. The manual also includes over 200 specific manual techniques that the therapist must learn and later demonstrate with proficiency before attaining CPT certification.

After studying the manual, the applicant receives an intensive two-week clinical internship which includes testing, training, and review with our top staff. Having passed that phase, s/he is tested again before final certification. Applicants take two written tests — one before and one at the end of the two-week intensive training. These tests are designed to assess knowledge of anatomy, theory, and overview of patient care, and to find any areas where we may need to fill in gaps, or hone the therapist's treatment skills before certification.

If the therapist passes all of these tests, s/he can be certified for one year. We re-test assessment and treatment skills during that year, and take the therapist through any re-certification training we feel is needed, around year-end. All of our therapists receive regular updated instruction and training in the Wurn Technique®.

When Treatment becomes an Art

The Wurn Technique® originated out of our desire to treat Belinda's pain, to help others with chronic pain and dysfunction, and to return patients to an active, fulfilling lifestyle. Over the years it has evolved into a treatment offering much more.

Over the decades that we developed the Wurn Technique®, we witnessed improvements in areas we expected – joints and organs that were glued down by adhesions. But we witnessed often dramatic improvements in unexpected areas such as digestion, hormonal balance, pituitary function, endometriosis and intercourse pain, female sexual function, small bowel obstruction, chronic headache, PCOS, and early surgical trauma (such as female genital mutilation).

As we have done with patient reports in the past, we follow the scientific method to investigate each new claim. That is, we will move from anecdotal reports (e.g., "This area feels and works so much better.") to pilot studies (tracking the same symptoms and results in other patients), to clinical trials (retrospective, then prospective tests before and after therapy), to controlled studies suitable for publication in peer-reviewed medical journals.

The ideas and stories in this book represent a photograph in time, as our work continues to evolve. We have already published scientific studies or citations on many of the diagnoses presented in the chapters ahead. Others are in an earlier stage of investigation.

We invite you to join us on a remarkable adventure through the remaining chapters of this book. There, we will examine what can happen when a skilled therapist listens well, works closely with his or her patient, and using hands, heart, and intuition, begins to unravel adhesive bonds that form in all of our bodies, throughout life. We invite you also to witness many of the heart-rending and sometimes miraculous stories, told by patients in their own words — of lives changed, seemingly impossible conditions reversed, and bodies and spirits healed.

Section Two

Miracle Moms

A new, non-surgical approach to treat female infertility

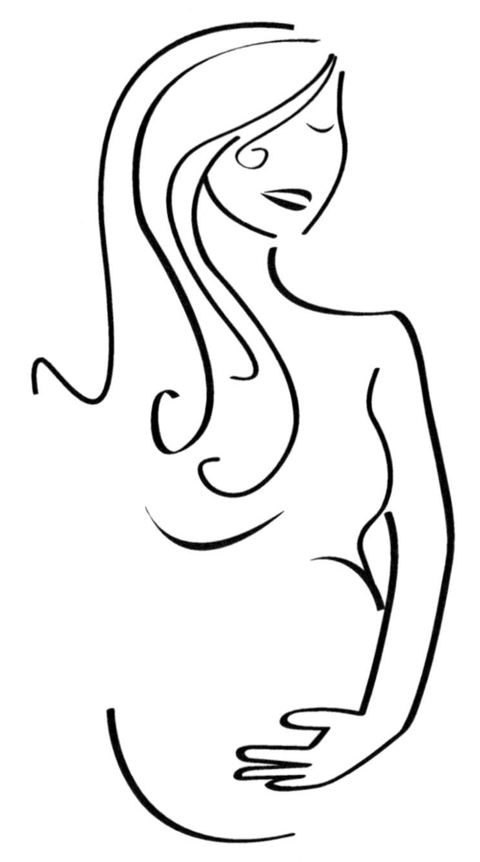

"People who say 'it cannot be done'
should not interrupt those who are doing it."
George Bernard Shaw

There are many diagnoses and treatments for female infertility available to women. It is not the intent of this section of this book to give an in-depth analysis of all of these treatment methods. Rather, it is our intent to take you with us in our voyage of discovery as we uncovered the facts about a new manual physical therapy.

As you will see, in many cases we found answers for which we were not really searching. We never thought to open blocked fallopian tubes. This was just something that happened in the course of treating pelvic adhesions. Once that happened, we felt obliged to create a scientific investigation for the potential benefit the findings could bring to women, their spouses, and physicians. That study has now been published and cited in two respected peer-reviewed journals.[2]

We certainly had no intention of addressing hormone or age-related infertility. This was the furthest thing from our minds. In fact, we actively discouraged women who were approaching menopause and those whose hormone levels indicated they were unacceptable for IVF (FSH levels over 10) from applying for therapy. Yet over time, we have treated many women who were diagnosed menopausal who subsequently had natural full-term pregnancies after therapy (and some now with second natural pregnancies) that we are now investigating that phenomenon as well.

It appears that adhesions and the mechanical gluing down of tissues that happens to all of us as we age is a process which is at work in all of these cases. In the following chapters, we invite you to join us on our journey as we investigate various ways that the natural process of healing — the laying down of adhesions — causes problems for so many women diagnosed infertile. Further, this laying down of adhesions is a process which is apparently reversible by non-invasive, non-surgical, and non-pharmaceutical therapy. This discovery and journey, grouped by diagnoses, is the subject of the chapters in this section of the book.

Chapter Five

Fertility Basics

Five thousand years ago, the diagnosis of infertility was presumably much easier to make than it is today. Since women bear children, early civilizations generally assumed that infertility indicated a problem with the woman. In fact, we do not know the date that humankind began to understand that conception required sexual intercourse. Even after early civilizations came to realize that conception required a man, most cultures still considered the woman at fault if no pregnancy occurred.

Early Egyptians appeared to log the first recorded diagnosis for infertility on papyri scribed between 2200 and 1500 BC. The early papers listed several diagnostic tests. Among these was one that was based on the principal of "Clear Passage."[3] The theory was that in order to be fertile, a woman had to have a clear passage from her mouth to her vulva. A common way that early Egyptians tested a woman's fertility was to place a clove of garlic in her vagina. They would wait a few minutes and determine whether they could smell the garlic on her breath. When they could, it indicated that the woman was fertile, with a "clear passage" throughout her system.

Today, only a part of that theory remains valid. There must be a clear passage between the fallopian tube, uterus, cervix, and vagina for natural conception to occur.

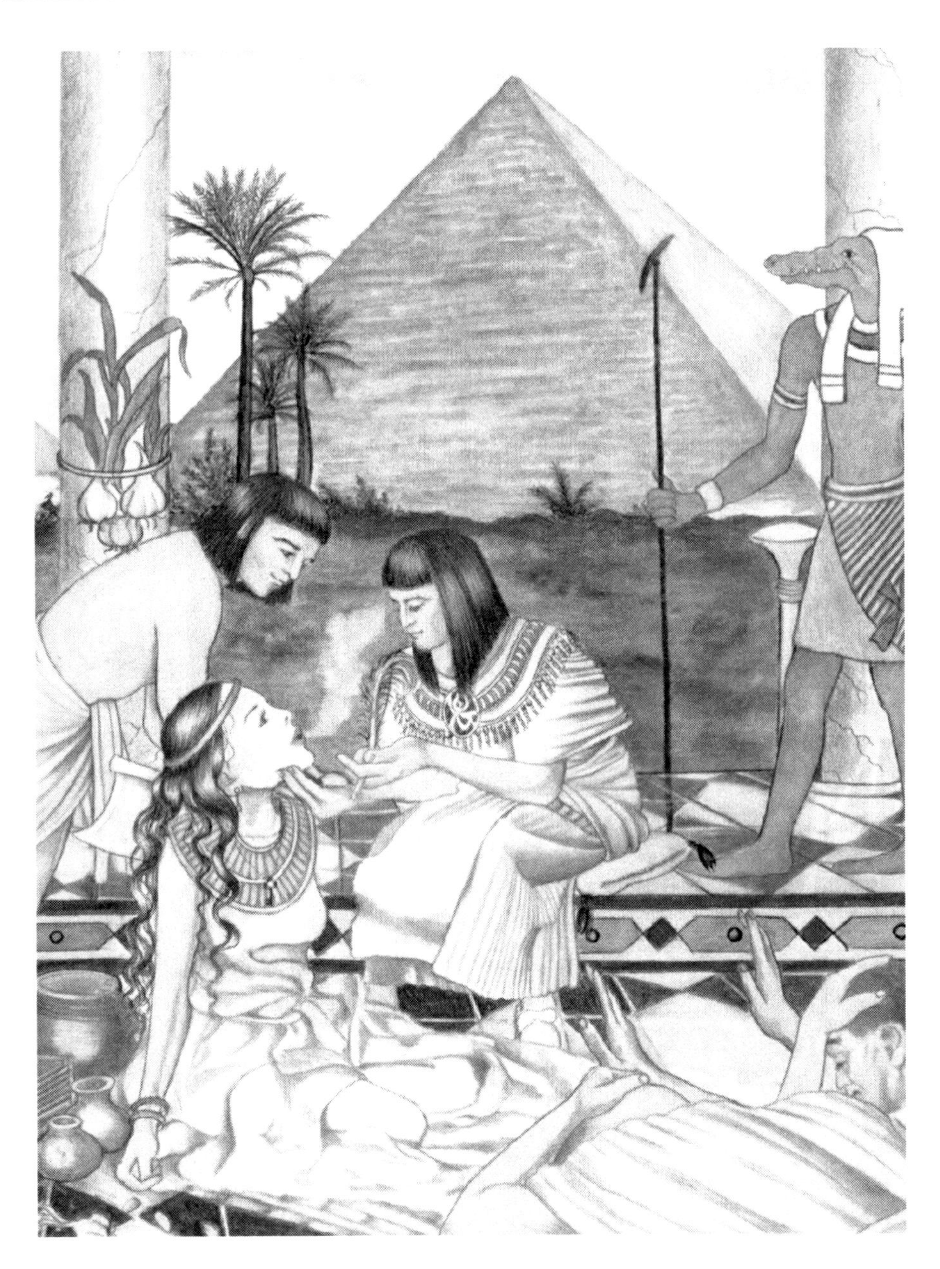

The first diagnosis of infertility was in ancient Egypt. Physicians placed a garlic clove in a woman's vagina. If they could detect it on her breath, she had a "clear passage" through her body, and was considered fertile.

Modern day research shows that about 40% of infertility is due to problems in the male, with an equal amount attributed to the female. The final 20% is considered unexplained, or a combination of the two.

Infertility in men is fairly straightforward and relatively easy to diagnose with tests regarding erectile function, as well as quantity, quality, mobility, and motility of sperm. Male infertility is not a subject of this book.

For most reproductive physicians, female infertility remains a much more complicated area to diagnose and to treat.

Female infertility is divided into three general categories:

- Mechanical infertility (adhesions, blocked fallopian tubes, cervical stenosis, etc.)
- Hormonal or medical conditions (such as age- and disease-related conditions)
- Idiopathic (no known cause)

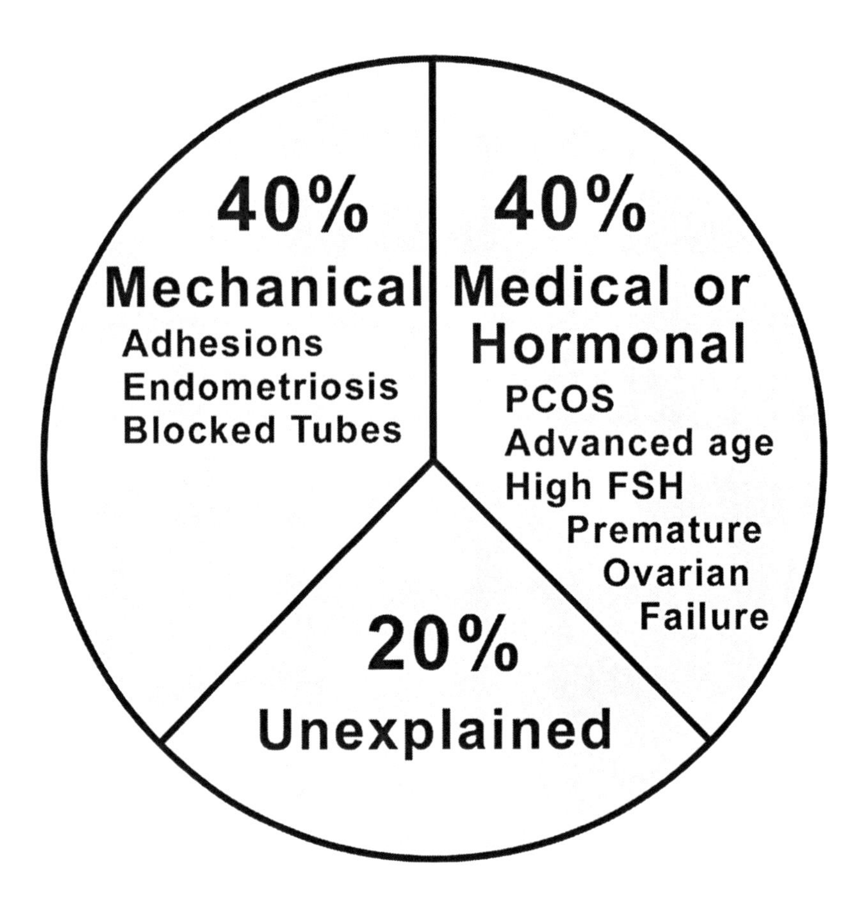

INCIDENCE OF FEMALE INFERTILITY IN THE UNITED STATES

Diagnosis

The diagnosis of female infertility can be a lengthy process, and one that is generally approached systematically and conservatively. Following the Hippocratic Oath, most physicians start with a review of history, along with visual examination and palpation of the reproductive structures to search for any abnormalities

Mechanical Causes of Infertility

If there is no pain and no obvious cause for the infertility, the conservative physician will move on to minimally invasive diagnostic tests and procedures, such as ultrasound or sonogram.

If those tests are inconclusive, or do not show an obvious cause, the physician may prescribe a more invasive procedure, such as a hysterosalpingogram (HSG). In this test, radiographic dye is injected into the uterus via the cervix.

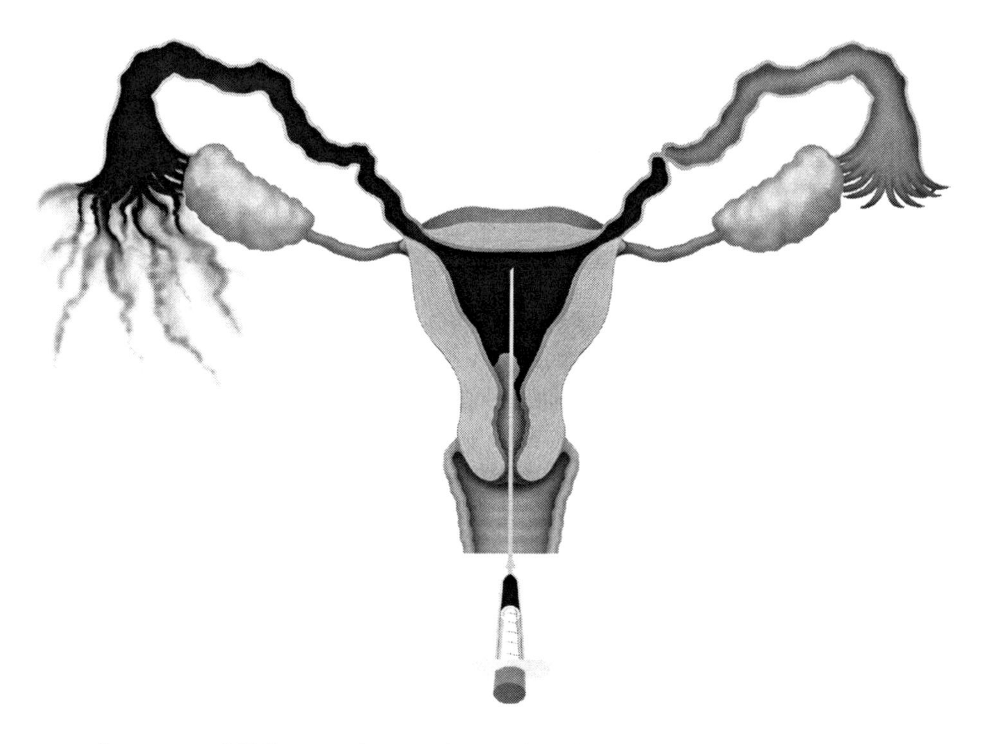

During an HSG procedure, radiographic dye is inserted via the cervix into the uterus. The physician views the dye's progress through both tubes. Here, dye flows freely through the left fallopian tube, but cannot pass the mid-tubal area of the right tube.

The physician will observe (and usually photograph) the course of the dye. Both doctor and patient can watch on a television monitor that follows and photographs the course of the dye as it enters the uterus to determine:

- if the dye proceeds unhindered into the fallopian tube,
- the shape, physical structure, and symmetry of the inner wall of the uterus and fallopian tubes, and
- if each tube is unobstructed and patent (clear) and whether "free spillage" of the dye occurs, which is the most desirable state.

The physician may also deduce whether or not there is any swelling within the tube (hydrosalpinx) which indicates a present or former inflammatory process. In addition, some physicians can deduce whether there is scarring or adhesive activity, due to an unusually circuitous or erratic path of the dye as it proceeds through the fallopian tube on its way to the ovary.

If this and other minimally invasive procedures fail to demonstrate a physical cause of infertility, some physicians may reconsider events in the patient's medical history. For example, if the patient has a history of chronic pelvic or low back pain, intercourse or menstrual pain, or prior surgeries or infections, the physician may begin to suspect that adhesions formed within, around, or between some of the reproductive structures. Other conditions may be considered, such as endometriosis, in which the lining of the uterus is found outside of the uterus, often interfering with delicate reproductive structures such as the ovaries or fallopian tubes.

Adhesions and endometriosis do not generally show-up on x-rays and can only be inferred by HSG, ultrasound, or medical history. They can be definitively diagnosed only by direct visualization during surgery such as a laparoscopy or a laparotomy (open surgery). Complicating some diagnoses is the fact that adhesions can form within structures (as can happen between muscle cells within the cervix or uterine wall), thus they cannot always be visualized by surgery. In addition, we believe that microscopic collagenous cross-links (the building blocks of adhesions) may decrease mobility and function even though they are too small to be visualized during surgery.

As surgical procedures go, most physicians consider a laparoscopy to be much less invasive than an open surgery (laparotomy).

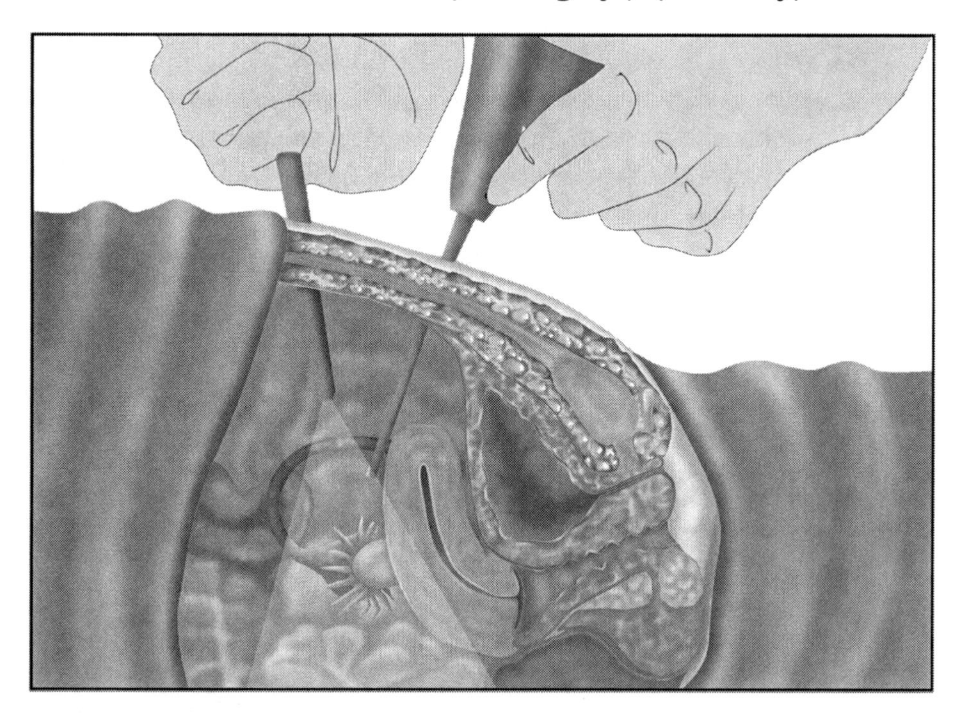

Laparoscopy is performed under general anesthesia. The abdomen and pelvis are filled with gas to separate the organs. The physician uses a light and scope to visualize conditions of the internal structures.

With a laparoscopy, the physician inserts a tube in or near the umbilicus (belly button), then pumps carbon dioxide under pressure into the pelvic cavity. As the gas expands, it creates a space between all of the pelvic organs. The surgeon then inserts a tiny camera to observe and film any mechanical anomalies, such as cysts, fibroids, endometriosis, adhesions or disease processes. If s/he sees any of these, s/he may cut or burn (lyse) some of the mechanical anomalies with a scalpel or a laser. For example, the surgeon may cut accessible adhesions to free the structures bound by strong adhesive bonds. S/he will generally avoid cutting adhesions in areas that could cause further problems, such as those that attach to compromising locations of the fallopian tubes, ovaries, bladder, or delicate walls of the intestines.

If the adhesions are severe or if the physician cannot safely and effectively access them laparoscopically, s/he may elect to change procedures and go directly into an open surgery, called a laparotomy. This is the most invasive level of surgery, usually reserved for those times when the surgeon feels laparoscopy cannot do an effective job.

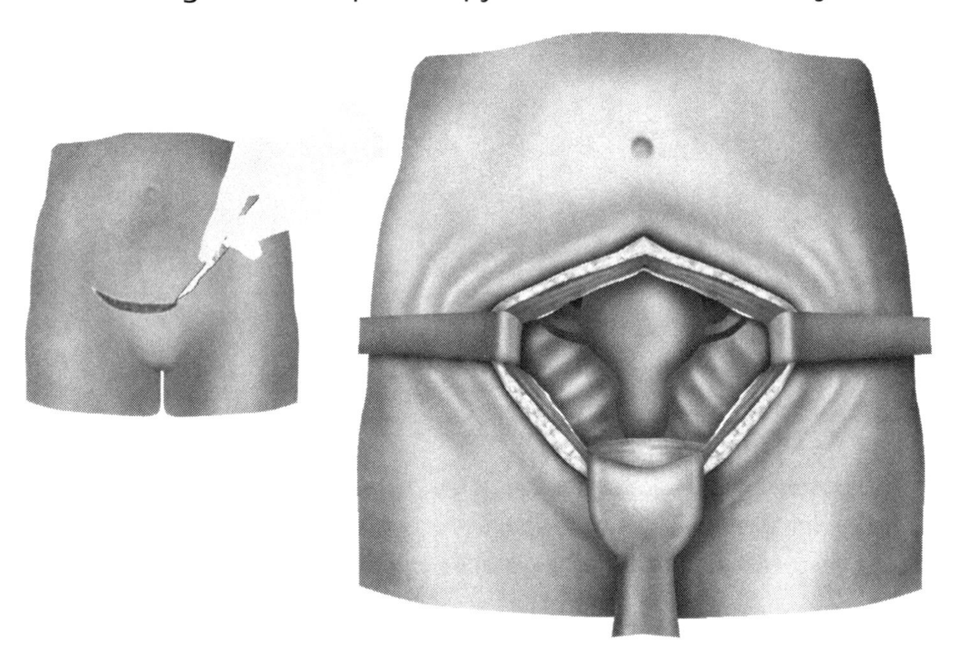

The most invasive of all abdominopelvic surgeries, laparotomy (open surgery) lets the physician observe and repair internal structures directly.

Laparotomy provides the physician and patient with significant advantages and disadvantages. A primary advantage of open surgery is that the physician can see and access everything directly. Unhindered by a camera, small instruments, or a tiny space, the doctor can visualize the exact nature, size, and structure of fibroids and cysts. The surgeon can often see the full extent of any adhesions that formed as a healing response in their patient's life. Furthermore, the physician can clearly see where adhesions join to the bowel, fallopian tubes, uterus, or other delicate abdominal or pelvic structures. Thus s/he can do the least amount of damage in removing adhesions or abnormal structures in those areas.

The problems that arise with open surgery include exposure to the elements in the surgical suite (being exposed to airborne infections) and a significantly increased rate and geography of post-surgical scarring (adhesions).

The scarring inherent in open surgery is generally higher than that in laparoscopy for several reasons. As the surgeon cuts the skin, through layer upon layer to access the target areas, each of those layers has to reattach to its former position in order to heal. As cut tissues reattach, the process requires collagen repair (scarring). While scarring repairs cut tissues, it can also adhere layers that were previously mobile and independent from neighboring layers or structures. Unfortunately, the irritation and inflammation of normal movement on newly adhered tissues may cause additional inflammation — with subsequent post-surgical adhesions. When these bonds draw previously mobile tissue together, they can cause pain, decrease mobility, and restrict normal organ function (including reproduction).

Over the past 20 years, physicians have introduced adhesive barriers (often a fine mesh) in hopes of decreasing the scarring that forms between layers of tissue. Notwithstanding the skill and best intentions of the surgeon, the body heals by creating adhesive collagenous bonds. Thus, surgeries create adhesions or scarring as the body repairs from the surgical trauma to the tissues. For more information on post-surgical pain and dysfunction, please see Chapter Sixteen.

Hormonal Infertility

During the diagnostic process, the physician will also test for hormonal factors that may decrease a woman's ability to conceive or experience a full-term pregnancy. Various hormones can be tested at different times during the menstrual cycle. During days 2 or 3 of the menstrual cycle, a physician may test FSH and LH levels. These will be measured against normal levels and against each other. A panel of estradiol and progesterone levels may also be ordered to check for polycystic ovarian disease and/or an androgen panel may be run to check the levels of free testosterone and dehydroepiandrosterone (DHEA).

Some hormone tests may be done at any time during the menstrual cycle. These include thyroid stimulating hormone (TSH), free T3, T4, free testosterone, DHEA, androstenedione, and prolactin. Physicians and reproductive endocrinologists decide which tests are appropriate for their patients, and may individually consider different hormone levels acceptable. For example, many reproductive endocrinologists will not proceed with IVF stimulation unless FSH levels of day 1 through 3 are below 10. Others accept women with somewhat higher FSH levels.

If the physician cannot find mechanical or hormonal problems, the patient may be diagnosed with unexplained infertility (see Chapter Eleven).

Medical Treatment Options

Mechanical Infertility

Treatments for female infertility depend on the diagnosis. In addition, treatments may overlap depending on the physician and the patient's goals. Mechanical infertility is generally treated mechanically, or with techniques designed to bypass poorly functioning structures.

Intrauterine Insemination (IUI) and Clomid®

As noted above, many physicians suggest procedures to medically bypass the causes of mechanical infertility problems. Intrauterine insemination (IUI) is one of the least invasive of all of these procedures.

In an IUI, the physician inserts a catheter into the woman's uterus via the cervix. S/he then injects the partner's sperm directly into the uterus. This method allows sperm to bypass the vagina and negates the need for the sperm to find the cervix and swim into the uterus.

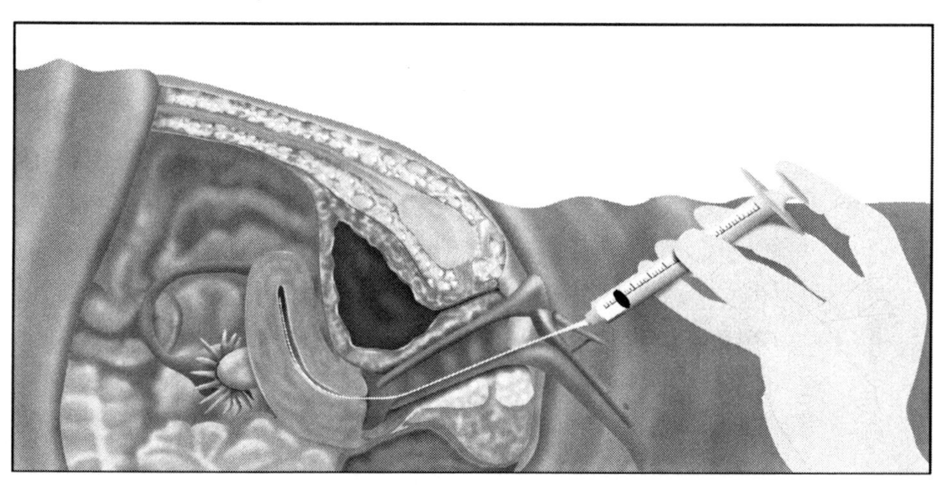

During an Intrauterine Insemination (IUI) the physician injects sperm directly into the uterus.

Clomid or other fertility drugs are often coupled with an IUI. Clomid works to increase the production of eggs in the ovary. Thus, reproductive surgeons and gynecologists have found it to be a useful adjunct to fertility treatment in some cases. An IUI procedure is designed to be administered for a single menstrual cycle. If it fails to produce a clinical pregnancy, it must be repeated at one or more subsequent cycles.

In Vitro Fertilization (IVF)

Patients are sometimes encouraged to move to in vitro fertilization (IVF), if IUI does not produce a full-term pregnancy or the fallopian tubes are swollen, impaired, or totally blocked, or for any of numerous other reasons. IVF procedures are conducted by gynecologists with advanced training in fertility diagnosis and treatment or (more commonly) by reproductive endocrinologists (REs). All REs who are licensed to practice in the United States undergo several years of specialized training in diagnosing and treating infertility, after they receive their gynecology credentials.

While IVF protocols vary widely among physicians and depend upon patient diagnosis and treatment responses, most physicians who perform IVFs first conduct physical and medical diagnostic tests to determine:

- whether the woman has a reasonable chance to implant, carry, and nurture a fertilized egg to birth,
- whether the woman is likely to respond positively to ovarian stimulation and other medication,
- if there are any other issues which may impact fertilization, and
- if there is an optimum site to place the transferred embryo(s).

Most physicians will start an IVF cycle by giving the woman pharmaceuticals such as birth control pills to totally shut down the process of natural menstruation. The RE or infertility specialist thus starts with a "clean slate" in which s/he can totally control the woman's reproductive cycle, as much as possible.

The next step often involves giving the patient ovarian stimulating drugs to increase egg production. The initiation of stimulating drugs marks the official "start" of the IVF cycle. Success rates determined by the American Society for Reproductive Medicine (ASRM) and the US

Center for Disease Control (CDC) are published for all participating US infertility clinics, based on this "starting point." These success rates are available at www. cdc.gov/ART.

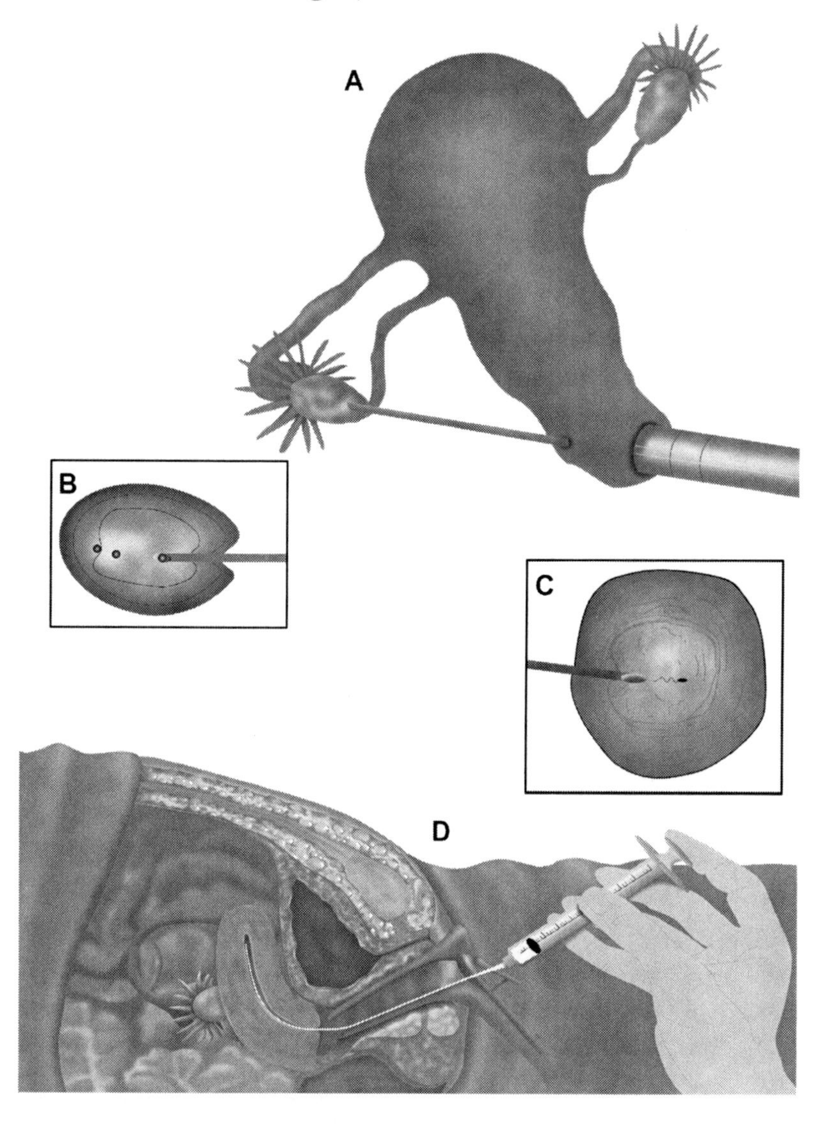

IVF is a series of procedures in which (A,B) one or more eggs are surgically retrieved from the ovary, (C) united with the partner's sperm, then (D) re-inserted into the woman's reproductive tract (uterus or fallopian tube).

The surgeon then surgically removes eggs from the ovaries while the patient is under anesthesia. One or more eggs are chosen and joined with the partner's sperm in a laboratory. Finally, the best of these fertilized eggs are placed inside the woman's uterus.

Like IUI, IVF has one chance to work each menstrual cycle. Many reproductive physicians suggest saving and freezing some eggs for follow-up IVF procedures. If it is unsuccessful, the entire transfer process must be repeated or frozen embryos must be used.

Hormonal Infertility Treatment

Pharmaceuticals such as Clomid® have been shown to increase egg production. Hormones such as FSH, LH, estrogen, estradiol, testosterone, progesterone and TSH may be administered by the physician in order to help normalize or increase a woman's natural ability to conceive. With the assistance of these medications or other options mentioned later in this book, some patients with hormonal factor infertility may be able to conceive naturally, or pursue the IVF process explained above. We discuss hormonal dysfunction in greater detail in Chapter Eight.

Idiopathic (Unexplained) Infertility Treatment

Once a woman and her partner have both been thoroughly tested and the cause of infertility is still unexplained, physicians may review the ovulation cycle with both partners to make certain they understand how to best work with the menstrual cycle. This review will include a thorough explanation of the window of time available in each cycle for natural pregnancy to occur. Since the prime time for conception generally begins four days before ovulation and lasts until the day ovulation starts, it may be necessary for the couple to track ovulation for several months before they get a good sense of when that four-day window of opportunity occurs.

Once that knowledge has been achieved, and if there still is no pregnancy after six months, physicians generally recommend some form of fertility enhancing pharmaceuticals such as Clomid (as noted above). The physician may order a sonogram or pelvic ultrasound to make sure that the ovaries are producing eggs. Another possible suggestion is an IUI (as noted above), sometimes with a course of fertility enhancing drugs.

Alternative and Complementary Treatment Options

We have only found three natural treatments for increasing fertility that are backed by scientific evidence, with quantitative studies published in peer-reviewed western medical journals. These include group therapy, acupuncture, and our manual physical therapy, the Wurn Technique®. Other techniques have been suggested as fertility enhancements, but to date, none of these have published results in peer-reviewed scientific journals.

Various herbs and traditional Chinese medicine (TCM) have been credited with enhancing fertility by many patients and practitioners, but to date there are no controlled studies published in western journals to support those theories. To date, we have not found science to confirm and quantify, or to deny, success rates for these claims.

Mayan abdominal massage, a technique which was developed and passed down through the Mayan civilization, has been suggested as a self-treatment technique. Mayan abdominal massage differs significantly from manual physical therapy. The intent with Mayan massage is to improve the placement and alignment of the uterus. Because the treatment addresses only the placement and alignment of the uterus, most practitioners do not feel that it can help women with hormonal infertility, blocked fallopian tubes, and conditions outside the uterus. No published scientific studies show that Mayan massage increases fertility or decreases pain.

The list of fertility enhancing "potions," positions, and adjunct techniques is long. As long as a technique is not injuring someone, our feeling is to follow the Hippocratic Oath: "Above all, do no harm."

That is to say, if it is not going to harm you, there is likely no danger in trying something that makes sense to you. As always, we suggest consulting your physician before attempting anything that might interfere negatively with your fertility, or with your physician's treatment.

Behavioral Therapy

In 2000, Harvard psychologist Alice Domar, PhD, published a study in which she found that women who participated in group therapy were 30% more likely to experience spontaneous conception and medically-assisted conception than those in the control group. Participants in the group therapy received relaxation training, cognitive restructuring, methods for emotional expression, and nutrition and exercise information related to infertility.[4]

Acupuncture

A German study published in 2002[5] showed that patients who received acupuncture at specific points on their bodies 25 minutes prior to and 25 minutes after IVF transfer had increased pregnancy rates versus the control group. In 2007, a similar study conducted by the University of South Australia[6] found that fertility rates were also higher in participants who received acupuncture prior to and after IVF transfers.

Some physicians note that the final success rate for the acupuncture group was relatively low compared to the norm throughout the US. While no explanation was given for this in the study, it has been suggested that participants were perhaps more challenging cases who had previously had no success with IVF transfers. However, the success rates between the non-treatment control and the acupuncture group were high enough to surmise that acupuncture improved the IVF pregnancy rates significantly for the participants.

Manual Physical Therapy (Wurn Technique®)

We approached the prospect of affecting fertility with a great deal of caution. Raised as we were in traditional medicine, and dealing with physicians every day for many years before our initial infertility successes, we harbored our own skepticism at the same time that women were telling us, "My doctor told me I would never become pregnant. Since you have treated me, I'm now going to be a mom."

On the one hand, we realized that if this were true, this would be a real boon to womankind. To find a non-surgical, non-pharmaceutical adjunct infertility treatment would be a tremendous benefit to many women, their spouses, and their physicians. On the other hand, we realized that even if scientific investigation confirmed that we had achieved positive results, we would still be met with a great deal of skepticism.

In the end, Dr. King, along with several other physicians coached us through creating scientific trials and studies to determine whether or not we were able to reproduce our positive treatment results. Part of our intent was to try to delineate the specific success rates for various types of female infertility, as well as noting any risks or adverse side effects.

In 2004, the first definitive studies of our work with women diagnosed infertile were published in *Medscape General Medicine.* To date, we have completed seven published studies and abstracts. All studies were conducted under the direction and guidance of independent physicians and scientists at our Clear Passage Therapies® clinic in Gainesville, Florida. In each chapter of this book, we discuss the relevant studies we conducted along with data from studies we have published in peer-reviewed medical journals.

In the 2004 *Medscape* study[7], 71% of women who had been infertile for an average of five years became pregnant naturally after receiving 20 hours of the Wurn Technique®, and 64% produced full-term births. Subsequent review showed that 33% of the new mothers had a subsequent natural pregnancy and birth, suggesting the therapy has lasting effects for some women.

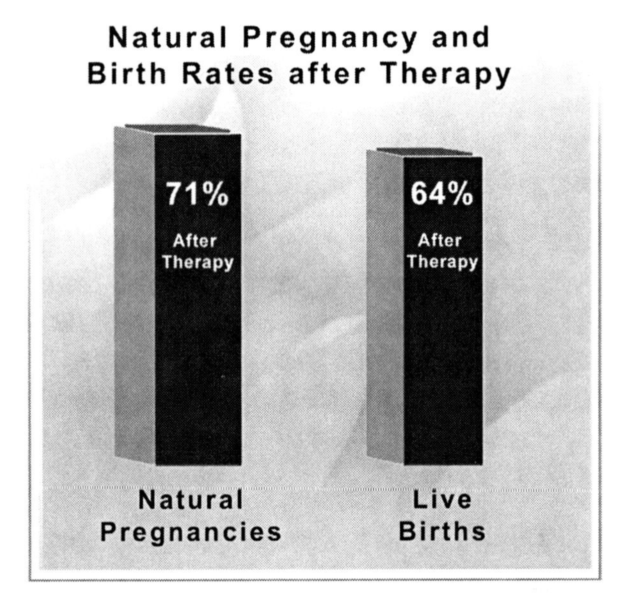

In a concurrently published study, 67% of women undergoing IVF after receiving the therapy had clinical pregnancies after embryo transfer, versus the 41% national average, used as a control. (We used the national "transfer success rate" of 41% rather than the "start of cycle" success rate of 28% because at that time we had no idea that we could improve hormone levels. Thus we were testing the "mechanical" aspects of IVF after embryo transfer, exclusive of the hormonal aspects that affect the ability of a woman to proceed to transfer.)

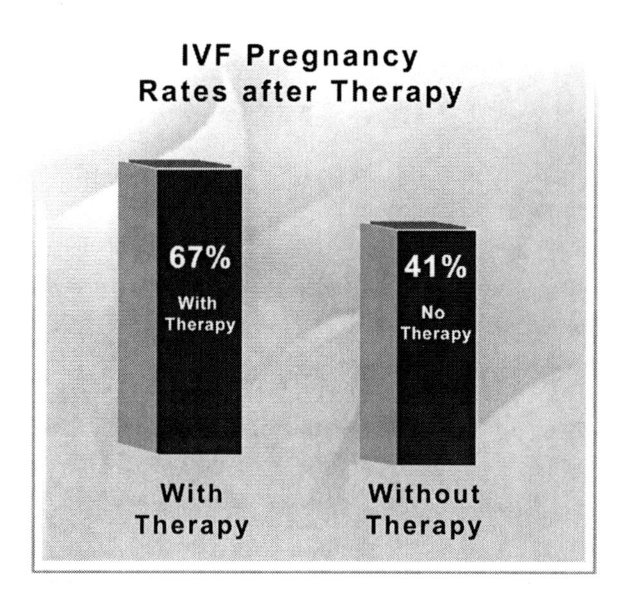

While the number of participants in these studies was small, we've been told it is often that way in pioneering studies. The fact that we were able to conduct these studies under the direction of independent physicians, that the facts and methods passed peer review (the scrutiny and review of physicians and scientists assigned anonymously by the journals), and that the results were found compelling enough to be worthy of publication and/or presentation to large physician groups speaks to the credibility of the data we obtained.

Endometriosis and Multiple Failed Surgeries, IUIs, and IVFs

- Madison's Story

I was shocked when I could not become pregnant. My husband and I had always assumed we would be able to have children when we wanted. But after trying for a year, we finally sought the help of my gynecologist.

Because infertility tests are less intrusive for men, my husband was the first to be tested. When his tests came back normal, my personal struggle with infertility began.

HSG (Hysterosalpingogram)

My physician immediately suggested I have a hysterosalpingogram (HSG) — a test to determine if there was any blockage in my fallopian tubes. I was relieved when the HSG revealed that my tubes appeared to be functioning properly.

I knew something else had to be wrong. Since the onset of puberty, I had experienced excruciating pain during my periods. My doctors had never been able to find the source of my pain. I thought that pain might be tied to my infertility.

I consulted another physician who suspected I had endometriosis — a condition in which endometrial tissue grows outside of the uterus, and can cause severe pain and infertility.

Laparoscopic surgery

Unfortunately, the only way to diagnose endometriosis is through laparoscopic surgery. My physician found severe endometriosis encasing the majority of my reproductive system and bladder. During the surgery, he removed any endometrial tissue he could access. However, the surgery caused my bladder to shut down and a bladder specialist had to be called in. I had to spend considerable time healing, due to these post-surgical complications.

Fertility drugs

Even after the surgery, we found we were still unable to become pregnant. My doctor then prescribed Clomid®, to enhance my fertility. Because this drug affects the hormonal system, I experienced side effects, such as having little control over my emotions. I continued taking Clomid for six months. But after no success, our doctor decided to refer us to a specialist.

IUI (Intra-Uterine Insemination)

The specialist we consulted thought an intrauterine insemination (IUI) was our best option. During the IUI, a thin catheter was inserted through my cervix and my husband's washed sperm was injected into my uterus. Because an IUI has to be performed within six hours of ovulation, I was given hormonal shots. I was prescribed Paxil®, an anti-depressant, to help with emotional swings, but I still felt like I was going through menopause. I would wake up in the middle of the night and want to strip off all my clothes.

Because my menstrual pain was back, my specialist recommended I have another laparoscopic surgery.

My frustration increased when the IUI wasn't successful and two subsequent IUIs also did not work. Because my menstrual pain was back, my specialist recommended I have another laparoscopic surgery. I was hesitant to undergo the procedure again, so I sought a second opinion.

Our new specialist agreed that a laparoscopic surgery would be beneficial. I decided to go through with the surgery, but it turned out far worse than the first. This surgeon accidentally nicked my intestines while removing endometrial tissues — causing me to stay in the hospital for a week.

IVF (In Vitro Fertilization)

After the disappointing results of both surgeries, my husband and I decided to try in vitro fertilization (IVF). For ten days, I gave myself injections that made me sick with an upset stomach. Then, while I was under sedation, the specialists used an ultrasound-guided needle to reach my ovaries, and retrieve my follicles. They were then incubated with my husband's sperm. After an egg was fertilized, the embryo was transferred to my uterus.

I had to wait two excruciating weeks before I could return to the clinic for a pregnancy test. When we were finally told the results, we were devastated to learn the IVF was unsuccessful. Three months later, my husband and I decided to try another IVF transfer. Once again, our transfer ended as a "failure." Grasping thin threads of hope, we schedule a third IVF transfer.

Manual physical therapy

Before the procedure, our superintendent asked me and my husband if we had ever heard of Clear Passage

Therapies (CPT), a clinic that offers manual physical therapy to help relieve pain and improve fertility. My husband and I researched CPT, and read their website and medical studies. Because it had proven success without the drugs and surgery that had caused me so many problems, we knew this was something that I should do. We felt it would not only increase my chances of pregnancy, but would also help my body heal from all I had undergone to that point.

When I arrived for my week of treatment, the therapists first explained that when the body heals from trauma (surgery, abuse, etc.), scar tissue forms and can turn into adhesions that cause pain and prevent proper function within the body. During my twenty hours of treatment, the therapists worked to loosen adhesions and restore proper function to my body.

Afterwards, my body felt looser and healthier. When I returned home, my husband and I were elated to find that there was no longer any pain with sex. My husband joked that he would send me back for more treatment in a heartbeat. Another amazing outcome was that I no longer experienced pain from my endometriosis.

Another amazing outcome was that I no longer experienced pain from my endometriosis.

We completed our third IVF just one month later. When my pregnancy test came back positive, I was so excited! I knew it had to be the manual physical therapy that made the difference.

We were so happy when our beautiful baby girl was born. Five months after her birth, we discovered another surprise. I found out I was pregnant again! After struggling with infertility so long, my husband and I never considered using any form of birth control. It was then that I knew CPT had healed and restored proper function to my body.

Looking back, I wish I had gone to CPT sooner. After all the drugs, the painful, unnecessary surgeries and treatments, it was a natural, drug-free treatment that finally enabled me to become a mother.

Chapter Six

Blocked Fallopian Tubes

"That's impossible!" the doctor practically yelled. "There is just no way you can open fallopian tubes — or do anything to reduce adhesions with your hands."

He was clearly upset.

We had called him for advice. As Chief of Reproductive Medicine at a large medical school, we hoped he might give us some guidance about unusual findings we were witnessing in patients diagnosed infertile. Among the most puzzling of these were full-term natural pregnancies in women who came to us with a history showing several years of totally blocked fallopian tubes. Since blocked fallopian tubes do not generally re-open spontaneously, this was very unusual indeed.

We were also seeing spontaneous natural pregnancies in an unusually high percentage of women who had been infertile for several years, despite medical attempts to achieve pregnancy. We thought the head of a research and learning institution would be pleased to hear of our clinical findings, and give us some guidance as to how to apply a greater measure of scientific inquiry to our findings. Instead, he seemed upset, and intent on giving us a piece of his mind.

Between the lines, we felt he was almost saying, "You cannot treat infertility; that is the sole purview of gynecologists and reproductive endocrinologists." He did not seem to understand that as physical therapists, our group worked regularly with physicians as an adjunct to their regular care. Given the positive reputation we already enjoyed with hundreds of physicians with whom we were affiliated, this was a scary introduction to the world of assisting infertile women.

Still, women were coming to us for treatment, and based on our results to date, we could hardly refuse, or even discourage them. In all events, we approached treatment with caution, but always with a focus on success for each patient.

Eventually, things would become even more strained between us and this physician. His feelings intensified when some of his own patients were successful with us after treatment with him failed.

Over the years, we have been pleased to find that attitudes like his are diminishing, due in part to several published citations about the Wurn Technique® in scientific and gynecologic journals. We believe that most physicians are primarily interested in seeing success for their patients. More and more, infertility specialists are becoming open to working with adjunct therapies to help their patients achieve their goals.

The Three Types of Blockages

The fallopian tubes are among the smallest organs in the female body. Charged with the task of capturing a one-celled egg and then providing the environment for its union with a single sperm, the fallopian tube is truly the place where life begins.

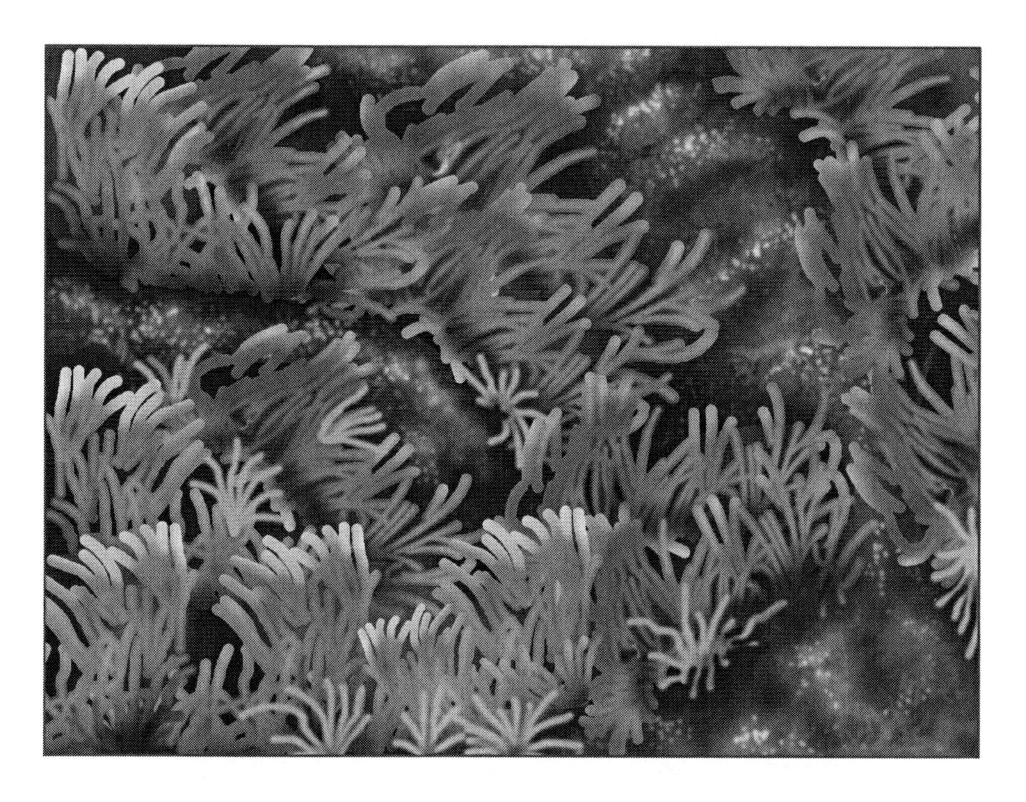

The inner wall of a fallopian tube is truly remarkable, with thousands of tiny cilia, like a lush underwater garden.

The structure and function of each fallopian tube is complex, almost beyond belief. As small as a strand of spaghetti, the inside of the tube is extremely delicate. The walls of the tube are lined with thousands of delicate hair-like structures called cilia. In fact, more than one person has noted that the internal walls of the fallopian tube appear to resemble a lush and supple coral bed, when viewed under an electron microscope.

Due to the tiny size of the inside of the tube and the delicate garden-like structure within, the fallopian tube is poorly prepared for the invasion of collagen cross-links that form as a response to inflammation or infection. As the body heals, and collagen lies down within the tube, it covers and adheres the cilia and the garden of support structures within the tube, blanketing them in a glue that constricts their movement and function. Continual adhesion formation can finally bind one side of the tube to the other, resulting in total tubal occlusion (blockage).

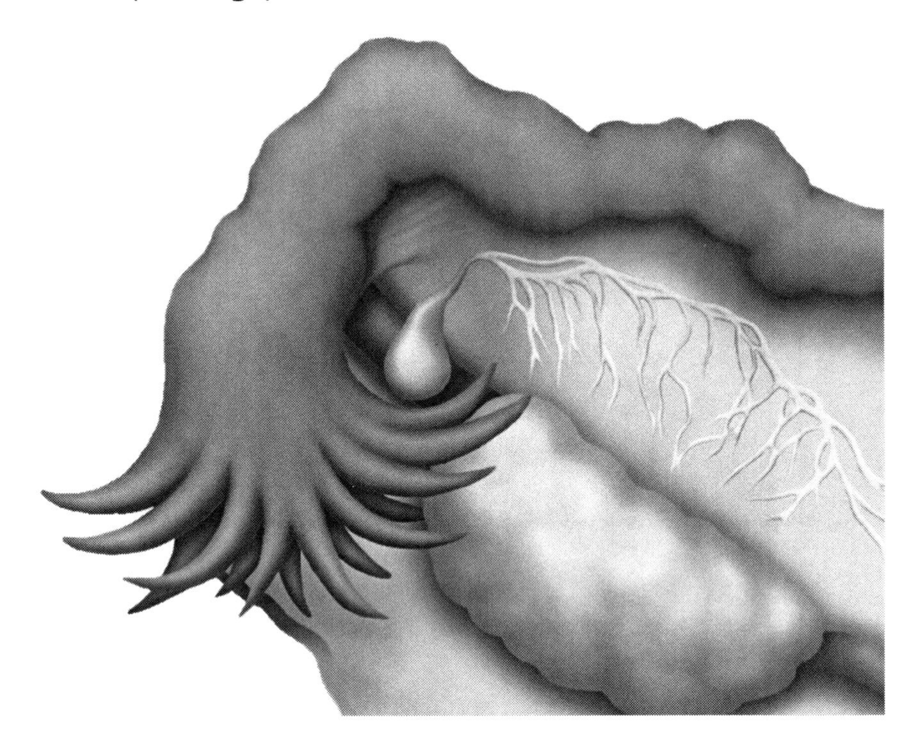

The end of the tube near the ovary has delicate finger-like projections designed to grasp the one-celled egg released by the ovary.

At the end of the fallopian tube, the delicate finger-like fimbriae are designed to grasp the single-celled egg as it emerges from the ovary each month. In appearance, the fimbriae are like the petals of the finest flower imaginable. These tiny but magnificent structures must be free floating in order to function properly. But after inflammation, infection, surgery, or injury in the pelvis, collagenous cross-links can form and bind the fimbriae together, creating a structure which is adhered by tiny collagenous glue-like adhesions. These cause the tube to lose its delicacy, mobility, and ability to grasp the egg. In severe cases, these cross-links can draw the fimbriae together into a blunt structure resembling a closed fist – a condition sometimes referred to as "clubbed fimbriae."

The diagnosis of "blocked fallopian tubes" is one of the most difficult diagnoses for a woman to hear and for a gynecologist to treat. Blockages may be found in the following areas:

- Proximal: near the uterus, called the isthmus
- Mid-tubal: in the middle portion of the tube, called the ampulla
- Distal: at the end of the tube, by the ovary and fimbriae (the fingerlike projections that create the end of each tube)

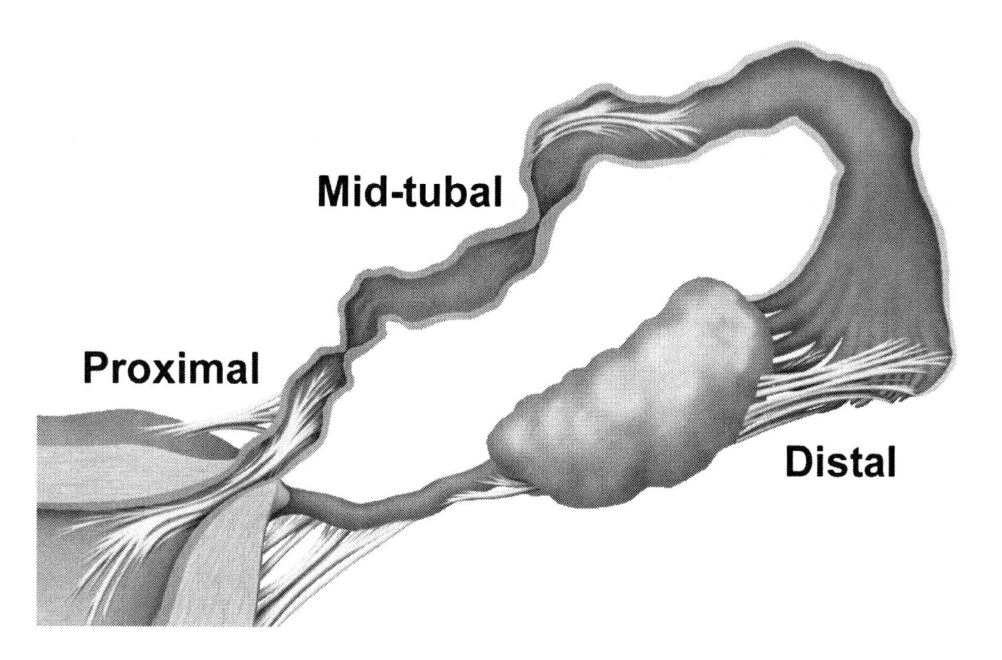

Fallopian tubes may become blocked in any of a number of places.

Either the left or right tube can be blocked in one or more of these three places, or both may be partially or totally blocked anywhere along their length. While most blockages occur in only one of these locations, occasionally bipolar blockage (blocked at both ends of the tubes) can occur.

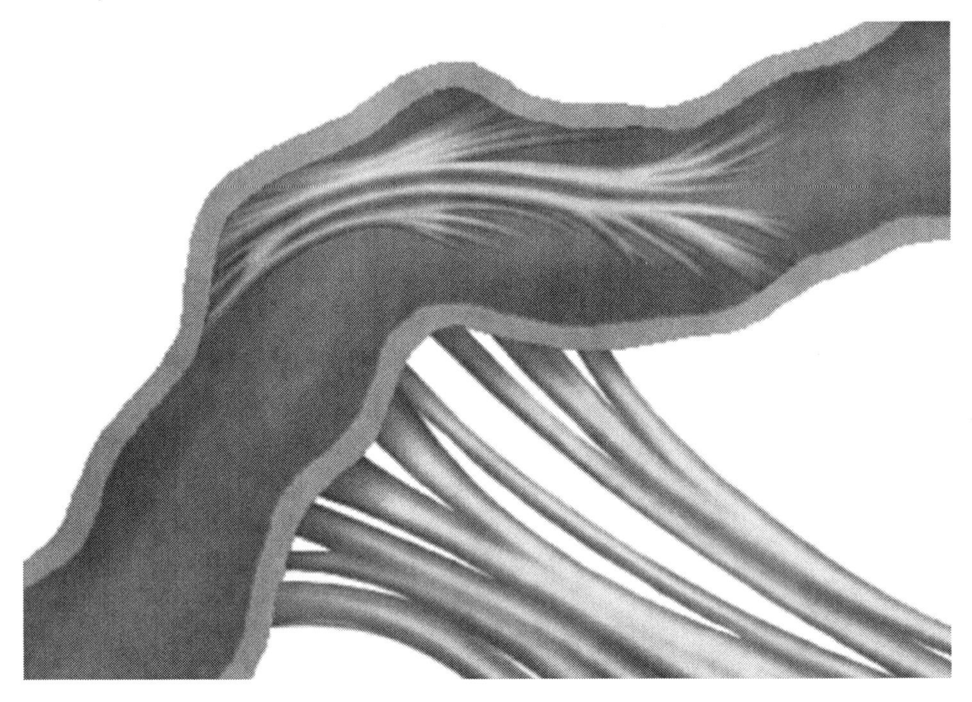

Adhesions can block fallopian tubes from the inside, or may pinch them from the outside, like a kink in a garden hose.

In some women, the reason for the blockage may be unclear. For some patients, tubal occlusion is thought to be related to adhesions that form after a C-section or pelvic surgery, such as the repair of a ruptured appendix. In a large number of cases, sexually transmitted diseases (e.g., Chlamydia or PID), pelvic infection or inflammation (e.g., salpingitis) cause adhesions that can block a tube. In most cases, adhesions are the primary cause, or are intimately involved in tubal occlusion.

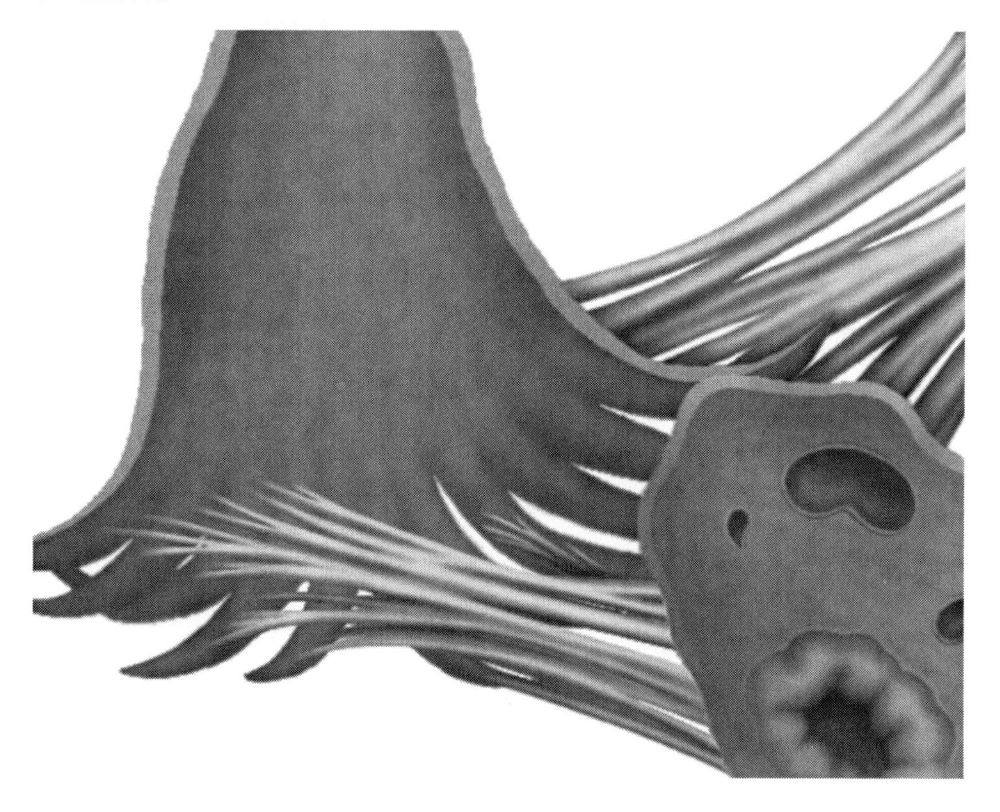

Adhesions at the fimbriae are a major problem for patients with distal occlusion, impairing transfer of the egg from the ovary to the tube.

Secondary causes of blocked fallopian tubes include tubal spasm and mucous plugs. Spasm of the fallopian tubes is considered to block the tube, but only when it is in spasm. While some physicians feel that this does not represent true blockage, others acknowledge that spasm represents a pathological state which can interfere with fertility.

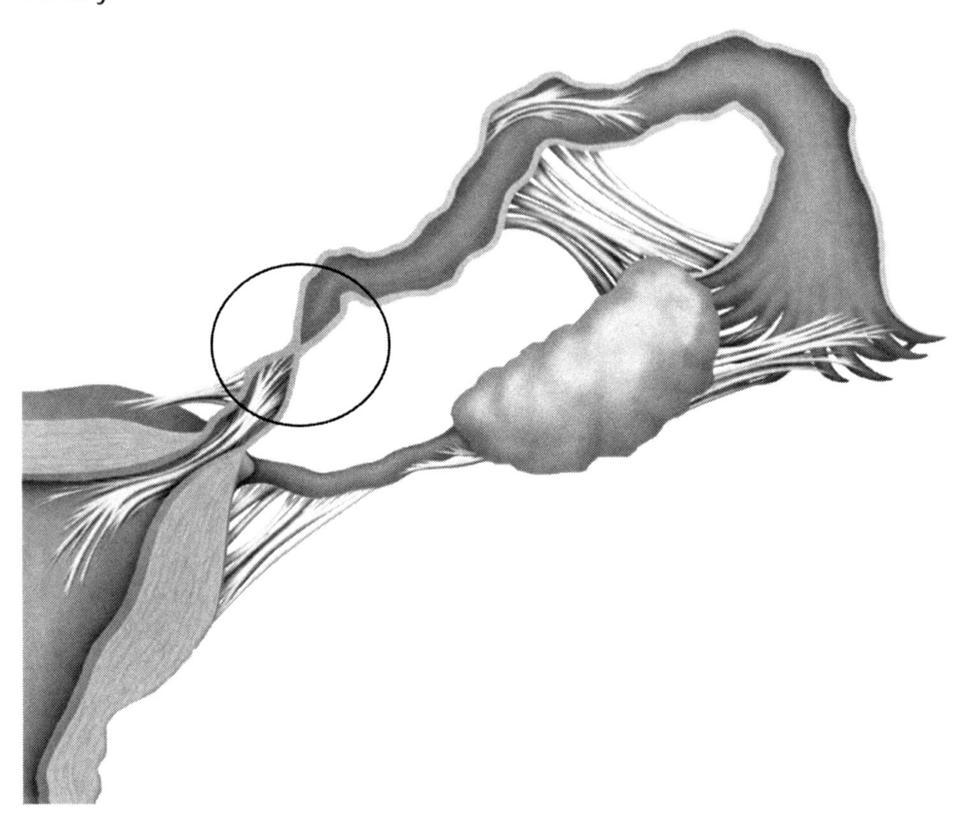

Spasm in the tube represents a dysfunctional state that may interfere with fertility.

Mucous plugs are generally thought to form as a response to inflammation or tissue injury.

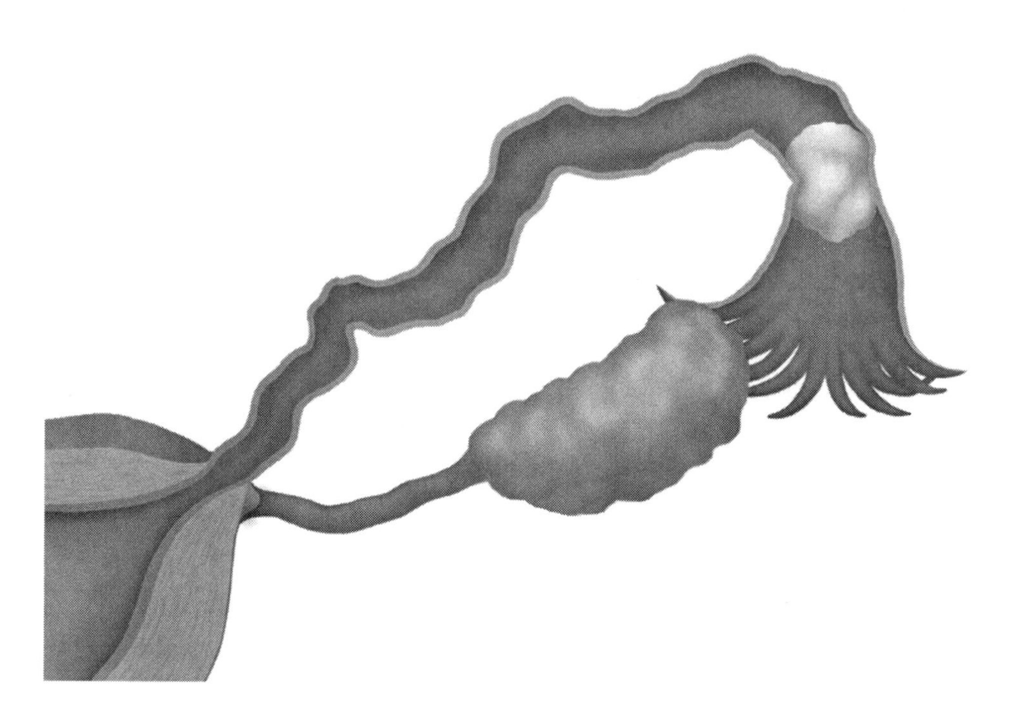

Mucous plugs can block tubes, and may be "blown out" by the dye to clear tubes during an HSG procedure.

Just as your knee might swell if you've received a trauma to that area, the body sends white blood cells and repair mechanisms to the fallopian tube that has become inflamed or infected to help the area heal. As tissues repair and the body's immune system starts to fight infection, adhesions may form within the tube.

The initial inflammation sometimes creates a thickened mucous plug, similar to pus. This plug indicates that a healing process has taken place, or is still taking place. A long-term concern is that adhesion formation often accompanies healing, placing the tube at risk of closing due to adhesions. Another concern is that the plug can act like a bottle-stopper, also blocking the tube. When a diagnostic physician applies extra pressure to the injected dye during an HSG procedure, the doctor is often trying to expel any mucous that may be blocking the fallopian tube. If the dye will not pass through after increased pressure, the tube is generally thought to be blocked due to adhesions.

In severe cases, there is partial or complete blockage at the end of the tube, coupled with dilation within the fallopian tube. This indicates the presence of a hydrosalpinx.

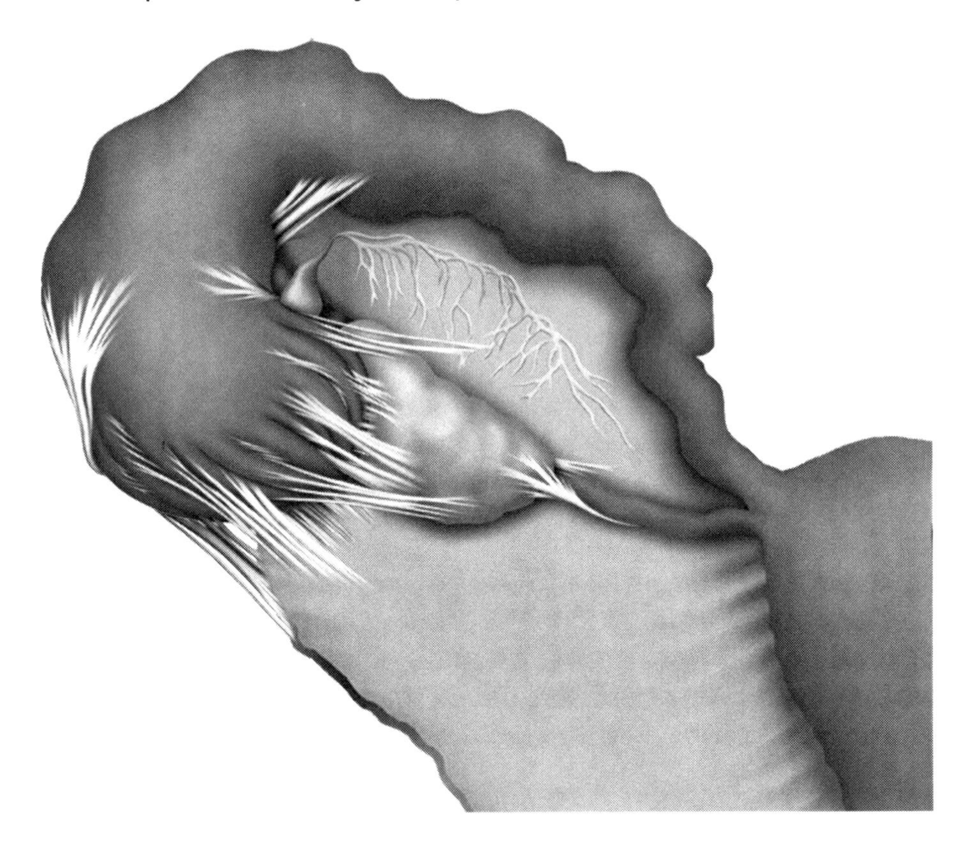

In a hydrosalpinx, the distal end of the tube closes and the tube swells with a liquid that may be toxic to an implanted embryo.

In this case, the tube has not only blocked at the distal end (by the fimbriae and ovary), it has also become swollen and engorged with a fluid that is considered by some reproductive endocrinologists (REs) to be toxic to a recently fertilized egg. You can read some remarkable success stories for women with hydrosalpinx and our study results later in this chapter.

Making the Diagnosis

There are two ways to diagnose a blocked tube: hysterosalpingogram (HSG) and surgical chromotubation. Both use a liquid dye to determine whether or not the tube is patent (open) and functional.

Hysterosalpingogram (HSG)

The least invasive method of determining if the tubes are open is to perform a hysterosalpingogram (HSG). This dye test is generally conducted in the radiology department of a hospital, but without the need for anesthesia (although some physicians recommend valium or another relaxant about an hour prior to the procedure).

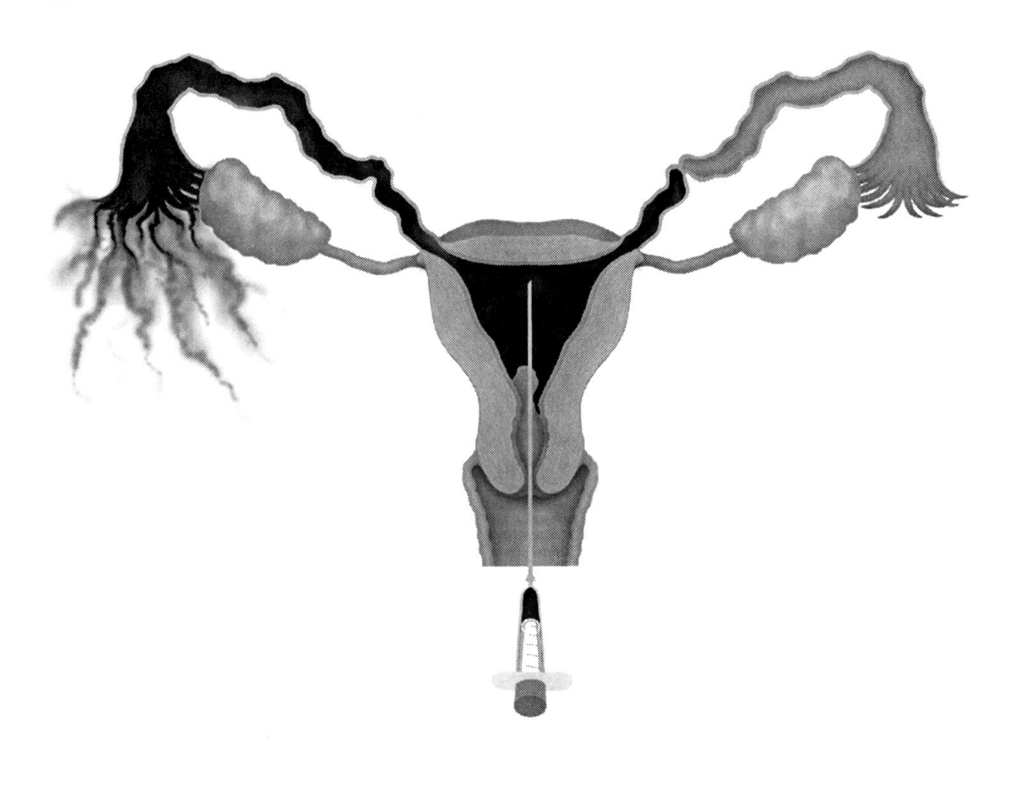

In the HSG above, "free spillage" of dye is noted from the left tube, indicating the tube is free and clear of obstruction. However, the dye does not exit the right tube, indicating total blockage on that side.

In an HSG, a catheter (a mobile straw) is inserted into the uterus via the cervix. The physician then injects a radiological dye through the catheter, and films the process of the dye as it goes into the uterus, and hopefully through the fallopian tubes. Thus, the physician can then tell whether there is "free spillage" of the dye (the preferable outcome), partial blockage (delayed or minimal spill), or total blockage (no spill into the abdominal cavity), and whether the blockage occurs proximally, mid-tubally, or distally. The physician can also tell by the shape of the dye within the tube if there is any swelling, indicating hydrosalpinx.

Physicians who are experts at reading HSG films can get a sense by the shape and course of the dye of the effects of adhesions, uterine fibroids, and other factors that might present a problem to fertility. In doing so, they can generally determine if there is an easy and clear passage for sperm and egg to travel through the tube, or if any restriction exists.

Surgical Chromotubation

Chromotubation is performed during a surgical procedure, either laparoscopy or laparotomy. During the surgery, dye is injected through the cervix and into the uterus. The surgeon observes directly whether the dye exits from the end of the tubes, by the ovary and fimbriae.

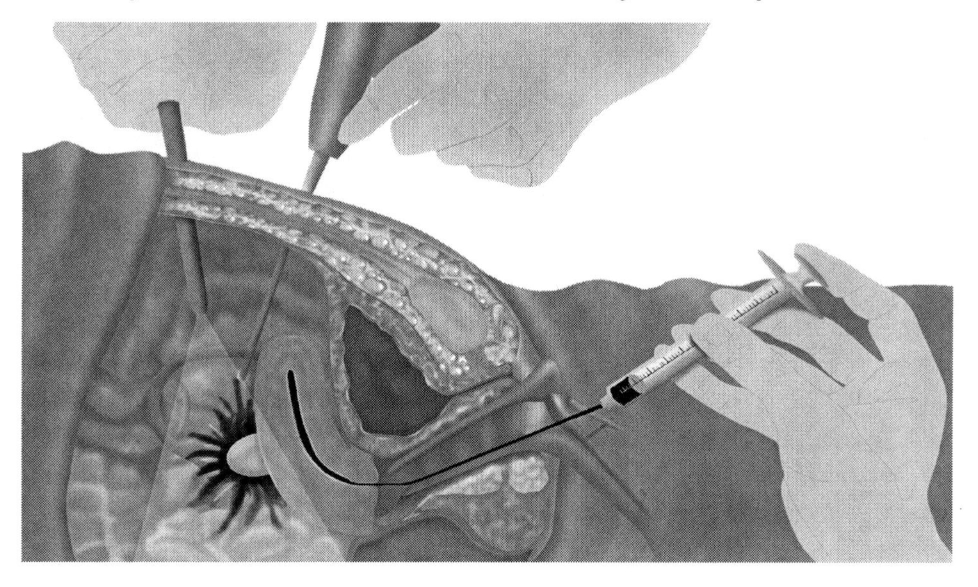

A physician can also test and view the course of dye through the end of a fallopian tube during a surgical procedure.

If the dye exits copiously (called "free spillage") the tube is open (patent) and generally considered functional. Surgery has the advantage (or disadvantage) of excluding spasm as a cause of tubal occlusion because the tubes and reproductive tract are totally relaxed, with the patient unconscious, under general anesthesia.

Hysteroscopy

Hysteroscopy uses a thin optical device that is inserted through the vagina into the uterus. It may be performed before or simultaneously with a laparoscopy. The physician uses saline or carbon dioxide to fill the uterus. A light at the end of the instrument allows the doctor to see the uterine walls, the opening of the fallopian tubes at the top of the uterus, and any fibroids or polyps. A camera is attached to the end of the scope to broadcast the image of the inside of the uterus onto a video screen. Hysteroscopy is considered non-invasive, but some women report pain with the procedure.

Treatment Options: Surgical and Non-Surgical

Surgical Treatment

Surgeons may choose to surgically repair a tube in any of several ways. When the blockage is proximal (near the uterus), they can insert a wire, catheter, or balloon into the tube to try to open it. Most physicians find their greatest success when the tube is blocked proximally — close to the uterus. This surgical site can be accessed from inside the uterus with cannulation, sometimes accompanied by a balloon to widen the channel — a procedure involving the insertion of a flexible catheter or tube into the fallopian tube. Other physicians choose to cut or burn the adhesions with a laser.

The success rate for surgically opening proximally occluded tubes is high, but unfortunately, over 80% re-block six months after surgery, according to published medical literature.[15] Thus, more often than not, the surgery grants the patient a brief window in which to conceive naturally. (For more information on adhesion formation after surgery, see Chapter Sixteen.)

Tubes that are blocked mid-tubally require a more complicated surgical intervention via laparoscopy or open surgery performed under general anesthesia. A tube that is blocked in its mid-portion can be cut (resected), and the adhesions cut or burned. Then the ends of the tubes are rejoined via tiny sutures (stitches) or by laser cauterization.

The long-term success rate for these patients has not been measured. Because it is a much more complicated surgery than cannulation and it involves cutting the fallopian tube wall, some physicians assume success rates may be lower than cannulation due to the delicacy of the tube and the post-surgical scarring that occurs in this area. However, we have found no published data on the long-term follow-up to these more invasive surgical procedures.

Perhaps the most difficult tubal occlusion to treat is a tube that is blocked at the distal end, by the ovary. As noted earlier, the end of the fallopian tube has very delicate fimbriae. These are finger-like projections whose job is to grasp the egg when it is released from the ovary. It is very difficult to surgically free fimbriae that are adhered from scarring, endometriosis, or infection, and to prevent these structures from scarring again.

With distal occlusion, physicians have no choice but to perform laparoscopy or laparotomy to attempt to clear the blockage. A gynecologist can cut the tube and surgically separate the fimbriae in an attempt to recreate the delicate flower-like petals at the ends of the fallopian tubes, but the physician cannot keep the body from laying down more cross-links and adhesions as the fimbriae recover from the surgery. Success rates for subsequent full-term pregnancies in patients with fallopian tubes blocked at the distal end are extremely low.[9]

Non-Surgical Treatment — The Wurn Technique®

Understanding the complexities and often poor outcomes of surgery on the fallopian tubes, you can understand the surprise and delight of our patients (and the shock of our therapists and our referring physicians) when they found that the manual physical therapy techniques we had developed to treat pelvic adhesions were opening blocked fallopian tubes at all three sites, followed by natural full-term pregnancies.

Over time, we have come to understand that by slowly peeling away adhesions cross-link by cross-link, we appear to free the underlying tissues and return them closer to their original shape, structure, and function. As such, even the most adhered and seemingly impossible cases often surprised us with resulting open tubes, full-term pregnancies, and in several cases subsequent pregnancies from the previously blocked tubes and clubbed fimbriae.

Scientific Investigation of Non-Surgical Treatment to Open Blocked Fallopian Tubes

The results of a multi-year study of treating women with total bilateral tubal occlusion using the Wurn Technique® was published in *Alternative Therapies in Health and Medicine* and summarized in *Contemporary Ob-Gyn*, both respected peer-reviewed journals. Most of the 61% of women whose tubes we opened with this therapy became pregnant naturally, and some have now had second full-term pregnancies.

The women in the published study had total occlusion before therapy because either:

- one tube had been removed and the remaining tube was totally blocked, or
- both tubes were totally blocked.

Research Methods

Our scientific inquiry began after we witnessed several initial successes. We felt an obligation to examine and quantify the results we were seeing in the clinic every month.

Luckily, a large highly-respected medical school is located in our town. We consulted several physician-researchers to help us design a scientifically valid method to test and measure our ability to open and improve the function of blocked fallopian tubes.

At the urging of several local gynecologists and scientists, we decided to conduct clinical research to determine the effectiveness (if any) of our treatment in opening blocked fallopian tubes at all areas of the tube (proximal, mid-tubal, and distal). The general consensus was that, if we could improve function of these tiny structures, which are arguably the smallest, deepest organs in the female body, we should by extension be able to improve the function of other structures affected by adhesions, which were larger and more accessible. For example, the ovaries and uterus are larger and much easier to access, as are other structures in the pelvis and abdomen which are affected by adhesions such as the bladder, intestines, liver, and kidneys.

Even before Dr. King came on board, Belinda and I consulted an infertility expert, who also happened to be Chief of Staff of a large local hospital. She was a gynecologist with a research background and a practice that was focused largely on female infertility.

As a scientist, she discounted the notion that we could open tubes based on anecdotal reports of pregnancies and births from past patients we had treated. Instead, she proposed we conduct a pilot study, a prospective clinical trial in which we would treat a woman whose tubes were scientifically diagnosed as 100% occluded (totally blocked) by an independent physician using radiological testing, or direct visualization. After therapy, the physician would order an independent dye test to see what, if anything, had happened. She was sure that nothing would.

We had no idea whether we would be successful, but based on prior results, we decided to start the study. The physician sent Marsha to us; Marsha was arguably the most challenging case of blocked fallopian tubes this physician had ever treated.

Our First Scientific Test Case: Two Blocked Fallopian Tubes, Despite Laparoscopy and Open Surgery

- Marsha's Story

Marsha was diagnosed with two totally blocked fallopian tubes by HSG, laparoscopy, and laparotomy (open surgery). Her pelvis was so adhered with scar tissue that she was diagnosed with "frozen pelvis." That is, she had no normal mobility in the pelvis because her organs and tissues were tightly adhered together in a mass.

"It's like glue was poured into her pelvis," the physician said. "I am sorry to send you such a difficult case, but she certainly fits the criteria of your study."

"It's like glue was poured into her pelvis," the physician said.

Marsha had undergone both laparoscopy and open surgery (laparotomy) in hopes of correcting her tubal problems and decreasing her pelvic pain. Despite all medical attempts, post-surgical diagnostic tests confirmed that both of her tubes remained totally closed, and even after the pelvic surgeries, she still had significant pain. We resolved to do our best to help her.

When Marsha came in for therapy, her situation was nothing short of severe. Years of inflammation, infection, and multiple surgeries had left her pelvis feeling like a rock. The skin was deeply sucked-in at her surgical scars.

Guided by nothing but the determination and skills we had developed over years of treating Belinda and others with adhesion pain, we embarked into unknown territory, hoping to help a woman whose (Chief of Staff) physician had told us was an "impossible case."

We began slowly and steadily to engage our hands into the tissues of Marsha's pelvis. In the beginning, it felt as if we were pushing against a small boulder, immobile and impassive. However, as the hours passed and the outer layers of adhesions began to detach, we noticed that the boulder began to move some upon palpation. Before long we were able to move Marsha's boulder a bit from side to side, then top to bottom, then diagonally.

Working both externally and internally, we slowly peeled away layer after layer of adhesions until the boulder began to divide into smaller structures which we called her "rocks and pebbles." Eventually, most of these dissolved as well and we were able to actually palpate specific organs within her pelvis. About this time, she reported that her back and intercourse pain, both of which had been severe, had dissipated significantly.

At the time, we had absolutely no idea how many hours of treatment we should render if we were to open either of her tubes. We were just going by touch, feel, and patient feedback. In the end, after 23 hours of the manual therapy, we felt Marsha was ready for a repeat dye test.

We held our breaths as we sent our test patient for an independent follow up dye test. To the utter surprise of everyone, the test results were nothing short of remarkable. The diagnostic physician reported that one of Marsha's tubes was now completely free, clear, and open with "free spillage" of the dye. In addition, the dye went measurably further through the other tube. We had done it! We had improved both tubes and totally opened one, when two different surgeries had failed to achieve any results at all!

Marsha's case provided the first scientific proof that the work we had developed over the course of many years of study, using Belinda as a test patient, had benefit for some very complicated and adhered infertility patients. We had discovered a new non-invasive treatment for adhesions and blocked fallopian tubes, that decreased pain as a side-effect. To commemorate the event, we created a concept and clinic with a name befitting our origins. Clear Passage Therapies® was born.

Perhaps as a testament to the difficulty of discovering, developing, testing, and finally proving the worth of a new treatment capable of resolving major health problems, it took us 16 years to develop and publish scientific data on the work that started long before we treated Marsha.

Looking back, it was a long and difficult, but exciting adventure, from early 1990 when our first patient with blocked fallopian tubes became pregnant, until January 2008, when our first in-depth study of opening blocked fallopian tubes was published in a respected peer-reviewed medical journal. While the project was incredibly time and labor intensive, we felt compelled to investigate a phenomenon that, but for our research, would have been known to us alone.

In the end, the physicians and scientists who worked on this study with us were pleased to find that fallopian tubes opened in 61% of the women we treated with total tubal occlusion.[12] Adding to the difficulty, we excluded no subject; we included every woman we had ever treated with both tubes completely blocked. This included women who only had one tube (one tube having been surgically removed and the remaining tube totally blocked), as well as overweight women whose structures were difficult to palpate.

The 61% success rate was considered very significant, as was the 53% pregnancy/birth rate of our successes (32% of the entire study group). Most of the women who had thier tubles cleared went on to have natural full term pregnancies.

This success rate compares well with surgical techniques to return function to blocked fallopian tubes. In fact, we achieved about three times the pregnancy rate for all fallopian tube occlusions, including the much more challenging mid-tubal and distal occlusions when we compared our results with minimally invasive surgery. For example, a surgical technique to open only the proximal portion of fallopian tubes (the simplest to access) opened 64% of the tubes, but only 11% became pregnant.[13] Other studies of surgical techniques sometimes showed a high rate in opening tubes, but most showed very low rates for patients actually achieving pregnancy or birth.

Part of our high natural pregnancy (and birth) success rate is likely due to the fact that the results of our therapy appear to last for years. While we have seen several women who have now had more than one child naturally after therapy (examples follow), surgery appears to carry an inherent timeline before tubes close again, presumably from adhesions that form due to the surgery.

According to our study, the adhesions that form as a byproduct of healing from the various invasive procedures may themselves be a cause of the high rates of reocclusion over time, even from the simplest of surgeries.[14] For example, a repeat HSG six months after an ambulatory, minimally invasive catheter procedure showed a total reocclusion rate of 35/43 (81%) of patients.[15]

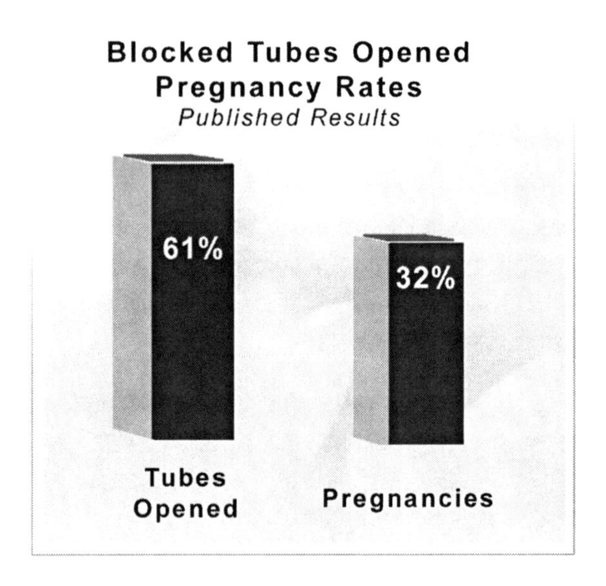

Opening blocked fallopian tubes was a happy discovery for us in part because by their very nature, they created a perfect venue for scientific investigation. Tubes could be examined by independent radiologists (as all of ours were) before and after therapy. The pre-therapy reports were then compared and measured against the post-therapy results for each woman to give us a clear yes/no answer as to whether or not a tube opened.

Knowing that tubes generally block from adhesions, by implication we were able to move on from blocked tubes to discover the ramifications of detaching, deforming and decreasing adhesions in the rest of the body for women with infertility, and for patients of both sexes who had adhesion-related conditions.

Two Blocked Fallopian Tubes and Then Unsuccessful IVF

- Roxanne's Story

In 1999, after seven years of marriage, my husband Justin and I realized that we wanted a family. However, it soon became apparent that the effortless quest for a family that so many couples experienced was not to be ours.

Not in my nature to give up or accept less than my dream, I resolved to heal my own body using holistic techniques.

I had an appendectomy when I was 10 years old growing up in Germany. The doctor warned that there was some internal scarring that could interfere with pregnancy later in life. Whether a self-fulfilling prophecy or an unusually prescient prognosis, at 30 years old, I found that indeed I could not get pregnant.

The sense of despair began after we sought assistance through the traditional medical system. I underwent several painful procedures to diagnose the problem and a laparoscopic procedure intended to hopefully clear two blocked fallopian tubes. That day was the low point of our struggle. The surgery was not successful, and that chapter ended with my doctor's very brusque statement to Justin that "she will never get pregnant through natural means."

After going through all of those procedures, we resolved to try a round of in vitro fertilization, courtesy of Justin's parents, who were eager to see a grandchild born.

Our fertility clinic had a good reputation, but the IVF resulted in no pregnancy.

Not in my nature to give up (or accept less than my dream), I resolved to heal my own body using holistic techniques. I was seeing an excellent naturopathic doctor and did quite a bit of research on my own.

About this time, a massage therapist friend from northern California sent us an article she found in a magazine about Clear Passage Therapies (CPT), in Florida. The therapy sounded so promising and reasonable, even to my skeptical husband. Coincidentally, when Justin's parents were vacationing in Florida that spring, we all made plans to send me to Gainesville a week ahead for the therapy; then I would join the rest of the family afterward. The treatment was wonderful and I loved everything about it! I felt empowered again.

I will never forget the moment I found out I was pregnant naturally, just three months after treatment. I was one week late with my period. I took a pregnancy test, feeling quite silly to think it could be true, and yes, it indicated a positive test.

The next day I had an ultrasound. Afraid to look at the picture, I saw my doctor's face with a smile and a nod — yes, I was pregnant!

What a day! I was so shaky with happiness that I hardly had a voice to tell my husband the results over the phone. He was just ecstatic. We cried when our daughter came into this world nine months later, one of the best moments of our lives.

We were very happy to have a small family, but later had another surprise. I became pregnant again naturally, six years later! I am amazed that the positive results of the therapy lasted all that time. It is wonderful to think that Justin and I went from two people in a scary and depressing search through the medical maze of infertility treatments to our present family of four — all naturally!

I would urge other women who face infertility to not give up! I would definitely recommend CPT, as I credit the therapists with breaking up the adhesions that were interfering with my fallopian tubes, and blocking my fertility.

Surgically "Unopenable" Fallopian Tubes

- Autumn's Story

Six years ago my partner and I made the decision to start trying to have a baby. She already had a son she had conceived thru artificial insemination, and he was two years old at the time. I had always wanted children and thought it would be an easy process. Boy…if I'd only known then what I know now.

We made an appointment with a reproductive specialist to start the process. After undergoing a battery of blood tests, they said I had to have an HSG performed. The specialist told me, "It's standard procedure and we don't predict any problems."

I immediately felt my stomach drop, then the tears started flowing.

But when the test was over, the specialist said, "There's a problem," and proceeded to tell me point-blank that my tubes were blocked. I immediately felt my stomach drop and then the tears started flowing. He told me to go home and when

I was ready, to call his office and schedule a follow-up; he would go over the results with me in detail then.

He had a nurse help me get my clothes on and in between sobs I asked her if I would ever be able to have babies and she said, "I don't know, but you need to know that, even with the predicament you are in, you have one of the best doctors in the state."

I knew at that moment that my predicament was VERY bad. The next week and a half waiting for my appointment with him was torture. My family and friends kept telling me that it probably wasn't as bad as it sounded, and to just wait for my follow-up and see what he said.

My partner and I went to the follow-up and I was sick to my stomach with fear. The specialist came in, looked at my papers, and started talking about the process of artificial insemination and what we needed to do to get started.

I was in shock, and in my mind I was thinking maybe it wasn't as bad as I thought. I asked the specialist, "I thought after the test you said my tubes were blocked?"

He looked at me questionably and then looked at my test results and said, "No, there may have been a little blockage, but nothing that should cause any problems."

I thought I was imagining things and my friends said, "See, we told you." But I just didn't understand.

The following month we started inseminations. I was excited, but scared because I felt like something was wrong. We tried for two months with no luck. It was then close to the holidays and we decided to take a break. During this time I thought a lot about the HSG and decided to find a different doctor for a second opinion.

My partner and I went to our appointment with the new doctor and told him everything that had happened. He said, "I would like to do a laparoscopy, so we can visualize the area directly, and test your fallopian tubes again."

My mom, who is a nurse, came the day of the surgery because my partner had to work. When I was in pre-op, the doctor came to see me and said, "I won't be able to talk to you after the surgery because you will still be under medication, but I will tell your mother what I find."

I remember waking up in great pain and asking the nurse what the doctor found. She told me she didn't know and that I couldn't see my mom until I got back to my room. I acted like I was in less pain so they would let me out of the recovery room.

When I got in my room they let my mom come back. I asked, "What did he say?"

She replied, "Just wait, he'll come in and talk to you."

"No, that's why he talked to you. He's not going to be coming to the room." My mom insisted she wait until my partner arrived. "Mom, just tell me," I begged her.

At that point I already knew it was bad news. She looked at me with a lot of sadness in her eyes and said, "He said your tubes are totally blocked and he could not open them surgically. There was no way you would have ever become pregnant through artificial insemination."

I was in total shock. I know it was very hard for my mom to have to be the one to tell me that. I cannot imagine being a mother and having to tell your daughter she can't have children.

Then my partner arrived. My mom had already called her and told her the news, so she was really upset too. I felt like my dream of having children was over, because I knew I could never afford IVF, which was the only way I could ever become pregnant, the doctor said.

I went through a couple of years of not knowing what to do. It is such a lonely feeling, and although everyone hurts for you, you know no one really understands because they already have children.

It is such a lonely feeling, and although everyone hurts for you, you know no one really understands because they already have children.

I never imagined how much anger I would feel when I heard about someone I knew being pregnant and then how much guilt I would have for feeling that way. I never knew how empty I would feel after having my baby nephew for a weekend. He would go home and I would lie in bed at night crying, holding onto this baby tweety bird shoe I bought when I first decided to start trying. It was just incredibly heartbreaking and lonely.

I started looking around on the Internet and came across the Clear Passage Therapies (CPT) website. It sounded too good to be true and I didn't understand it, so I kept looking.

But my mind kept going back to CPT, so finally I called and requested information. When it arrived, I watched the DVD and was surprised that their patients sounded very much like my situation. But the CP treatment was very different from any I had heard of, so I was quite skeptical.

I was going to Florida for vacation that summer, so I made an appointment to stop by the office and speak with a therapist. I wanted to make sure that this place was real.

I remember standing, reading all the articles on the walls and feeling my hope grow. But I was still scared because all I had was $4000 in a 401k account I could withdraw and use on either this or IVF. I knew it would be hard for me to come up with $15,000 for the IVF, and even if I did, it would only be once and knowing the chances of IVF working the first time, I was scared.

I took a leap and decided to withdraw my money and start getting things together to come to Florida and have the therapy. Although in my gut I felt like it was the right thing, I was very scared because I felt like I was putting all of my eggs in one basket. If this didn't work, my dream of having children would be over. Still, something about following my gut instinct rang true for me.

When I told my mom what I was doing she was very skeptical — even more so because she is a nurse. She also knew how devastated I would be if it didn't work.

I attended the first ten hours in December of 2006 and the second ten hours in March of 2007. My mom came to Florida with me in December and she wanted to know exactly what they were doing. It was hard to explain the treatment to her, and the only thing I could tell her was that it felt like it was working.

When I got done with my therapy in March, I scheduled a consultation with my infertility doctor. I wanted to schedule an HSG to see if the therapy worked.

I hadn't told my doctor about attending CPT before because I was afraid he would try to change my mind. When I went to the appointment, I explained to him my treatment. He looked at me like I was totally crazy. He said to me "You have completely blocked fallopian tubes; they couldn't even be opened in surgery. There is no way that treatment could have worked." Even though I had gotten back almost 75% of the treatment cost from my insurance, the doctor still insisted, "Whatever they did, it was overpriced."

Naturally, he didn't think there was a need for an HSG, but he reluctantly agreed to do one, even though he felt very strongly that there would be no change. I left his office very upset and feeling like a fool. All I kept thinking was, "If it sounds too good to be true, it probably is."

The day of the test, I had never been so scared in all my life. After my consultation, I refused to tell my mother when I was having my HSG. "There is no sense in both of us worrying," I thought. But the morning of the test I called her because I was very upset and when she asked what was wrong, all I could say was, "It's today."

My partner and I went to my appointment and the doctor came in and said, "Well let's see if they did any good down in Florida." I could tell he thought it was a total waste of time.

As soon as he was done, I sat up and asked, "Well?"

"I'm shocked," he stammered. "It's amazing."

"You mean my tubes are clear?" I asked.

"Yes! You can start trying to conceive next month."

My partner looked him in the eyes and said, "Go ahead, say it…"

He replied, "I was wrong, I admit it. I was wrong. It's a miracle."

I cannot tell you the joy I felt — and for the first time in my entire journey I was crying tears of joy. I went to get my clothes on and my partner pulled out the tweety bird shoe I always held on to when I was upset. It meant so much to me and we were both very happy.

For the first time in my entire journey, I was crying tears of joy.

When I got to the car I called my mom and when she answered she said, "Hey." She didn't sound good because she thought I would be calling with bad news.

I said, "IT WORKED!!"

"WHAT?" she asked with excitement.

"IT WORKED, IT WORKED, IT WORKED!!!" I screamed.

She then started crying and telling everyone at her work. It was the best day of my life!

I have not started trying to get pregnant yet because "life" keeps happening. The doctor immediately took blood work and discovered that I had thyroid problems. It took several months to get the medications leveled and then I hurt my back and was off work for four months.

I am now back to work and will hopefully be able to start trying in the next few months.

I had such a wonderful experience with CPT. I cannot even begin to thank them enough. They are truly changing people's lives and words cannot express what I feel for them. Their therapy gave me hope and that's something I have not had in a long time.

Fallopian Tubes Blocked Near Uterus

- Valerie's Story

For two successive years, Valerie and her husband, Bill, tried to have a baby. They were confounded at their inability to conceive because they were each just 25 years old.

Valerie consulted her gynecologist. Because of her history of ovarian cysts (one of which required hospitalization), severe endometriosis, and abdominal, pelvic, and low back pain, the doctor suspected she had pelvic adhesions and possibly blocked fallopian tubes.

Valerie was scheduled for an HSG dye test to determine if her tubes were open or blocked. When the procedure was over, the doctor informed her that both of her tubes were blocked near the uterus. She recommended Valerie have laparoscopic surgery to remove the pelvic adhesions and hopefully open her tubes.

Over the next couple of months, Valerie and Bill discussed their options. If they did not have the surgery, or if the surgery did not work, their only options would be adoption or in vitro fertilization (IVF).

By mid-summer they had resolved to move forward with the doctor's suggestion. Valerie proceeded with laparoscopic surgery.

If they did not have the surgery, or if the surgery did not work, their only options would be adoption or in vitro fertilization.

Once again, Valerie and Bill weighed their options. They considered IVF treatment, but it was going to be a huge financial burden for them. Valerie remembered that her mother had mentioned a non-surgical treatment designed to open blocked fallopian tubes.

Valerie called our clinic and scheduled an appointment. After completing the patient consultation, she decided to complete the one-week therapy program.

Two weeks after her treatment, Valerie returned to her doctor to have an HSG and see if the therapy had opened her tubes. She could barely believe it when the doctor told her one of her tubes was open.

Nine months later, Valerie became pregnant naturally, and nine months later she gave birth to her baby. After all they had been through, Bill and Valerie decided to name their baby Grace.

After Grace was born, it only took six months and Valerie was pregnant again with her second daughter, whom she named Reese. She considers them her two miracles.

Four Years Infertile with Blocked Tube

- Michelle's Story

I had been trying to get pregnant for two years when I sought the help of several doctors to determine the cause of my apparent infertility. I was told that I should have a surgery to remove multiple uterine fibroids because that might be the cause of the problem.

In 2003 I underwent a myomectomy to remove fifteen fibroids. During my recovery, the doctor revealed to me that one of my fallopian tubes was also blocked, which was contributing to my problems getting pregnant.

Two months later, I began fertility injections and pills to be able to conceive through intrauterine inseminations (IUI). After three rounds of IUI accompanied by a lot of hormonal changes, mood swings, and discomfort, the results always came back negative.

After three rounds of IUI accompanied by a lot of hormonal changes, mood swings, and discomfort, the results always came back negative.

At that point, I decided to give my body a break and take a different approach. Fertility requires peace and a sound mind — which was very difficult for me with all the infertility drugs. I decided to join a six month outreach program with my bible ministry which helped me focus on helping other people enrich their lives by developing a personal relationship with God. My life was blossoming with joy and peace. My belief was stronger than ever.

It was during that time that I started learning about natural treatments. While at a health food store one day, I found a magazine with a small paragraph entitled, "New Natural Technique Increases Fertility Rate." I found it very interesting, so I kept it and put it away. Later on, I went online to search on natural remedies to unblock fallopian tubes and I came across "Clear Passage Therapies (CPT)." What I did not realize was that this was the same place to which the magazine referred. When I went on their website and read their information, I learned the detrimental affects of surgery and the possibility that I could be full of scars. I was convinced that God was leading me to them.

I contacted them a few months later and obtained some literature and a video which my husband and I read and watched very carefully. The treatment and procedure made perfect sense to me because as a Christian I am fully aware of how God designed the human body in a way that all the joints and ligaments are interconnected with each other.

We decided to spend a week in the Florida clinic. During the treatment, I felt as if the muscles in my lower abdomen were hard and stuck together. I also felt great release, stretching, and relaxation practically immediately. The personnel were very

This time around my tubes were both totally opened!

professional, kind, and genuinely concerned about my well being.

After my treatment, I went to an infertility specialist who suggested I have another HSG. This time around my tubes were both totally opened! The next step would be to perform another IUI, using only Clomid.

Finally after a total of four years of trying to conceive, the result was positive and I am currently enjoying motherhood with my (now one year old) healthy and strong baby. I thank God for CPT. I hope their treatment will be promoted by physicians so that many other women can be successful with childbearing while utilizing a non-invasive, natural treatment.

Hydrosalpinx: A Unique Situation

Reproductive endocrinologists have generally felt that a tube swollen and filled with liquid (called hydrosalpinx) rendered that tube beyond repair and non-functional for life. One concern is that the liquid within the tube will spill down into the uterus after implantation of a fertilized egg, bathing the egg in a substance that could be toxic, thus decreasing the chances for a full-term pregnancy. The general consensus among REs is to surgically remove any tube with a hydrosalpinx, and proceed directly to IVF.

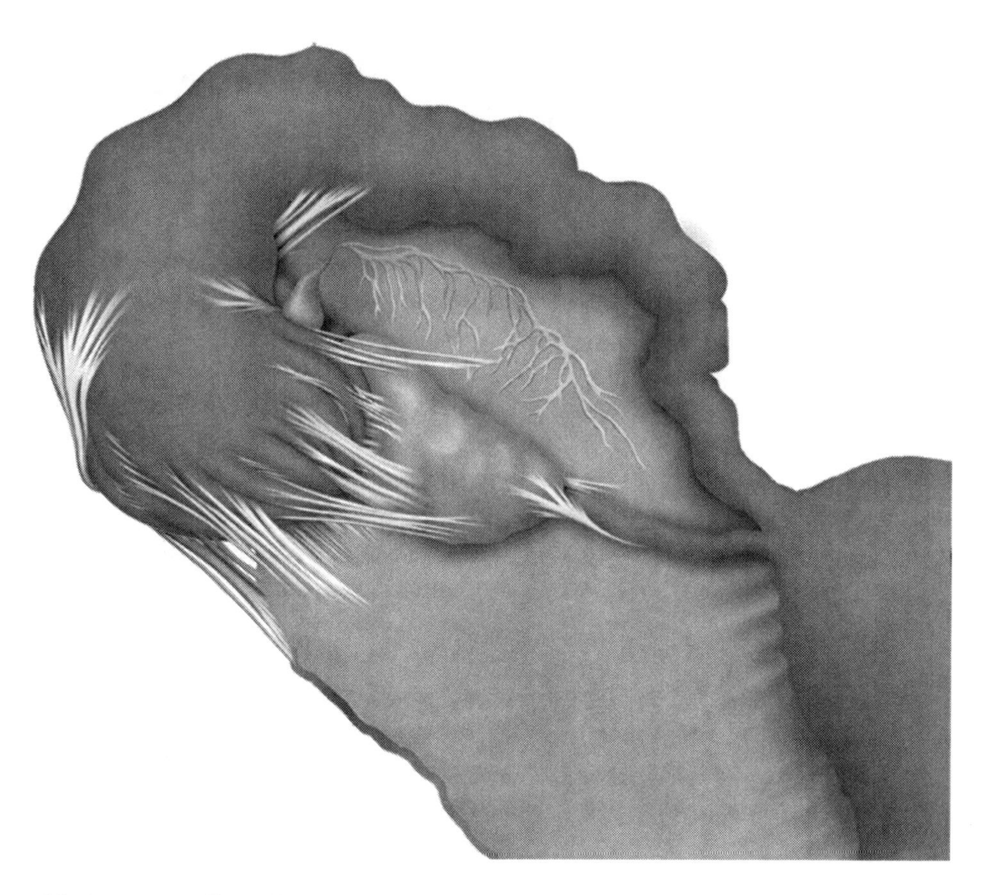

Hydrosalpinx (fluid filled tube) was considered beyond repair, but we started seeing natural pregnancies and births after we treated them.

We understood from our physician advisors that hydrosalpinx rendered a tube totally useless, irreparable, and damaged for life. However, we were also originally told that we could not open blocked fallopian tubes non-surgically, yet our patients kept proving the experts wrong. Similarly, we originally believed our physician advisors who felt we could never return function to a tube that was blocked with hydrosalpinx. Then Jen came to see us.

Hormonal Menopause, Only Remaining Tube Blocked with Hydrosalpinx

- Jen's Story

I've always been a healthy, positive person with big dreams. I knew some day I would meet that special someone and start a family.

From an early age, I always knew I wanted children. I come from a long line of fertility. My grandmother gave birth to 15 children, my mother 4, and my brothers and sister have 7 more kids among them, who I love dearly and who are a big part of my life. My love of children even drew me to my occupation as an early learning Spanish teacher working with the cutest little students ages three to eight.

When I was 26, a misdiagnosed appendicitis left me hospitalized for a week with an infection. I recovered from the ruptured appendix, but 15 months later I was hospitalized again and had another major abdominal surgery. It almost took my life and left me trying to figure out if I would ever have children.

I lost my right ovary, fallopian tube, and parts of my intestine to surgery. My remaining left tube was damaged. The medical diagnosis was that it was blocked and filled with fluid, a hydrosalpinx.

The doctors said that I had so much infection and disease that my ovary and tube weren't even recognizable. It was mush. They said I was going to have a lot of scar tissue and adhesions, leaving my insides "like concrete."

I was confused and afraid and while I was thankful to be alive, I had to ask the doctors a simple question ... "Will I ever be able to have kids?" His answer was, "Not naturally. It would have to be through IVF. You're young and healthy and you have your left ovary."

I lost my right ovary, fallopian tube, and parts of my intestine to surgery. My remaining tube was blocked and filled with fluid.

Now flash forward, I've met the man of my dreams, we're in a financial position to afford IVF and excited to start our family. Everyone advised me to get started with IVF early, since there can always be complications and it takes longer than you think. My biological clock was ticking and I wanted to have several shots at this before I turned 35.

While IVF wasn't exactly what I had planned when I dreamed of getting pregnant, with all the shots, hormones, and invasive procedures, I was thankful for all the progress in the field because for me, it was the only way for me to get pregnant.

At our first consultation the doctor told me I would be a good candidate as long as I had high quality eggs. She also recommended that before we do IVF, we should remove my remaining unhealthy tube because it had a hydrosalpinx — it was blocked with fluid that could be toxic to the embryo. I thought sure, whatever it takes because this is my only chance and every single doctor I asked said the same thing — that there was no way to repair my damaged tube. So according to all medical sources I checked, IVF would be my only chance, and I had to remove my only tube, which was beyond repair.

First I had to do blood work, and then we could get on with it. Another devastating blow came when our nurse called and said my hormone levels of FSH (which helps the egg mature) was abnormal. The normal and acceptable range is between 2 to 10. Mine was 26.2, indicating that my body wasn't producing quality eggs. In fact, I was officially diagnosed as menopausal. I was newly married and ready to start a family and our doctor was telling my husband and me that if we wanted to have children we would need a donor egg, or to adopt.

We were crushed. I took the news hard. This wasn't supposed to be happening to me. I was young and felt healthy other than the fact that I was "infertile." I felt so bad; it was my fault we couldn't have kids. I was mad at the doctors who first misdiagnosed my appendicitis, and I was heartbroken as I watched many friends and family around me get pregnant so easily. "So now what?" I asked myself.

I was open to new possibilities and I wasn't ready to give up on my hope of conceiving naturally, so I did a lot of research and I found Clear Passage Therapies (CPT). While I had my doubts, it seemed like the best fit for me since they said they had shown success opening blocked fallopian tubes. The therapy didn't involve surgery; it seemed therapeutic and nurturing and that made sense to me. I was following through on my instinct to find some alternative to surgery. Basically, I was following my heart.

I was following through on my instinct to find some alternative to surgery. Basically, I was following my heart.

With the love and support of my husband, we made plans to drive six hours to their clinic in Florida. We felt we had nothing to lose and we looked forward to the trip as a chance to get away for the week where we could be together, and I could concentrate on healing my body.

I had so much to be thankful for — a loving husband, a supportive family, a great job, and wonderful friends. I wrote in my journal, "I feel empowered because I am doing everything possible to better my chances. If it doesn't happen, I will know I tried. I'm a believer. I'm also feeling a little vulnerable because tomorrow starts the beginning of a new journey. Whether pregnancy is a result or not, I know Eddie and I will be able to deal with it."

Once I got there, any doubts I had disappeared. I felt good about the staff, their ability, and their professionalism and care. I knew I was being treated by experienced professionals who actually listened to me and what I had to say about my body. I received 20 hours of therapy. Eddie and I left there believing it worked, but the moment of truth would come a month later when I did the HSG dye test, to see if my tube had opened.

The day it was scheduled was an emotional day for me. I was nervous and anxious. Just a few years ago when I had the same test done, I fell apart in my mother's arms watching the dye collect in my tube, marking the beginning of infertility. Now I was holding my husband's hand watching the dye spill out of my tube — which was now open! We hugged and cried and immediately went home to try to get pregnant, the old-fashioned way!

We got pregnant naturally the next month with our first redheaded miracle, Maria Rose.

When Maria was seven months old we drove down to CPT again to thank everyone and have everyone meet Maria. I also received four more hours of therapy to address some pain issues from the vaginal delivery I had at Maria's birth. I have to say that once again, the positive changes from just those few hours were extraordinary!

Five months later I found out we were pregnant again naturally, this time with twins! I gave birth to two healthy babies, Edward and Katherine, in May, 2006. We now have three beautiful redheads completing this miraculous journey!

We got pregnant naturally the next month with our first redheaded miracle.

The significance of Jen's story is overwhelming. Once again, our patients were leading us into areas of exploration and demonstrating powerful, positive results. The potential benefits for other patients in need were beyond what we could imagine in our wildest dreams.

Some physicians feel that blocked fallopian tubes greatly decrease the opportunity to have a pregnancy, even when reopened surgically. In addition, most feel that tubes with hydrosalpinx should be removed.

But our patients and experiences seemed to be dispelling these theories. For example, here we had a totally impossible case; Jen had only one fallopian tube (the other had been removed). The only tube she had was totally blocked and filled with toxic liquid — hydrosalpinx. In addition, her hormone levels were so elevated that she was judged to be menopausal. Her physicians were sure that she would never become pregnant naturally.

Going by her history, our palpatory skills, and her goals, we treated the hydrosalpinx and blocked fallopian tube. Then, to address the hormonal issues, we also treated the ovaries, pituitary, and hypothalamus glands in her head (more on this in Chapter Eight). We hoped we could either open a fallopian tube or improve her hormone levels. If we opened a tube, her body could at least expel the toxic fluid, we thought; if we improved her hormone levels, at least it might provide her the opportunity for an in vitro fertilization, to have the child of her dreams.

Yet after we treated her, she not only became pregnant naturally and had a beautiful little girl, she went on to become pregnant again naturally, and delivered a set of gorgeous twins! All of this in a woman who had been diagnosed with total tubal occlusion — and menopause.

Stories like Jen's still give us chills and inspire us to go on, despite the nay-sayers. Honestly, we were nay-sayers in the beginning, or at least skeptical of our abilities to repeat these successes. But our patients and clinical results have proven that attitude wrong, again and again.

There, in living flesh, we were able to see, talk, and play with the positive results that none of us expected to come so naturally and so easily. And they did come easily! Jen became pregnant within a month after therapy and became pregnant again naturally 12 months after her first child's birth.

As the data continued to mount, blocked tubes continued to open and "impossible cases" continued to report open tubes and natural pregnancies. We felt two things at once. First, we were in awe of the positive reports women continued to send. Second, we felt certain that the deleterious effects of naturally occurring adhesions could be reversed in many patients. And when that happened, the body often returned to the pain-free functional state it enjoyed before the adhesions formed.

Until our manual therapy came along, reproductive physicians routinely recommended removal of any tube that was swollen with hydrosalpinx in a procedure called a salpingectomy. Then we presented a pilot study at the invitation of the American Society for Reproductive Medicine (ASRM) at their annual meeting in 2006. That citation published in the conference supplement of *Fertility and Sterility* (September, 2006) is considered a pioneering document in the non-surgical treatment of blocked fallopian tubes that are swollen with a hydrosalpinx.

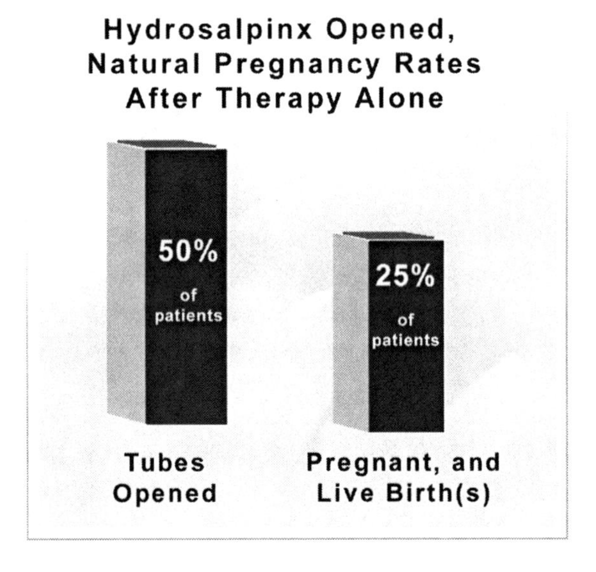

Hydrosalpinx with "Ovaries and Fallopian Tubes Buried by Adhesions"

- Jacqueline's Story

"Is this going to impact my fertility?" I asked my doctor. I was just 22 and my doctor wanted to surgically remove complex cysts from both of my ovaries.

She told me, "We will do our best to save as much of your ovaries as possible."

I was still scared she would have to remove my ovaries and fallopian tubes, but I knew the surgery was necessary.

When I woke up, my doctor told me the news was good. "You lost 10% of one ovary and 60% of the other. I am very happy with the results. You can go home and become pregnant."

Although the news didn't sound good to me, I was happy she thought I could still conceive. A lot of my friends were starting to become pregnant and I wanted to share their joy.

My husband and I tried for a year, but we still couldn't become pregnant. I started to become withdrawn from my social circles because it was hard to be around my friends who became pregnant effortlessly and didn't understand my struggle with infertility.

About that time I began experiencing severe pain in my abdomen and went to the hospital. My doctors discovered I had a large peritoneal cyst, and I was rushed to emergency surgery.

After the surgery, my surgeon told me, "We were able to remove the cysts, but your ovaries and fallopian tubes were buried by adhesions." He suspected that the adhesions were a result of my previous surgery.

My doctor recommended they remove my tubes ....

I knew I needed a natural treatment for the adhesions, and I began to see an acupuncturist. I continued searching for other treatment forms and finally found Clear Passage Therapies (CPT) on the Internet. Although my doctor was extremely discouraging and told me she didn't believe it would work, I felt their therapy for adhesions could help me and I immediately scheduled an intensive week of therapy.

My week at treatment went well. I found the atmosphere to be very calming. But 3/4ths through my treatment, I had a family emergency and had to return home. My therapists were understanding, but cautioned me I might need to return and finish my hours in the future for the treatment to be successful.

I hoped that the time I spent there would be enough and I continued trying to conceive on my own. Two years passed and I became frustrated and worried. I was in my early 30s and I knew my time was slipping by. To make matters worse, I worked with children and people would always tell me, "You're so good with children, you should have some of your own."

I decided to see another Ob/Gyn for help. He sent me for an ultrasound, which showed I was fine — no visible adhesions! He gave me a fertility monitor to help me track my ovulation, but it didn't help me become pregnant.

I then returned to the doctor for an HSG test. Afterwards, I was so nervous about the result that I didn't return for months. I finally called for the results and I was told that both of my fallopian tubes were blocked with hydrosalpinx. My doctor recommended they remove my tubes and do in vitro fertilization.

I thought surgery would be far too invasive and removing my fallopian tubes was a big risk — what if IVF didn't work? I was also uncomfortable with taking the hormones required for IVF.

After his diagnosis, I was sure my chances of conceiving were totally diminished.

I sent the results of my HSG to CPT. They felt they could help me and encouraged me to return and complete my treatment program. My time there was very relaxing. It was like going to a spa.

When I returned home, I wanted to do everything possible to increase my chances for fertility, and saw an acupuncturist. When I explained my condition and that I underwent treatment at CPT, my acupuncturist told me, "I am familiar with CPT, and if they cannot help you, I don't think we can either."

I then sought the help of another infertility specialist, who only offered IVF. Again, I chose not to undergo IVF because I felt it was too invasive.

That month I began experiencing pain in my abdomen. I missed my menstrual cycle and I was concerned I was going into early menopause. I went to see my doctor immediately and he thought I had a large fibroid. He told me, "We need to head to the OR." After his diagnosis, I was sure that my chances of conceiving were totally diminished.

I wanted one more opinion before I underwent another surgery. I went home and took a pregnancy test before I went to see another doctor. I couldn't believe it — it was positive! It was just my second cycle after my treatment at CPT and I was pregnant!

I went to see a midwife and she confirmed my pregnancy with a blood test. I had no complications with my pregnancy and I gave birth to a beautiful full-term baby.

I am so happy I decided to return to CPT. I could have gone through years of invasive treatment. Instead, I went to them and because of their hands, I got pregnant almost instantly.

Only Remaining Tube Blocked with Hydrosalpinx

- Gabriel's Story

Joseph and I met at the hospital where I work. I am a surgical technologist and he is a sales representative for an orthopedic/sales company. After dating for a year, we were married in 2003. Since we were both in our mid thirties, we wanted to start our family. After being unsuccessful for a year, we became concerned and talked to my gynecologist. He then scheduled several tests to check FSH levels, sperm count, and progesterone levels. We also had an HSG to see if there was blockage in my left tube. I had my right rube removed years before because of adhesions that formed after a nephrectomy (removal of kidney) at age two.

I had my right rube removed years before because of adhesions... (Now) our doctor wanted to schedule surgery to remove my left tube.

Our doctor studied our test results and advised us to try IVF. We were sent to a fertility clinic and were hopeful for a positive outcome. Months passed by with fertility shots, weekly blood tests, and ultrasounds to ensure no cysts had formed due to the daily injections.

The emotions during the ride home were unbearable. We shared tears, anger, and frustration. When we arrived home, I broke.

Our last visit to the clinic was April 14, 2004. Our journey ended because the ultrasound showed fluid in the tube. Our doctor advised us to stop treatment immediately and wanted to schedule surgery to remove my left tube. He was concerned that the fluid might fill the uterus after implantation via IVF had taken place and destroy the embryo.

That day I faced the thought and heart wrenching feeling that we may never become pregnant. The emotions during the ride home were unbearable. We shared tears, anger, and frustration. When we arrived home with our family waiting, I broke. That night I told myself tomorrow would be a new day.

As Christians, our decision was to give it to God, His will be done. I needed help and understanding and Joseph needed guidance. Six months went by as we prayed every night and I trusted our faith. I asked for God to take away my desire for a child, if it was not His will. Throughout it all, my want never weakened and I began to feel at peace. I knew it was God's plan, I just didn't know how it was going to happen.

It had been eight months since our last clinic visit and one night I was on my laptop, reading medical websites. I came across statistics about Clear Passage Therapies. As I sat in amazement, I read story after familiar story of women just like me (some better, some worse). I had my husband read the history of Clear Passage and he was puzzled, but amazed. He just didn't understand how adhesions could be "free" without surgery. I didn't know either, but what I did know is that a little voice in my heart was letting me know I had my answer. The success stories were too amazing not to believe.

I called the office and the staff was so nice and helpful. I received the information packet within days and filled out the medical history questionnaire. We made our trip to the clinic in February of 2005 for an intensive week of treatment.

Clear Passage was truly an experience of a lifetime. It was a vacation for the mind, body, and soul. Results came fast, within two days. Joseph and I began to see visible changes in my abdomen scar from surgery. My incision site began to flatten and I had a belly button … wow! Our week went by so fast, and when Friday came I hated to leave.

With my clear mind and new body, we settled home and back into our normal routine. While Joseph was on a business trip in March, I became really ill. I knew it had to be more serious than the flu, maybe food poisoning. I called my mother and she drove me to the ER. They wanted to run blood tests and I asked if they would also do a pregnancy test. He looked at me strange and told me he didn't think that was what was wrong. I insisted. To his surprise and ours, he informed me with a congratulations. I was pregnant!

He just looked at me with tear filled eyes and asked softly, "You are pregnant?" I said, "Yes." I have never heard anyone cry for joy the way we did.

My thoughts quickly turned to my husband. Because of a plane delay, he would not be home until the next afternoon. I swore my mother to secrecy and she took me home. After the longest twenty-four hours of my life — he was finally home! Before he took his bath, I handed him a present. I had wrapped baby items as a way of telling him the news. Our anniversary was the next month, so I just said it was an early present.

After opening the gift, his eyes were fixed on the baby things for what seemed like forever. He just looked at me with tear-filled eyes and asked softly, "You are pregnant?" I said, "Yes." I have never heard anyone cry for joy the way we did.

> Our pregnancy was beautiful. I just loved being pregnant. The delivery was magical and more tears of joy flowed. A big, healthy baby boy was born to us in November 2005 — eight pounds, five ounces, and 22 inches long. He was perfect! He is still the joy of our lives and the miracle God gave us through Clear Passage.

Ectopic Pregnancies: Concern and Hope

As mentioned earlier, blocked fallopian tubes are considered by many physicians to permanently compromise the integrity of the fallopian tube. Adhesions that form inside or outside of the fallopian tube can seal the tube, or kink it like a garden hose, partially or totally obstructing the easy flow of sperm and egg through that tube. In some areas, these obstructions or kinks can create eddies or pockets within the normal course of the fallopian tube, creating the opportunity for an ectopic pregnancy (a pregnancy within the tube). This signals the end of that pregnancy and represents a dangerous, potentially life-threatening condition for the mother. Thus, as too many women and their physicians know, the union of sperm and egg does not always create the desired outcome.

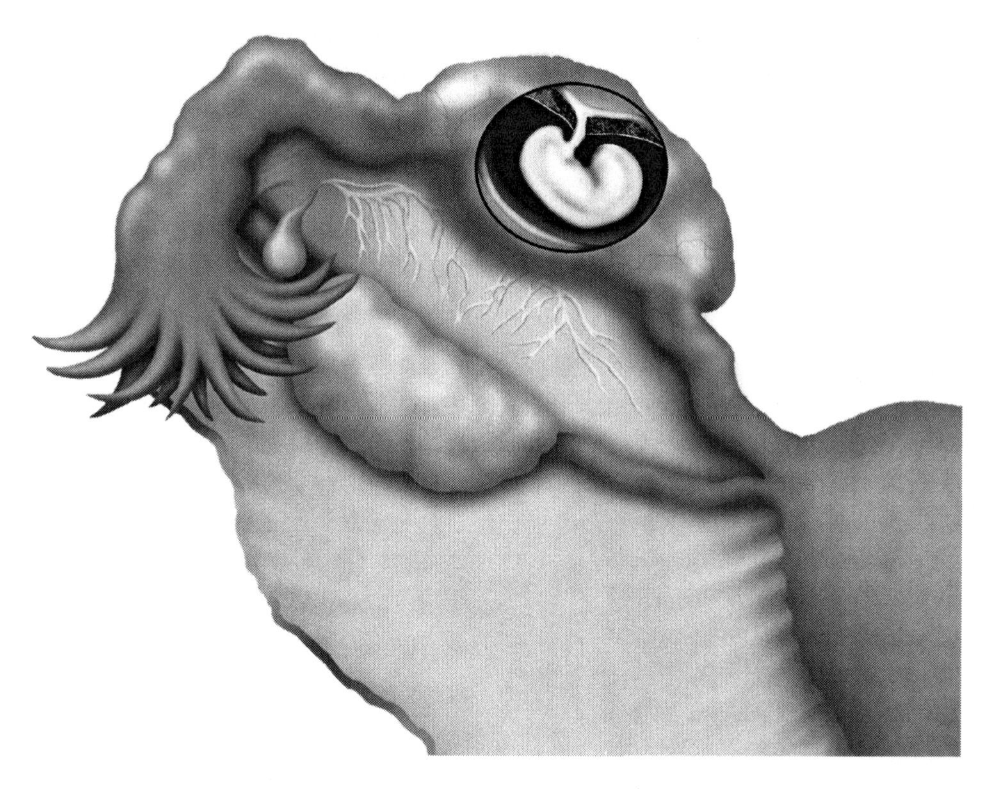

Ectopic pregnancy occurs when the fertilized egg cannot escape the fallopian tube. It must be dealt with quickly in all cases.

Physicians caution that all women who have had tubal problems in their life (adhesions, inflammation, blockage, or tubal pregnancy) are at higher risk for ectopic pregnancy. There is no known method to rescue a fertilized egg that has been trapped within the confines of the tube. Of greater concern, if left there, the pregnancy can continue to grow and become life-threatening to the mother.

Caught early, a tubal pregnancy can be treated with an injection such as methotrexate. This drug dissolves the attached egg, and leaves the tube with a minimal amount of damage.

Tubal pregnancies that persist for more than a few days may have grown too large to be dissolved pharmaceutically. In that case, an emergency laparoscopy or laparotomy (open surgery) will be required. Once s/he locates the ectopic, the surgeon will perform a salpingostomy or salpingotomy — a surgery in which the tube is cut open with a scalpel or laser — remove the attached embryo, then re-stitch, repair, or (in some cases) remove the tube or close it permantly at the site of surgical repair. Thus, besides the pregnancy loss, the tube has now been damaged or removed during emergency surgery.

We were pleased to find that in the participants of our published study, "Treating fallopian tube occlusion with a manual physical therapy," published January, 2008 in *Alternative Therapies in Health and Medicine*, we had only one ectopic pregnancy despite significant adhesions and surgeries in the women we treated. Since the study contained a relatively large number of women (28) with total tubal occlusion, physicians tell us they would have expected several ectopic pregnancies in the group. We are encouraged that the slow decrease of adhesions by manually pulling them apart, cross-link by cross-link, may help reverse the risk of ectopic pregnancies among the women we treat with blocked fallopian tubes.

I went to the hospital and the doctor discovered one of the embryos had implanted in my right tube causing an ectopic pregnancy. He immediately scheduled me for surgery to remove the tube. After the surgery, the doctor told me I had a lot of scar tissue at my right tube and that I probably had scar tissue surrounding my left tube, as well.

– Faith, who later became naturally pregnant and delivered a baby boy after CPT

Two Children after Ectopic and Adhesions

- Savannah's Story

In early 2004, I became pregnant for the first time. But my husband and I were soon devastated when we learned it was an ectopic pregnancy. My doctor recommended laparoscopic surgery to find the cause. During the procedure, he noted adhesions around my ovaries and fallopian tubes.

I went online right away to learn more about adhesions. I wanted to do everything I could to reduce adhesions and avoid another ectopic pregnancy. While searching for treatment options, I found Clear Passage Therapies (CPT). Their therapy focused on reducing adhesions and I thought they had a good chance to help me.

After researching the treatment for a few weeks, I decided to schedule therapy. I completed the program in one week of intensive therapy. It was a very positive experience and it was immediately obvious to me that they could help me.

During my initial evaluation, the therapists examined my body and palpated my organs. Although my doctor's report had not arrived at the clinic yet, they explained the different areas where they felt tension, decreased mobility, and possible lack of function. My therapists gave me a whole new level of awareness about my body and how it works than I had ever experienced before.

Later that afternoon, the doctor's report arrived and everything they told me correlated with my doctor's findings!

Areas that were once so tight had become far more supple and mobile . . . areas that were tender were now pain-free.

As the week progressed, I could feel changes in my body. At first, they couldn't sink their hands very deeply into my body. They also found areas of stiffness when they checked for mobility in my body. By the end of treatment, their hands could sink much deeper into my body without tension. The areas that were once originally so tight had become far more supple and mobile. Furthermore, areas that were tender at the start of therapy were now mobile and pain-free.

I returned home on Friday and my husband and I tried to conceive on Saturday. Incredibly, that was all it took — we became pregnant right away! An ultrasound showed that everything was progressing normally. I gave birth to my beautiful son, Daniel, who is now three years old.

Last summer, we had another surprise — I became pregnant again! Now, Daniel has a baby brother to play with.

I believe anyone with pregnancy issues should consider this therapy prior to trying to conceive.

One Ectopic Pregnancy, One Miscarriage, and Multiple Unsuccessful IUIs

- Isabella's Story

My journey to become a mom was not an easy one. My husband and I tried for a family soon after getting married in February of 2003. Our first setback came in June of 2003 when I suffered a ruptured ectopic pregnancy in my right fallopian tube. The physicians removed the tube, and as a result, I was left with only my left fallopian tube.

In September of 2004, I became pregnant again, only to have a miscarriage. As difficult and emotionally draining as these setbacks were, my husband and I tried to remain positive in that at least we could get pregnant.

This soon changed as months of trying turned into a year with no luck of becoming pregnant again.

At that point I was referred to a fertility specialist. We went through a battery of tests and the only thing that made any sense as to why this wasn't happening for us was that I was left with one tube and I likely had scarring or scar tissue from the ectopic pregnancy.

We tried four months of Clomid and IUIs with no luck. We then had to take a couple months off as my cycle became "out of whack." Next we tried three cycles of injectables and IUIs, but again had no success. Finally we decided to move on to IVF.

In the meantime, my mom had read an article about Clear Passage Therapies (CPT). I decided to see if I might be a good candidate. When they determined I would be a good candidate for therapy, I decided I would attend before my IVF transfer. Six weeks before I was scheduled to start IVF, I went to the CPT clinic, where I was treated for 20 hours over five days.

Four months of Clomid and IUIs... then (two) months off as my cycle became "out of whack." Next we tried three cycles of injectables and IUIs, but again had no success.

My IVF cycle was a bumpy one. The injectables weren't taking and in the end, I only produced three mature follicles — not enough to go through IVF, they told me.

My doctor suggested we try an IUI so that the past six weeks of medication, doctor visits, etc. wouldn't all be for nothing. Two of the three mature follicles were on my right side, where I do not have a fallopian tube, so the odds were really against us this cycle.

I went through with the IUI on July 15th and to our shock and amazement (as well as the doctor's) I was pregnant! Whereas this was my seventh IUI, the only reason I can imagine why this time was successful was because I had undergone the manual physical therapy at CPT. It was just too much of a coincidence that I had just had therapy, and that this cycle worked.

My doctor was also amazed. She admitted after the fact that in all the patients they treat, they had only seen one or two patients have success with IUI after a canceled IVF cycle.

My doctor was amazed.

We welcomed our little bundle of joy, Jacob, on April 1st weighing in at 6 lbs. 5 oz., 20 inches long. He is a happy, healthy baby and when my husband and I look at him we turn to each other and say how blessed we are.

Ectopic Pregnancy and Laparoscopic Surgery

- Norah's Story

There was nothing remarkable about the room. It was outfitted with the typical hotel décor — peach and teal floral-print bedspreads and plastic gold-framed prints adorning the walls. Yet somehow, this room, this trip, held more promise than I could handle. Though my journey through infertility began a year earlier with an inexplicable ectopic pregnancy, I knew my ten-hour drive to Clear Passage Therapies (CPT) was the beginning of the path that would lead me out of that dark loneliness.

Bags unpacked and calls of my safe arrival placed, I settled in with a book, though my mind wandered back to another time and place.

Warm and softly lit, an ultrasound machine consumed the intimate space. "I'm not sure ..." whispered the ultrasound tech in response to the doctor's question. Hearing only fractured words from their conversation, my heart raced. "It isn't thickened," she said again, and then "Here . . . by the ovary." The technician and doctor continued to discuss the "abnormalities" they were seeing, while I lay there clutching my husband's hand with a white-knuckled grasp. Nine weeks earlier, I'd felt a flood of excitement flow through me knowing that I was pregnant. Now, I felt that same rush of adrenaline. But this time it was cold, the tingling almost painful as it spread from the center, where my child should have been, throughout my entire being. As if suddenly realizing our presence, the doctor asked us to meet him in the examination room to discuss our options.

I heard the medical terminology for what was ultimately an ectopic pregnancy. I was ashamed of myself, of my body. Confused and heart-broken, I rode home silently, allowing the gravity of the circumstances to wash over me, in hopes of some cleansing. Yet I found none. Instead, I was greeted by a grim reality. In order to protect my life, I had to be the willing recipient of a drug that would dissolve my child.

Sleepily, I set my book on the nightstand and clicked off the light. Curling up, I could feel the exhaustion from the day's drive, but anticipation about my CPT treatment kept me from fully relaxing. My physical

> ***The technician and doctor continued to discuss the "abnormalities" they were seeing, while I lay there, clutching my husband's hand with a white-knuckled grasp.***

trip began early that morning, but my emotional journey into motherhood started long before.

Never in all my daydreams about pregnancy and motherhood, did I envision such uncertainty, confusion and turmoil. Had it really been seven months since I sat in the hospital, waiting for surgery after my ectopic pregnancy?

As we walked through the sterile corridors of the hospital, I couldn't help but think of the morbid irony. I felt completely empty in every sense of the word as I waited in the hospital room for the nurse to wheel me downstairs for surgery.

"Do you think they'll take the blocked tube?" I asked my husband for the hundredth time, knowing full well that he would never say "Yes," even if he thought so. I knew he was nervous because he was even more reserved than usual this morning. For the first time, I thought about how this might feel for him. And that's when I realized the startling difference between us, and why we needed each other more than ever. I couldn't have cared less about my own body, my own safety. I was angry and frustrated with my infertility. What did it matter if I was hurt or harmed? All I thought about was the child I so desperately longed to hold.

I felt empty in every sense of the word as I waited for the nurse to wheel me downstairs for surgery.

He, on the other hand, was thinking of me. Perhaps he had thoughts of an angel-faced baby and fantasies about playing catch with his boy in the backyard. But sitting there pretending to be interested in the news report on the television, his anxiety reached me and strangely enough, calmed my fears. He responded, "Na, I told 'em I couldn't take having you around the house for six weeks, so I'm pretty sure it'll just be a scope today."

Grinning, I half-heartedly turned my attention to the magazine I'd grabbed from the waiting room. Sitting cross-legged in the hospital bed, I began flipping absent-mindedly through the pages. I found myself expecting the worst — the loss of a tube or ovary — and yet hoping for the best. As if on cue, my eyes came to rest on an article about infertility. Reading intently, I was encouraged to read about a unique physical therapy that had helped several women facing infertility.

"Miss? We just got word that they're ready for you." The nurse's voice brought me back to my surroundings.

"Great. I think I'm ready now too," I replied, closing the magazine and thinking once again about the perfection of God's timing. I was still nervous, but now saw a glimmer of possibility regardless of the day's outcome.

Perhaps it was the unfamiliar bed, the absence of my hubby, or the butterflies flying around in my belly that caused me to wake before the alarm the following morning. Whatever the reason, I was in blissful disbelief that the hours of pre-authorization, planning and preparation were finally going to pay off.

Unlike my surgery, my apprehension about treatment was more exciting and exhilarating. As I left the hotel on my way to the treatment center, I found a sense of peace that confirmed I was where I was supposed to be and that I'd found the answer for which I'd been searching.

I arrived at the treatment center ahead of schedule and found the therapist who greeted me with a handshake and friendly smile. She showed me around the small office and then to my treatment room. "Have a seat and I'll be right in, I'm just going to grab your file," she said cheerfully, indicating the armchairs by the shuttered bay window. Celtic music played softly in the background, as we discussed my diagnosis. I was struck by her genuine interest in all aspects of my condition, and not just what the medical records indicated.

It was finally time for therapy to begin. In my gym shorts and T-shirt, I completed several range of motion exercises and made myself comfortable on the hydraulic massage table. For four hours each day, we shared stories about family, work, hobbies and interests while she worked on my body. Each evening, I found comfort in my solitude by visiting nearby gardens, movie theaters, restaurants or coffee shops.

I was struck by her genuine interest in all aspects of my condition, and not just the medical records.

As my final session ended, I was ready to see my family, and couldn't wait for enough time to pass to test the success of the treatment. Comparing results of the same range of motion exercises from earlier in the week, I could tell that significant changes had taken place. I felt taller, lighter. I appreciated my body's strength, embraced its resilience, and for the first time in a long time accepted its imperfect beauty.

Just two months after treatment, I woke very early that humid July morning, unable to resist checking my temp. Still elevated. This is the longest it's stayed up, I thought to myself as I padded down the stairs in quiet excitement. I dug out one of the several pregnancy tests housed under the bathroom sink. I kept it completely covered until the three minutes had passed. Breath held, the deafening pounding of my heart the only sound I heard, I slowly removed the towel and stared at the two pink lines.

Breath held, the deafening pounding of my heart the only sound I heard, I slowly removed the towel (to stare at the test).

"Honey..." I whispered. "Babe! We did it. We're pregnant!" I reported happily. Even in his sleepiness, I could feel his excitement as I snuggled in close.

A hoarse, "Really?" escaped his lips as he gently kissed me on the forehead. "We're really pregnant?"

"Yup. I just had a positive test about five minutes ago."

The following months were filled with the usual appointments, and once we were past the three-month mark we shared the news with friends and family. The pregnancy continued without incident and in March — just ten short months after my CPT treatment, I delivered a healthy baby boy at 36 weeks.

As if the arrival of our son didn't radically change our lives, the second addition to our family — whom I am now expecting just 17 months after the first, will certainly throw us into the deep end of parenting.

Ectopic Pregnancy After Surgery To Open Blocked Fallopian Tubes

- Melissa's Journey to Joy

My husband and I are blessed this year to be celebrating our 10th wedding anniversary and the first birthday of our sweet baby twins, Peter and Lydia. This last year has been the most joyful of our marriage as we have eagerly embraced the year of "firsts:" first Christmas, Thanksgiving, Mother's Day, Father's Day, and birthdays. It just seems to get better and better with each passing month. However, the road to this place of glee and joy was not an easy one.

Our struggle with infertility easily spans a period of over seven years. We were quite slow about catching onto the possibility there might be a problem. It was easy to make excuses, mostly timing, since I traveled for work. My gynecologist was in no hurry for me to get results either. I kept visiting her year after year but she took a very conservative approach and was slow to recommend any testing or treatment.

It wasn't until after one of my girlfriends relayed her struggle with infertility that I realized it sounded somewhat like mine, except that she had done something about it and now had two precious babies. Once I heard my story in the form of someone else's, I realized I needed the help of a specialist.

The next day I scheduled an appointment with a reproductive endocrinologist. Within a month of our first visit to the RE, we learned I had blocked fallopian tubes. Optimistically I had tried to think of it as "good news" when the doctor told me my tubes were blocked (at least there was a reason we hadn't gotten pregnant all those years), and it was possible our problem had been mechanical all along.

I chose to undergo the recommended surgery to attempt to open my tubes. Afterwards, she recommended trying natural conception, which we did and within three months we were pregnant! We couldn't have been more thrilled!! Unfortunately, this part of the story does not have a happy ending. Six weeks later we learned the embryo had not made it to my uterus — it was stuck in my fallopian tube. I was forced to have surgery to remove the very pregnancy we had hoped and prayed over for so long.

Just before the surgery, my doctor asked me, "Do you want us to try and save the fallopian tube?"

To rub salt in the wound, just before the surgery, my doctor asked me, "Do you want us to try and save the fallopian tube?" It seemed like a ridiculous question to me. Of course I wanted to preserve my fallopian tube, but she almost made me feel foolish for wanting to keep it. I wasn't ready to give up half of my chances to conceive on my own so quickly.

After the surgery, I was at a very low point. I had just turned 38 and was feeling the pressure of the clock ticking. And after two surgeries and an ectopic pregnancy, I was feeling quite discouraged and quickly losing hope.

While doing research on conceiving after an ectopic pregnancy, I stumbled upon some information regarding Clear Passage Therapies (CPT). I was encouraged by what I had read: A treatment that produced successful results without drugs or surgery! How refreshing! My husband, a nutritionist and practitioner of holistic healing, was also intrigued. After having gone through two recent surgeries, it was quite possible adhesions had contributed to my tubal blockage and could be preventing pregnancy. CPT also could increase my chances of a successful IVF transfer if I later decided I wanted to pursue that route. Based on all this, we felt we had nothing to lose and took steps to visit them.

I turned 40 a month and a half before our twins were born.

We visited CPT seven months after my ectopic pregnancy. The staff was extremely friendly and genuine and went the extra mile to ensure we received the proper physical treatment. Emotionally it was a place of renewal and restoration, particularly of my hope.

Soon after coming home from CPT I "celebrated" another birthday, 39. I was hopeful but had clearly lost the luxury of time. My husband and I then decided six months after visiting CPT that it was time to pursue IVF. This was a big step for us but we felt we had done everything possible to ensure a natural conception and this was the obvious next step for us in our journey of pursuing parenthood.

We got pregnant after the first try and to our amazement, with twins!! We simply could not believe after all these years of hoping and wanting, it was actually coming true. Nine months later I gave birth (naturally, I might add, with NO drugs) to the sweetest and most precious babies I have ever laid eyes on! I turned 40 a month and a half before our twins were born.

During the (years of) despair and disappointment, I would have never believed what was in store for me.

Years ago, during the despair and disappointment of our pursuits, I would have never believed what was in store for me at this age — a beautiful baby boy and a sweet, precious baby girl! What an incredible double blessing — my hopes and dreams had been fulfilled!

Remarkable Patient Success Stories

Clear Passage Therapies® began when we observed several surprise pregnancies in women whose fallopian tubes were totally blocked. Using resources, scientists, and physicians from the nearby medical school, we were able to conduct scientific studies to determine that we could open fallopian tubes using only our hands. This in itself was remarkable.

Over time, we were able to document these results statistically to the extent that we can now measure our success rates of opening blocked fallopian tubes scientifically.

An exciting aspect is that therapy involves virtually no risks. In fact, the only side effects we have seen have been positive (decreased pain, increased sexual function, and increased mobility). With surgery, the simplest surgical technique to open proximally blocked tubes resulted in tubes closing again within six months in over 80% of patients. But we continue to see one or more pregnancies and babies born even years after giving therapy to women whose blockage may have occurred anywhere in the tube. Thus, as well as being non-invasive, the therapy appears to open a much wider window of opportunity for pregnancy in the women we treat who have blocked fallopian tubes.

We are thankful to our patients for their support and to the physicians and scientists who encouraged us to create a scientific investigation of this fascinating phenomenon. As Dr. King said to us, "So many of the patients you are seeing are the ones for whom there is virtually no hope. They are at the ends of their rope, or at least thought they were until you came along. Now, you have given them back hope, with an opportunity for their bodies to truly heal, and to return to a more functional condition."

We are excited and humbled by our success in opening blocked fallopian tubes. That first success opened a door in our lives and the lives of our patients to help heal fallopian tubes and other conditions associated with the adhesions that form naturally in each of us, as the body heals.

> ***The doctor (said), "I found severe endometriosis throughout your reproductive system. It is strangling your fallopian tubes from the outside and blocking them inside. Your case is the most severe I have seen in a long time."***
>
> *– Hannah, who later became naturally pregnant after treatment at CPT*

Blocked Fallopian Tubes, Three IVFs, and Multiple Miscarriages

- Nicole's Story

One year into their marriage, Nicole and her husband, Keith, still couldn't become pregnant. Nicole told us, "We dated for three years before becoming married. We never used protection. So when we had been married for a year, we realized I hadn't been able to become pregnant in four years."

Nicole expressed her concerns to her Ob/Gyn, who ran a series of tests. When everything came back normal, she suggested an intrauterine insemination (IUI). Nicole told us, "We tried that, but it failed. My doctor didn't know what else she could do to help us and referred us to a reproductive endocrinologist (RE)."

Their RE decided to perform more tests. "That's when I found out I had an undetected STD, Chlamydia," Nicole explained. "It had caused scar tissue to form around and block both of my fallopian tubes."

Nicole's RE gave her two options, "I suggest you see a doctor who specializes in surgically opening blocked fallopian tubes or consider IVF."

Nicole decided she wanted a second opinion and went to another Ob/Gyn who specialized in infertility. That physician suspected she had fibroids in her uterus that prevented an embryo from successfully implanting. He suggested she undergo a myomectomy to remove the fibroids, and he would also try to open her blocked fallopian tubes at the same time.

Nicole underwent the surgery and her doctor successfully removed numerous fibroids. But despite his best efforts, he could not open Nicole's blocked fallopian tubes.

Nicole then decided to move on to IVF. Her first IVF was successful, but she soon miscarried. They then tried another transfer using frozen eggs, but there was no pregnancy.

"We decided to do another fresh transfer and I became pregnant with twins," Nicole explained. "But, I lost one baby almost right away, and then the second one at 15 weeks when my water broke unexpectedly."

Disheartened by the miscarriages, Nicole and Keith stopped fertility treatments for one year. During this time, Nicole frequently visited infertility chat sites. On one of the sites, Nicole read about a woman who had become pregnant after treatment at Clear Passage Therapies (CPT).

Nicole immediately called CPT for more information. After reading the information she was sent, Nicole discussed the treatment with Keith and decided to pursue treatment.

She scheduled herself for an intensive 20 hours of treatment. Nicole told us, "I was scared at first when I came out to CPT, but everyone was friendly, and it turned out to be a good experience."

When Nicole returned home, she spoke with her doctor about having another HSG. "It took some persuading," Nicole explained. "Before I went to CPT, my doctor was very discouraging. When I told her I went for the treatment and wanted a follow-up HSG, she brushed me off. She told me she didn't think I needed another one. But I finally convinced her to perform the test."

Nicole went to see the HSG technician for the test. When the results came in, Nicole didn't even know the test was over. "During my last HSG, it was extremely painful and I had a lot of cramps. During this HSG, I felt nothing — I just assumed they weren't finished!" The results showed that both of Nicole's tubes were now clear.

Nicole returned to her doctor to discuss her results, but her Ob/Gyn remained concerned that her fimbriae were far too scarred to catch an egg. She encouraged Nicole and her husband to undergo IVF, and after thorough discussion, they agreed.

Despite his best efforts, he could not open Nicole's blocked fallopian tubes.

"That's when I got pregnant with my daughter," Nicole told us. "At nine weeks I discovered I had twins, but one passed away early in the pregnancy." Nicole later gave birth to her baby girl, Joy.

Nicole told us that after giving birth, she was asked about going on birth control. "I looked at them like they were crazy. I didn't believe for a second that I would be able to conceive naturally."

Upon returning home with her daughter, Nicole discovered that her breast milk was drying up and she wasn't feeling well. She told us, "I had been bit by a mosquito and I was convinced that I had West Nile Virus. For weeks I fretted and finally my husband made me sit down and research the symptoms of the virus. After learning that the symptoms were very serious, I realized I was okay."

But Nicole continued to put on weight and couldn't understand why. "I was supposed to be a bridesmaid in my cousin's wedding, but I couldn't fit in the dress! I was frustrated because I thought I would have lost some of the baby weight by then. I begged my cousin to let me out of the wedding, but she insisted I participate. So, I had to buy a girdle to fit in the dress!"

Shortly after the wedding, Nicole discovered she was nine weeks pregnant. She couldn't believe it and told us, "We didn't try anything and we got pregnant!"

I looked at them like they were crazy. I didn't believe for a second that I would be able to conceive naturally.

When Nicole told us her news, we weren't surprised. Sometimes it takes women's bodies six months to a year to adjust after our treatment. Many times, women feel pressured by the ticking of their "biological clock" and thus feel forced to pursue another treatment option. After they give birth, they forget about contraceptives and only then discover that their body is functioning naturally and properly.

This was exactly the case with Nicole. She gave birth to her second child, a healthy baby boy, at thirty-eight weeks. Now her daughter has a little brother.

Five Years Infertile with Two Blocked Tubes

- Sarah's Story

Infertility is a lonely road to walk down. My husband and I tried for over five years to have a child. Every time we received a friend's birth announcement or invitation to a baby shower, we were painfully reminded of our own struggles and felt isolated from our friends' joy.

When my husband and I suspected we had fertility problems, we decided to speak with a doctor. We had to skip around from doctor to doctor at first because we moved from Minnesota to New Hampshire. As a result, we were never able to spend much time with one doctor and always felt pressured to quickly make decisions.

We finally settled with an endocrinologist in New Hampshire who suggested I have a hysterosalpingogram (HSG) to see if my fallopian tubes were blocked. I was very hesitant at first, but I finally decided to go through with the procedure. We didn't expect anything to be wrong. Yet, the results showed that both of my tubes were blocked.

The endocrinologist suggested we proceed with laparoscopic surgery to attempt to open my tubes. If the surgery did not work, we could consider IVF or adoption.

I wasn't comfortable with having surgery and IVF wasn't an option for us because of personal and financial reasons, but adoption had always been in the back of our minds. We had even been accepted as parents at an adoption agency.

However, I still didn't feel ready to make a decision. I was the live-in caregiver for my grandmother at the time and under a lot of stress. I needed more time to think about our options.

Every time we received a friend's birth announcement or invitation to baby shower, we were painfully reminded of our own struggles and felt isolated from our friends' joy.

I wanted to tell my husband how I felt, but I was worried he would not understand. I finally decided to speak to him one night. I was surprised to find out he felt the same way I did and had been afraid to talk to me! After a lengthy discussion, we decided to put everything on hold for six months.

A few months later, my husband and I settled into the couch to watch the nightly news at 5 PM — a time we seldom watched. A report about Clear Passage Therapies (CPT), a clinic that had success relieving pain and increasing chances of fertility, aired on the news. They reported that the treatment used manual physical therapy, without drugs or surgery.

My husband and I were both intrigued, so I asked him to watch the news again at 6 PM — the time we normally watched. When the news report did not come on at 6 PM, we knew it wasn't a coincidence that we had sat down early to watch the five o'clock news.

I asked my sister-in-law, who had worked as a massage therapist, if massage could actually help with pain or infertility. She assured me that massage had the potential to help with many problems and that CPT might be worth my time. I sent my information in and was excited when they approved me for treatment.

The first day of treatment I felt nervous and uneasy. However, my anxiety dissipated when I met my therapists. They were so warm, friendly, and natural with me that I felt comfortable and relaxed.

Over the course of the week, I had ten hours of therapy. By the end of the week, my entire body felt healthier and I headed home to try and become pregnant. After five months, we still had no success. The therapists had told me that most of their patients experienced success after 20 hours of treatment, so I decided to return for ten more hours.

I was excited for my second round of treatment. It was comforting to be back in the relaxing atmosphere with encouraging therapists.

Following the treatment, my husband and I tried for six months to become pregnant. When we had no results, I called CPT to see if I should return for additional treatment. They urged me to complete another HSG so they could know my progress.

My husband and I went to the hospital together for the procedure. Afterwards, the doctor brought in the results and showed me that the dye had gone through my tubes — both of my tubes were clear! Tears of joy ran down my face and I couldn't wait to tell CPT.

However, we still did not become pregnant naturally. Because my tubes were open, the endocrinologist suggested we try Clomid® (a hormonal drug) with an intrauterine insemination (IUI). Although I was nervous about the entire process, my husband and I decided to try it.

After seven agonizing years of infertility, I was finally going to experience pregnancy and parenthood.

A few weeks after my IUI, I woke up in the middle of the night and decided to take an early pregnancy test. It showed I was pregnant! I woke up my husband, excited, "The test is positive! It's positive!" Because it was only three in the morning, he groggily asked, "What test? You took what? What is it?" I finally calmed down enough to explain I was pregnant.

The next day we had a blood test that confirmed my pregnancy. I was overwhelmed with joy. After seven agonizing years of infertility, I was finally going to experience pregnancy and parenthood.

Now, our beautiful baby girl is three years old. I am so grateful for CPT and the doctors who helped us overcome infertility.

Blocked Tubes after Myomectomy

- Tina's Story

Three years ago my struggle with infertility began. My husband and I were trying to get pregnant at the time, but finally decided we needed to talk to a doctor. My doctor recommended I try Clomid, a fertility drug that assists ovulation. However, after three months, we still did not have success.

About the same time, I began noticing some pain in my pelvis. I was not sure if the pain was related to my infertility, but I finally went to the hospital when the pain became severe. The doctors discovered I had a large uterine fibroid, which they removed during surgery.

Six months after the surgery, I thought, "Why am I still not pregnant?" I returned to my doctor to have an HSG and he discovered my tubes were blocked. I couldn't believe it. They suspected that my surgery to remove my fibroid had caused scar tissue to form that was now blocking my fallopian tubes.

My doctor immediately referred me to a fertility specialist. The specialist examined my HSG results and told me, "I would not advise surgery to open your tubes. Sometimes this type of surgery is not useful, and in your case, I recommend you move straight to IVF."

In April, 2008, I began IVF medications and everything seemed to be going well. The transfer was completed and I was anxious to hear the results. "I'm sorry, Tina," my doctor said. "Your results came back negative."

I told myself that I needed to look for other options and see if there was something that could help me. I went on the Internet and typed in "blocked fallopian tubes." Thousands of results came back, but one caught my attention. It was a physical therapy treatment to open blocked fallopian tubes. I read over their results and their patient stories and then decided to apply.

I broke down into tears. I felt hopeless at first, but I couldn't give up.

I attended therapy for an intensive week and my experience was very good. It was one of the less stressful treatments I had undergone in the past three years. My time there really encouraged me.

A month after treatment, I returned for an HSG. The HSG technician was very patronizing at first. "You were just here and your tubes were blocked. Why do you want to do this again?" I explained the treatment I had undergone and she reluctantly performed the procedure.

I watched her face as she looked at the results and her jaw dropped in shock. I turned to look at the screen and I saw free spill from my fallopian tube. It was beautiful. My right fallopian tube had opened completely and my left was now half open.

My doctor reviewed the results and told me, "Wow, if I hadn't seen this, I wouldn't have believed it."

She took a deep breath, smiled, and told me, "Tina, go make your baby."

It has been one month since she told me those glorious words and my husband and I plan to conceive in the next six months. I am so thankful I put my faith in God and that he saw me through. When I first discovered CPT, their treatment sounded too good to be true. But God enabled me to put my doubts aside and have faith in the treatment.

My doctor reviewed the results and told me, "If I hadn't seen this (myself), I wouldn't have believed it."

I hope that other women can find the peace I did because approaching fertility treatments with the right mindset is half the battle. It was faith that saw me through, and now I can finally become pregnant.

Chapter Seven

Endometriosis and Fertility

Endometriosis is a common and often painful disorder that is estimated to affect one in ten women of childbearing age in America.[16] In this condition, a specialized type of tissue that normally lines the inside of the uterus (the endometrium) is found outside of the uterus. Endometrial tissue responds to hormones during the menstrual cycle, thickening prior to a woman's period and then shrinking or dissipating during menstruation. Endometriosis can lead to debilitating pelvic pain, bowel conditions, bladder pain, painful sex, and numerous other pains or dysfunctions, which we discuss in Chapter Seventeen.

Endometriosis Stages

- **Stage One** - few endometrial implants, most often in the cul-de-sac (the space between the uterus and the rectum).
- **Stage Two** - mild to moderate levels of endometrial implants (usually with a few small areas of scar tissue or adhesions).
- **Stage Three** - moderate levels of superficial and deep endometrial implants in several reproductive areas (often with several areas of scar tissue or adhesions).
- **Stage Four** - widespread superficial and deep endometriosis implants often throughout the pelvic area (usually with large adhesions).

One of the most common and devastating results of endometriosis is infertility. Approximately 30 to 40 percent of women with endometriosis are infertile.[17] In fact, most women do not even discover they have endometriosis until they undergo diagnostic surgery to determine the cause of their infertility.

Physicians do not know the cause of endometriosis, or exactly how it contributes to infertility, especially in its early stages.

Endometriosis and Adhesions

Through our clinical experience, we theorize that a major part of endometriosis is adhesions. We suspect it occurs like this:

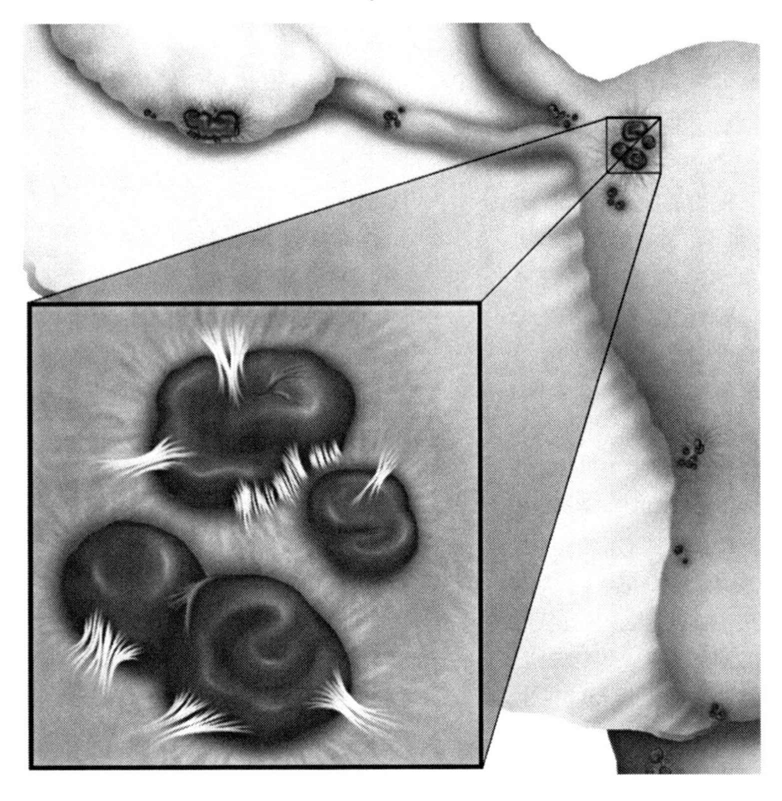

Tiny adhesive cross-links attach at sites of endometrial tissue because of the inflammation inherent to the condition.

When endometrial tissue outside the uterus responds to a woman's hormone cycle, it thickens and bleeds each month. Trapped within the pelvis, endometrial implants create inflammation wherever they exist. Like any other inflammation, the inflamed tissues associated with endometriosis cause tiny adhesions to occur. These adhesions attach the endometrial deposits to underlying tissues and structures.

When the endometrial tissue swells each month, it pulls on the attached adhesions, causing pain. The adhesions from inflamed tissue may also spread to other areas of inflammation.

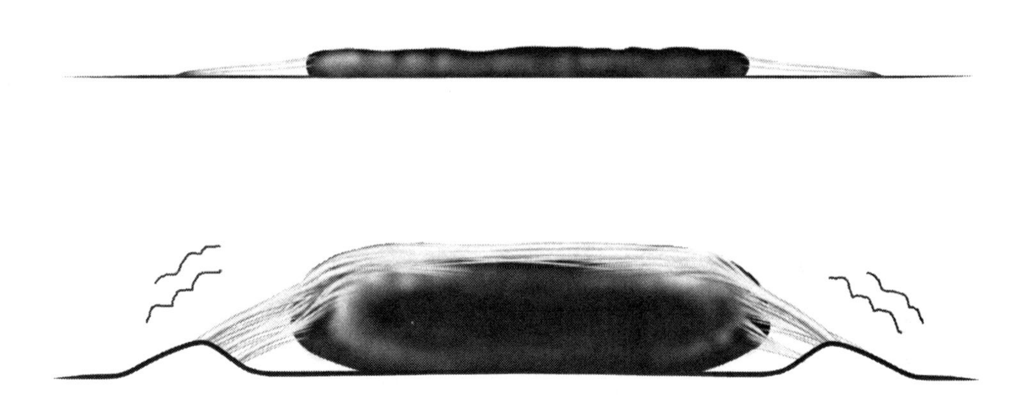

A side-view of an endometrial implant and its adhesions shows less pull during most of the menstrual cycle (top drawing) but significant pull on underlying tissues and structures during menstruation (bottom).

When adhesions form on or near nerves, pain occurs. When they form on the delicate tissues and organs of the female reproductive system, endometriosis and its related adhesions can glue the structures down, restricting normal mobility, reducing reproductive function, and sometimes causing pain.

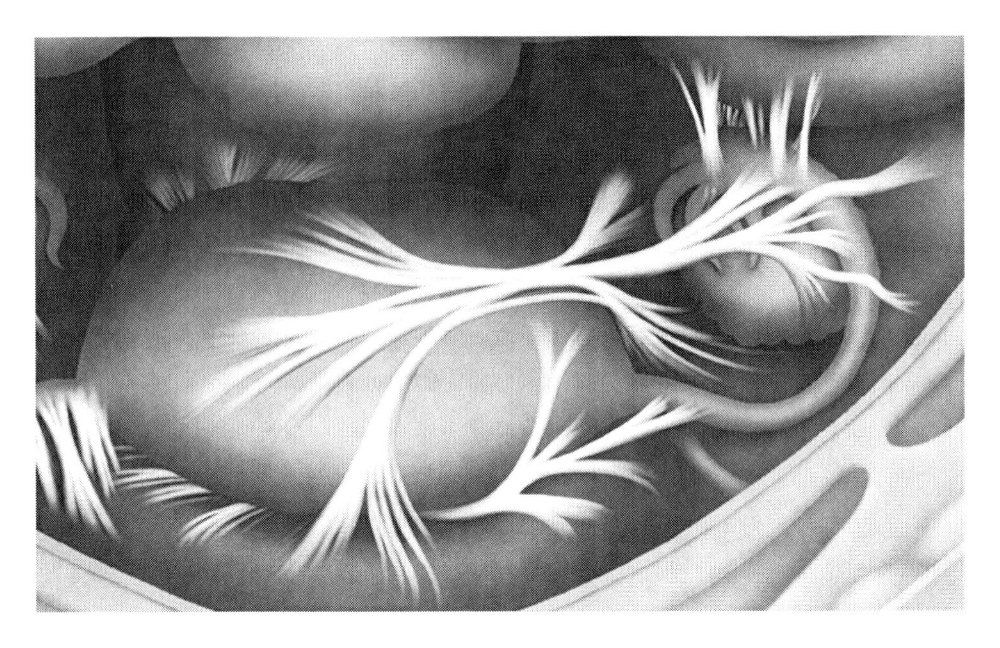

The female reproductive structures are among the most common sites for both endometriosis and adhesions to form.

The delicate tissues and organs of the female reproductive tract do not react well to being glued down. Their proper function relies on free movement within and among the various organs in order for conception to occur. The adhesions produced by endometriosis can trap the egg in the ovary, inhibit the mobility of the fallopian tubes, and impair the ability of the fimbriae to grasp an egg that has been released by the ovary. They can also decrease the function of the uterus by creating glue-like bonds with consequent spasm, decreased mobility and motility, and excess tension in the uterine walls, thus decreasing the possibility for egg implantation.

The Elusive Diagnosis

Many physicians feel that the only way to make a definitive diagnosis of endometriosis is by directly visualizing it through a surgical procedure, either a laparoscopy or a laparotomy (open surgery). In laparoscopic surgery, a tiny incision is made near the navel, where the physician fills the interstitial spaces (the areas between organs) using compressed carbon dioxide (which is considered non-toxic) to separate the organs from each other. Once that is accomplished, s/he inserts a slender viewing instrument (laparoscope). By moving the laparoscope around between the structures (which have been visually separated by the CO_2 gas) the surgeon can view and film the condition of the pelvic and abdominal organs.

In 2006, Belinda and I were invited to a conference of some of the world's foremost endometriosis experts, hosted by the US National Institute of Health (NIH) and the American Society for Reproductive Medicine (ASRM). There was heated debate on the most appropriate methods to diagnose endometriosis. Some physicians argued against the necessity for exploratory surgery. These physicians trusted their non-surgical diagnostic skills. If certain signs and symptoms were present as patient complaints, they felt it unnecessary to perform diagnostic laparoscopy that could create more adhesions.

Surgical Treatment

Because so many doctors feel that endometriosis can only be definitively diagnosed through surgical procedures (laparoscopy or laparotomy), physicians also use these procedures to remove the endometriosis. The surgical procedure is generally accompanied by a laser or scalpel to lyse (burn or cut) adhesions and endometrial tissue. Dr. King has found that in some cases, an electro-cauterizing device called Helica may be less damaging to underlying tissue than other methods. (See Chapter Seventeen for more information on the Helica.)

Whatever tool is chosen, the surgeon will take special note of any endometrial implants and adhesions that attach to areas that would be difficult to access without risking damage to the patient. For example, the bowels (intestines) are delicate structures that can be nicked by a scalpel or laser. If this happens, the contents of the bowel can spill into the pelvis and/or abdomen, causing severe internal infection called peritonitis. Surgeons are generally cautious in attempting to remove endometriosis or adhesions that are closely attached to the bowels, bladder, ovaries, or fallopian tubes.

The fallopian tubes and ovaries are extremely delicate structures. While cutting them is not usually considered dangerous or life threatening, addressing endometriosis adhesions on these delicate reproductive organs can either enhance or impair fertility depending upon the condition the physician finds, the location of the traumatized tissue, and the skills of the surgeon. While physicians can normally address adhesions and endometriosis on the muscular walls of the bladder, most surgeons are extremely cautious in addressing adhesions which are closely attached there.

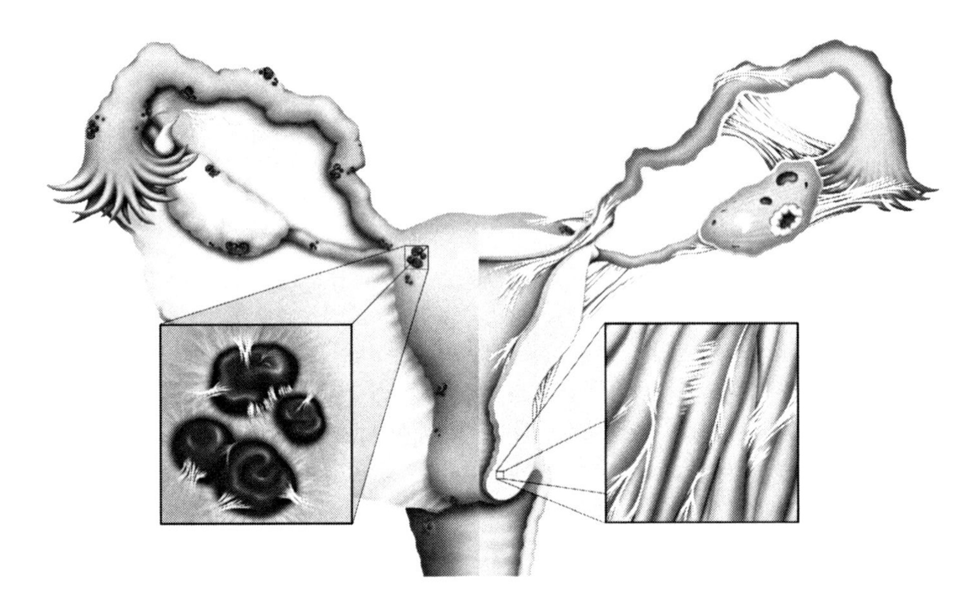

Endometriosis (left) and adhesions (right) act like glue affecting the delicate reproductive structures, causing infertility and sometimes pain.

A unique problem with endometriosis is that while it can be a surface condition, it can also be found deep within the tissues. Some physicians feel that they can often decrease pain and increase function by cauterizing (burning) endometriosis at the surface of structures. Others are firmly convinced that they need to dig deeply into the organ, cutting through the living tissue that forms the wall of that organ, in order to excise the full depth of endometrial implants or adhesive processes. Clearly, the deeper the cut, the greater the potential for surgical damage to the organ being cut.

In many cases, women undergo more than one surgery to decrease endometriosis pain and remove the adhered endometrial tissues. While surgery is often successful at removing endometrial tissue, the most gifted surgeon cannot prevent the adhesions that form as part of the healing process which occurs after surgery to treat endometriosis. As well as the surgical adhesions, endometriosis can and often does recur. Either occurrence may inspire the physician to suggest another surgery.

Pharmaceutical Treatment

Patients with endometriosis are often placed on birth control pills after surgery to limit stimulation to the endometrium, in hopes of decreasing bleeding and pain. A drug called Lupron puts the patient into temporary menopause to decrease endometriosis pain. Lupron normally is administered for a maximum of six months in hopes of retarding the growth of the endometriosis. Obviously, drugs which stop menstruation are contraindicated for any woman who is trying to conceive.

How Endometriosis Impacts IUI and IVF

Women who have already undergone surgery to remove endometriosis are often dismayed when they are still unable to become pregnant. Frequently, doctors recommend they try IUI or IVF to increase their chances. Although these procedures work for some women, for others, the endometriosis and adhesions continue to create a mechanical barrier to fertility.

Fourteen Unsuccessful IUIs and Endometriosis

- Andie's Story

Prior to finding Clear Passage Therapies (CPT), my husband and I had all but given up on conceiving. We had tried infertility treatments for three years with no success. I felt like my body had been through everything imaginable — months of Clomid®, laparoscopic surgery to remove endometriosis, Lupron shots, seven months of hormonal shots, and fourteen unsuccessful intrauterine inseminations (IUIs).

As you might imagine, I was on an emotional rollercoaster. The different medications and hormones made my body have extreme highs and lows. It was always hard to see my friends or even complete strangers with children. I knew I had this loving family and home to bring a child into, but for some reason, it just wasn't happening for me.

"What shot do I need to take today? How many days until I ovulate?" ...It slowly began to take its toll on me, my husband, and our marriage.

I tried not to live my life by the clock, but I was. I had no choice: What shot do I need to take today? How many days until I ovulate? When does my husband need to take off work for our next insemination? It slowly began to take its toll on me, my husband, and our marriage.

Finally, I decided enough was enough. I couldn't live my life that way. Our doctors wanted us to pursue in vitro fertilization (IVF), but we weren't comfortable with that option and I didn't want any more medications, surgeries, or invasive treatments.

My husband and I learned of CPT and were curious as to whether they could help me. We read that they had success treating endometriosis and we decided their therapy was worth a shot.

I was nervous on the first day, but my experience at CPT was wonderful. My husband and I drove up every week and the treatment was so relaxing that I would actually fall asleep on the car ride home.

My first ovulation after treatment was pain-free. I usually experienced one day of sharp pain because of endometriosis, but this time I didn't feel anything.

My first ovulation after treatment was pain-free.... That month, I became pregnant naturally!

That month, I became pregnant naturally! After the years of emotionally and physically taxing treatments — it was a natural, non-invasive treatment that enabled me to become pregnant. If we had known about CPT prior to everything we did, we would have saved ourselves a lot of time, money, and emotionally taxing years.

As we look at our daughter today, we are thankful that we can leave our years of infertility behind and enjoy our precious gift.

Ten Years Infertile and Four Surgeries for Endometriosis

- Amania's Story

I'll begin my story with a mantra that I have always held dear, "Clarify in your mind what it is that you want; hold it in your heart and never let go until you have it." I believe that faith is very important, but focused persistence is key to achieving what you want in life — in my case, fertility.

I am the second oldest of four girls. I grew up in a happy, close-knit family. I believed in the fairytale and was sure that I would fall in love, get married and have a family of my own someday.

At 18, I was having increasingly painful menstrual cramps. The diagnosis ended up being endometriosis and my doctor's suggestion to me was to "get pregnant as soon as possible because you may end up infertile." I was shocked at the suggestion to get pregnant when I had no boyfriend or husband, and had just started college.

So, I hoped he'd be wrong and went on with my life. During the next six years, my cramps grew more and more painful and the drugs I was given to handle the pain were stronger and stronger.

I met my husband in college and we got married when I was 24. We planned on starting our family right away, so I never took birth control. After two years of no pregnancy, we consulted a fertility specialist.

We tried six rounds of Clomid and double doses of Clomid with two artificial inseminations, with no success. We were discouraged and heart broken. My husband never thought it would be that difficult to get pregnant. I felt so sad and humiliated, as if I were less of a woman because my body wouldn't "produce" as it should.

Every time someone got pregnant, I would be filled with conflicting emotions. My sister already had two sons and my friends and sisters-in-law had children too. I was happy for them and excited about the babies, but also suffered terribly with bouts of depression over my inadequacy and empty nest. At times I felt extremely angry at pregnant women and mothers with their children. Other times, I would tell people that I had no desire to be burdened by babies, which was a defense mechanism, I guess.

I wanted to have faith, but it was hard when "specialists" were telling me there was no reason to feel hopeful.

I then underwent laparoscopic surgery and other invasive procedures to clear the endometriosis.

Well-meaning people were always quick to give their advice to help me. This advice ranged from standing on my head, to acupuncture, herbal remedies, adopting a baby so that I'd miraculously become pregnant and the old favorite, "Just relax and don't think about it, and POOF — you'll be pregnant before you know it!" How could I NOT think about it when with each passing menstrual cycle, there was a constant reminder? I would think to myself, "How can I relax when I want it so much and am reminded of it everyday?"

After that, we moved to Arizona and I was referred to a well known fertility specialist. After meeting with him and coming up with a plan of action, I was so renewed with hope!

I had an HSG and another laparoscopy, and underwent two failed IUIs with Clomid. My husband and I disliked how "un-romantic" and clinical this process was. And stressful!

I changed specialists three more times, and had a laparotomy that cleared 80% of the endometriosis but left scarring. We then did in vitro fertilization (IVF) with ICSI.

After that failed, we were told that I should consider donor eggs since my FSH level was beginning to get high and I was not a good candidate to retry IVF. A second specialist confirmed this diagnosis as well.

We were heartbroken. I became really depressed and underwent psychiatric therapy for six months. I was told to "have faith" by my family and I really WANTED to continue to have faith but it was hard when "specialists" were telling me there was no reason to feel hopeful.

During this time, I heard of Clear Passage Therapies (CPT) and discussed it as an option with my doctor. He discouraged me from pursuing it since his method was (according to him) the only proven successful option. (This may have been before they published any of their studies — or else he hadn't read them.)

After about six months in therapy for my depression, I felt better again. During a check-up with my primary care physician, I told her that I was feeling mentally better again and wanted to continue looking for options to get pregnant. She gave me a magazine containing various fertility methods, and in it, I read an article on CPT. I felt like it was a sign, and that I should pursue it since it was the second time I came across it. So, I looked into it, called the office and felt really positive by what I was presented with, by the friendly, caring, and knowledgeable staff.

I went to their clinic for four hours of therapy per day for five days. I arrived on a Sunday and had my sister stay overnight with me. We went to Disneyland on Sunday to kick off this exciting week and had so much fun! Then, I'd take a walk on the beach and meditate every morning before attending therapy.

I returned home in high spirits, feeling healthier, renewed and relaxed.

On the 2nd and 3rd day of my morning meditation on the beach, a baby seagull flew over to me and sat and watched me. I definitely felt like it was a sign that my baby was close to getting here!

My experience with CPT was extremely positive. Not only was my endometriosis addressed, but my therapist gave me more information and knowledge about my body and how it works than I could have ever hoped to know.

I returned home in high spirits, feeling healthier, renewed and relaxed. I started taking my basal temperature every morning with my next cycle and we tried once again to conceive via "the natural method."

Two weeks later, I was feeling "off." I had purchased some pregnancy tests since we would be "trying" for the next six months. Lo and behold — the test was positive!! I just stood there looking at myself in my bathroom mirror, not believing and yet believing that it had finally happened to me! And within two weeks of my therapy!

I am crying again now, as I remember this awesome moment. I had a wonderful, healthy pregnancy and our daughter, Mia Bella, is now 22 months old and the light of our lives.

In the end, it took 10 years before I got pregnant — too bad I didn't know about CPT sooner!

Whenever someone is wishing for a miracle, I always tell them my story, refer them to CPT and tell them to be persistent and patient, as it can pay off.

Two Failed IVFs and Endometriosis

- Samantha's Story

Two years into our marriage, my husband and I started trying to conceive. After a while, we realized that something wasn't right and I decided to talk to my gynecologist. She told me, "It takes most couples an average of one year to naturally conceive. If you and your husband do not conceive in a year, you can return and we will discuss your options."

I was happy to hear there was nothing to be concerned about. But when a year passed, I returned to my doctor for help. We tried a couple of rounds of intra-uterine inseminations, but they didn't work.

My doctor then referred me to an infertility specialist who recommended we try IVF. We did a fresh cycle right away, but none of the embryos implanted. We then tried a cycle using embryos they had frozen from my first cycle. When that also didn't work, I knew it was time we tried the holistic route.

I began seeing an acupuncturist who also put me on some special juice drinks. After a year with no success, I began searching for other treatments and read about Clear Passage Therapies (CPT) in a magazine.

I set up an appointment and began seeing CPT over the course of a year. My treatments were always very relaxing and it felt like they were helping everything in my pelvis to become more mobile. One of my therapists said she suspected I might have endometriosis from the way my pelvis felt, and suggested I discuss it further with my doctor.

I was discouraged (but) my disappointment didn't last long though — I found out I was pregnant on my own!

After treatment, my husband and I decided to sit back and not pursue any treatment for a while. We spoke with a new infertility specialist to discuss our options for the future, and he also suspected I had endometriosis. I underwent diagnostic surgery and the doctor confirmed what my CPT therapist had felt — endometriosis.

My doctor explained that IVF was in our best interest because endometriosis frequently returns and the surgery to diagnose and remove endometriosis can cause scar tissue to form that could impair my fertility.

We had a fresh IVF transfer right away and to our surprise, we became pregnant! My pregnancy went well and I later gave birth to our healthy, happy TWINS!

About two years after their birth, my husband and I decided to pursue IVF again. When it didn't work, I was discouraged. My disappointment didn't last long though — I later found out I was pregnant on my own! Our third child is now a year old and doing well.

It's hard to say which treatment "worked" for me. I think a large part of my success was learning to relax. My treatment at Clear Passage enabled me to become more familiar with my body and calm down. I know their treatment helped to restore balance in my body and mind, preparing me for my transfers and natural birth.

Manual Physical Therapy — Wurn Technique®

Our manual physical therapy, completed by therapists who are trained to decrease adhesions that bind organs, can be very effective at addressing the mechanical problems associated with endometriosis. As noted earlier, endometriosis and adhesions are often intimately related. That is, women with endometriosis frequently have the concurrent problem of adhesion formation. The body responds to the endometrial implants by laying down adhesions.

Our focus is to detach, decrease, and dissolve the bonds that create these adhesions, strand by strand. This slow, meticulous manual therapy is apparently much less invasive than surgical techniques, which carry some risk of tissue damage and more adhesion formation, as well as the usual risks of surgery.

As we slowly stretch, deform, and peel apart many of the endometrial adhesions, we believe that the tiny attachments between collagen fibers begin to dissolve, and adhesions detach. Thus, while we cannot break the entire rope all at once, we can slowly peel it apart, fiber by fiber.

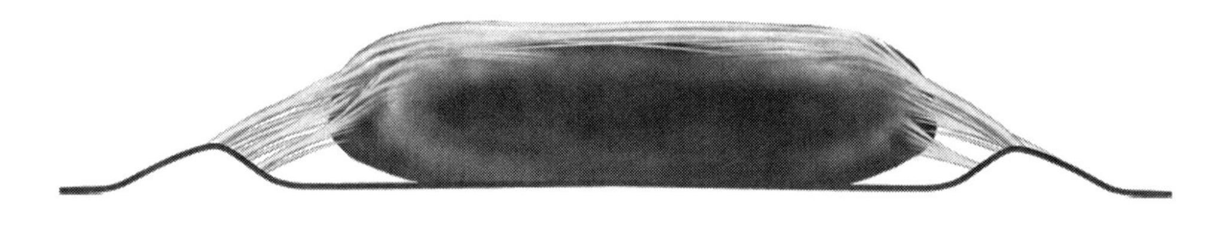

Adhesive cross-links can cause pain and infertility

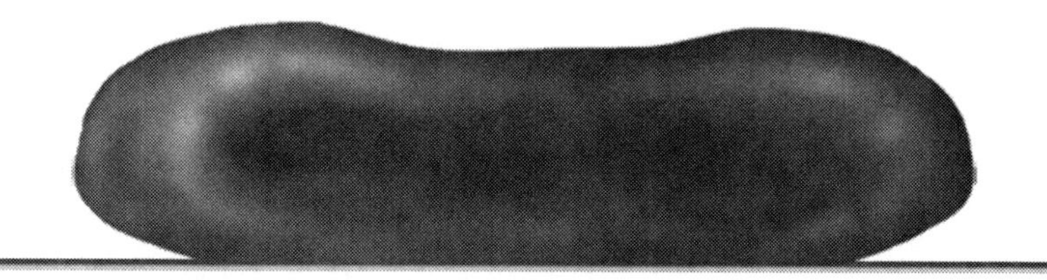

We believe this therapy detaches cross-links from swollen endometrial tissue attached to organs, improving the mobility and function of the underlying structures.

In doing so, we apparently release the powerful grip of these microscopic bonds between neighboring collagen fibers. Hour after hour, session after session, it feels to us like we are pulling out the run in a three-dimensional sweater of adhered tissues.

As the adhesions detach, the endometrial implants likely remain, but their mechanical attachments to the delicate reproductive structures upon which they have landed no longer bind the structures tightly together. Thus freed from their glue-like bonds, the reproductive structures can begin to move more freely and function as they did before the adhesions bound them in their vise-like grip.

Six Years of Infertility and Stage IV Endometriosis

- Liz's Story

When I was 24 years old, I was diagnosed with stage IV endometriosis. After I underwent surgery, my pain increased in severity and frequency.

Two years later, I married my long-time boyfriend, and we planned to have a perfect family. Because of my complications with endometriosis, I sought help from a fertility specialist and underwent another laparoscopic surgery. The surgeon drained a cyst, removed any endometriosis she found, and removed a stapled sac that was attached to the left ovary from my previous surgery.

The surgeon (said) we had a 1% chance of conceiving naturally.

Although the surgeon was optimistic that my endometriosis pain would be reduced, she told my husband and I we had a 1% chance of conceiving naturally. I was heartbroken; words cannot express the pain I endured in that moment.

I prayed for a miracle or sign of hope. Then, I received a phone call from my sister. On her local news, there was a feature about a manual physical therapy treatment that could help women with endometriosis and infertility.

My husband was skeptical at first, but I needed to try it out. I immediately called and received a packet of information about the therapy. What we read made sense to us, so my husband and I decided to sign me up for the treatment. We packed our bags and headed to Florida.

The rest is history. Ten days after the treatment and six years of battling with infertility, I was pregnant! My husband and I were so shocked that we had to administer the pregnancy test three times, to be sure.

I had a full-term pregnancy and gave birth to our beautiful baby boy. My son will be four at the end of this month and we also have another addition to the family. I was able to naturally conceive another baby three years later. She is almost a year old now. When we look at our children's faces and into their eyes, we are still amazed by our little miracles.

My husband and I were so shocked that we had to administer the pregnancy test three times, to be sure.

Endometriosis and Two Blocked Tubes

- Hannah's Story

"Your wife will never be able to conceive naturally," the doctor told my husband. I was still in recovery after a laparoscopic surgery to remove fibroid tumors from my uterus and endometriosis, but the doctor wanted to forewarn my husband.

When I finally woke, the doctor explained the results to me. "I was able to remove one fibroid tumor from your uterus, but there were two under the skin that I could not access without compromising your ability to carry a child." As we suspected, I also found severe endometriosis. Unfortunately, it is prevalent throughout your reproductive system. It is strangling your fallopian tubes from the outside, and blocking them from the inside. Your case is the most severe I have seen in a long time."

(Endometriosis) is strangling your fallopian tubes from the outside, and blocking them inside. Your case is the most severe I have seen in a long time.

He showed me an image taken during the procedure and it looked as if my fallopian tubes were a wrung towel. The endometriosis covered everything, and my ovaries did not look normal at all.

He immediately suggested I go on Lupron to prevent further growth of endometriosis. However, my husband

and I had been trying to conceive for nearly three and a half years and I wasn't ready to jump to a drug that would put me into a menopausal state. I wanted more time to educate myself about endometriosis and the different treatment options.

I had only recently heard of endometriosis when I went to see my doctor about pain I experienced during my periods and my inability to conceive. During that check-up, my doctor discovered I had fibroid tumors and scheduled me for laparoscopic surgery. He also suspected I had endometriosis and told me, "The good news is, I can diagnose and remove the endometriosis at the same time I remove your fibroid tumors."

However, my case was far worse than the doctor imagined and there was nothing he could do but offer pharmaceuticals. My husband wanted me to go on the medication right away so that I would be out of pain. He had given up hope that I would ever conceive.

I, on the other hand, still had hope. I devoted every spare minute I had to research and learned of the emotional and psychological side effects of Lupron.

I convinced my husband that I needed to find a more natural approach and continued researching. I purchased some books and started a new diet to help regulate my hormones and the growth of the endometriosis.

During my research, I came across Clear Passage Therapies (CPT). I requested more information and received a packet, along with a DVD. I spoke with my husband about it and we decided to give it a shot. Even if I wasn't able to become pregnant, at least it would help with the pain.

Because I reside in California, I needed my doctor to sign a referral form to see a physical therapist. My doctor scoffed at the treatment and refused to sign the paperwork. I didn't give up, and finally he reluctantly signed.

I drove south for a very intensive week of physical therapy. My therapist was absolutely amazing — her care and attentiveness were incredible. I will always remember her and how she was really there to help and listen to me.

After my treatment, I returned to my doctor and requested an HSG. He told me, "There would be no point. I performed one just five months ago during your surgery and your tubes were completely blocked." I insisted, and he finally allowed me to do the test.

Shortly thereafter, I went to see a technician for the procedure. After it was finished, I asked him, "How does it look?" I tried to lean my head forward to look at the screen.

He calmly replied, "It looks fine."

"What do you mean fine?"

"They're not blocked, it looks fine." I told him about my previous test and he looked at me like I was crazy. "No," he continued, "they both look fine."

(My doctor) said "I cannot believe what I am seeing. You have the tubes of a 20-year-old that has never had any problems."

I immediately called my husband and we tried not to get too excited before speaking with my doctor.

Finally, my appointment time came and my doctor walked in while looking at my chart. Without looking up at me, he said "I don't claim that medicine has all the answers, but I have to tell you, I cannot believe what I am seeing. You have the tubes of a 20-year-old that has never had any problems. There is no reason you cannot get pregnant." I will never forget that day.

Over the next few months, I began taking Chinese herbs to help regulate my hormones and improve my health.

In December of 2006, just seven months after my treatment at Clear Passage, the impossible happened — I was pregnant!

I delivered a beautiful and healthy baby boy, Riley, through C-section nine months later. As I held my little miracle baby in my arms, my husband had no words. We just looked at each other and smiled.

At Age 39, Four Years of Infertility Due to Endometriosis

- Michaeleena's Story

My name is Michaeleena. I am 39 years old and gave birth to a beautiful, healthy, and very alert little boy named Alex. I have no doubt that Clear Passage Therapies (CPT) helped my husband and me to conceive Alex, and carry him to term, but let me explain.

We had been trying to have a baby for about four years when Alex was conceived. Because we were both older (my husband had just turned 48), we knew we didn't have a lot of time to either conceive, or seriously consider adopting.

About two years into our trying, my husband and I were both tested. Everything appeared normal for me, but it appeared that my husband had very low sperm motility and morphology. He was seeing a different acupuncturist than I was when he was diagnosed. My acupuncturist, a Chinese herbologist and acupuncturist who teaches at a renowned alternative health school, convinced me that both my husband and I should go to her if we really wanted to have a baby. Our Chinese doctor said she could fix the motility but was unsure of the morphology. After about a year, he was tested again, and his motility had increased astronomically, but his morphology had not significantly improved. Consequently, when we began IUI treatments right after that, we weren't very optimistic that it would work.

After the fourth failed IUI, the doctors discovered I had developed endometriosis. In fact, my doctor told me that my left ovary and fallopian tube were covered with endometriosis.

Nevertheless, I started on IUI and Clomid treatments. After the fourth failed IUI treatment, the doctors discovered that I had developed endometriosis. In fact, my doctor told me that my left ovary and fallopian tube were covered with endometriosis; they were extremely inflexible, and blocked. During the hysterosalpingogram, the doctor said she was only able to get a few drops of the dye through my left fallopian tube, by persistent pushing and prodding. She also cauterized some endometriosis off of my uterus.

Her advice was to put me on medication to force early menopause, after which I would have a brief window in which to get pregnant. However, that was before she spoke with my fertility specialist. The specialist convinced her that I should start IVF right away because my FSH levels were pretty high and close to the unacceptable range.

My husband and I chose instead to wait a few more months and try naturally since we had often heard that right after surgery, pregnancy often occurs because the tubes have been moved around and loosened up. I did another IUI two months later — and had another failure.

A friend finally clued me into Clear Passage Therapies (CPT) in Florida. I began doing research on their treatment using manual physical therapy and was impressed and amazed by their success rate with helping infertile couples become pregnant. In addition, their methodology reflected my belief in using natural alternative methods to heal the body. After speaking to many massage therapists and physical therapists in other clinics, I decided to attend.

I attended the clinic for one week (20 hours of therapy). I really didn't feel any different after the treatment except that various tight spots on my body were looser (my left hip in particular was looser — it had become extremely tight and painful before therapy and I was sure yoga was the only thing enabling me to still have the use of it). I was doubtful that the treatment did any good. Nevertheless, the next month I decided to take Clomid "just in case"" it worked. To our great surprise and delight, I got pregnant the very first month after returning from CPT. Alex was born nine months later.

As healthcare professionals, we have always encouraged our patients to gather as much information as they can about various procedures, then follow their "gut instinct," intuition, or inner voice to choose the protocol that feels right to them. Some couples or women with infertility feel it helps if they ask themselves this question: "When this ordeal is over and I look back to see what I did, will I feel that I did my best to create a success?"

After we treat women for infertility, some decide to give themselves a few months to see if they become pregnant naturally. But the process of breaking down adhesions within the reproductive tract assists medical processes as well. Thus, while some women opt to wait for a natural pregnancy, others decide to move directly into Clomid, intrauterine insemination (IUI), or in vitro fertilization (IVF). For them, the process of manual physical therapy is a stepping stone to increase the chances for a success. In Chapter Nine, we will discuss how manual physical therapy appears to increase chances for a successful IVF transfer, evidenced by published scientific studies.

The next story is about a woman who decided to undergo therapy before in vitro fertilization. As you will read, it not only helped her to have a successful IVF transfer, but a natural pregnancy, as well.

Three Prior IUIS, One Prior IVF, and Endometriosis

- Danielle's Story

When we first heard Danielle's upbeat, southern accent, it was hard to imagine she had struggled with debilitating pain, infertility, and heartache for so many years.

Since the age of twelve, she had suffered from very painful menstrual cramps. Sometimes, her cramps were so painful that they would cause her to faint. At 21, she fainted from the pain while she was driving, and ended up in a serious automobile accident.

Danielle finally decided to have laparoscopic surgery to determine the cause of her pain. The surgeon found that she had endometriosis. He tried to remove whatever endometrial tissue he could access, but Danielle felt little relief from her pain after the procedure.

"At that point, I even considered getting a hysterectomy," Danielle told us. However, she decided to live with the pain because she wanted to experience pregnancy and parenthood one day.

Her cramps were so painful that they would cause her to faint.

When Danielle married, she was excited to finally start trying to conceive the child she had always wanted. But after a year of trying, she still wasn't pregnant. Danielle and her husband decided to consult a specialist.

After her husband was tested and his sperm rated of sufficient quality and quantity, the specialist recommended that Danielle have a hysterosalpingogram (HSG) to determine if her fallopian tubes were open and functional. When the test results showed that both tubes were clear and functional, the specialist recommended she try a hormonal drug called Clomid.

She and her husband were told they would probably have to use donor eggs if they wanted to have a successful pregnancy.

When that proved unsuccessful, Danielle and her husband decided to try an intrauterine insemination (IUI). Three IUIs later, there was still no pregnancy. "That really stunned me," Danielle said. "It was just so heartbreaking." Although her doctor could not determine why these attempts were unsuccessful, we felt it was likely that the inflammation and adhesions created by endometriosis prevented the fertilized egg from implanting onto the uterine wall.

Finally, Danielle and her husband decided to undergo in vitro fertilization (IVF). After the retrieval of her eggs, the surgeon fertilized some for immediate transfer and froze others.

"I miscarried two weeks after the IVF transfer," Danielle told us, "and I thought that was it." She and her husband were told they would probably have to use donor eggs if they wanted to have a successful pregnancy.

"When you're told that you cannot have your own children, you feel really isolated," Danielle explained. "I felt like it was somehow my fault — like I was less of a woman. Even with my husband, who is so wonderful, I still felt like he didn't understand, and that nobody understood."

My pain decreased precipitously during my menstrual cycle. In fact, I didn't even know I had started my period until I saw it!

A few months later Danielle read a magazine article that discussed our success reducing endometriosis pain and increasing fertility for some women.

She scheduled ten hours of treatment within one week. We focused on reducing tightness in her pelvis and returning normal mobility to her organs.

One month later, Danielle returned for her second 10-hour session of treatment. Because we had freed the surrounding areas, we were now able to focus on reducing adhesions and tightness in and around her reproductive tract.

She noticed the effects immediately, "My pain decreased precipitously during my menstrual cycle. In fact, I didn't even know I had started my period until I saw it!" She also experienced a significant decrease in pain during ovulation and intercourse.

Encouraged by the results of her treatment, Danielle and her husband decided to try a second IVF transfer with the frozen embryos.

However, she was cautious about getting her hopes up. "After all the disappointment I had been through," Danielle explained, "I just didn't think it was going to work." To their surprise and delight, this time the procedure was successful.

She gave birth to a baby girl nine months later. The real surprise came three months after that ... when she found she was pregnant again, naturally! "Clear Passage must have opened the floodgates!" Danielle exclaimed. She delivered a beautiful, healthy baby nine months later.

From Infertile to Miracle Mom

For many years, the only viable treatments for endometriosis-related pain, infertility, or adhesions were drugs or surgery. Now, this new non-surgical, non-pharmaceutical manual physical therapy technique has shown promising results in treating the pain and dysfunction of endometriosis, including infertility.

When a woman with endometriosis is diagnosed infertile, pharmaceutical solutions are of little use, because the most effective drugs for treating endometriosis pain and dysfunction work by shutting down the female reproductive process. Without periods, there is often decreased pain, but no pregnancy will result. Thus, until recently, the only treatment for endometriosis-related infertility was surgery.

We are actively investigating this new non-surgical, non-pharmaceutical approach to improve fertility and decrease pain in women with endometriosis. Two pilot studies we conducted on women with endometriosis were published in *Fertility and Sterility* and presented to The American Society of Reproductive Medicine (ARSM) at their national meeting in 2006[18]. While these studies showed excellent results treating endometriosis pain, and sexual dysfunction, infertility was not a focus of these studies.

Nevertheless, we see the same biomechanical process at work in endometriosis-related pain, sexual dysfunction, and infertility. Typically, the inflammation inherent in endometriosis creates an adhesive process that binds structures wherever it occurs. In doing so, glue-like adhesions form, decreasing mobility and function, and often causing pain. We and many of our referring physicians are pleased to find that a non-surgical approach to the pain and dysfunction of endometriosis is now available to decrease and detach endometrial adhesions for those who are interested in pursuing a more conservative treatment option.

Ten Years of Infertility, Four Miscarriages, One Ectopic Pregnancy, and Endometriosis

- Neveah's Story

The doctors could not determine why my first pregnancy had miscarried, why my second was ectopic, or why I continued to experience infertility for two years after the ectopic pregnancy. The nine days of spotting I experienced before my period was also a mystery to them.

I underwent several tests, including an HSG, uterine biopsy, and blood work, and everything came back normal. After seeing a reproductive endocrinologist, we were advised that our best chance of conceiving was through IVF.

We had concerns about pursuing that course, so I went back to my Ob/Gyn. He performed a laparoscopic surgery to ensure that all tissue from my ectopic pregnancy was gone and that nothing new had formed. He found moderate endometriosis and an ovarian cyst, both of which he removed. A couple of months after my surgery, I noticed that my nine days of spotting had shortened to four days, but the pain during my periods had increased dramatically. I had always experienced some discomfort in the lower back, but I never had the type of cramping in the uterus that I was experiencing. It became debilitating and no over-the-counter medication was strong enough to mitigate the cramping. I was miserable.

After searching the web for answers, I came across Clear Passage Therapies (CPT). I ordered the free DVD and materials and eagerly awaited their arrival. When they came, I read through them. I immediately got excited, but wanted to discuss it with my husband for a reality check. I respect his opinion because of his character and objectivity, but also because he has worked in scientific research and engineering. He understands the philosophies and theories that drive different treatment options.

I handed the information I had over to my husband and we watched the DVD together. The best way to describe our reaction to this therapy was to say, "It just makes sense." It seemed to work at all levels . . . scientifically, ethically, and practically. We understood that going through this therapy was not in any way a guarantee that we would have a baby, but we both thought that it would be worth doing to relieve my terrible monthly cramps. We were also very encouraged by CPT's willingness to help with our insurance issues and, as it turned out, our insurance did indeed reimburse us for the majority of the cost.

(The therapy) seemed to work at all levels... scientifically, ethically, and practically.

While my husband and I already had determined that we were going to pursue CPT, I decided to run it by my doctor out of curiosity. While he did not try to deter me from this therapy, he did not feel that I would be helped by it. Like many physicians, I suppose his skepticism was based on his concerns that he was not familiar with the treatment and results; yet I knew I had to at least give it a try.

All of my abdominal pain was gone without a trace!

My treatment went well and my last day of therapy was the first day of my period. Immediately, I felt a difference. All of my abdominal pain was gone without a trace! The therapy was totally worth doing to relieve my pain. The only symptom I still had was mild lower back pain. I started acupuncture and Traditional Chinese Medicine (herbs), which helped relieved that pain. Learning about other forms of healing had been an unexpected benefit from working with CPT. During my week of therapy, I borrowed several books and learned more about alternative and complementary treatments, diet, and how much of an impact they can have on reproductive health.

After my sessions at CPT, my pre-period spotting had been reduced to two days. Coupled with my acupuncture treatment, the spotting and mild lower back pain completely disappeared. Nowadays, during my period I feel a little bloated, but that is the extent of my problems.

Several months after my therapy, I wrote to CPT, "We thank you so much for the healing you have provided for me. Although we still very much hope to get pregnant we know that it is in God's hands and does not reflect poorly on CPT if

I do not. I consider my therapy a 100% success! Thank you so much!"

I now have to amend that statement because I am four months pregnant with what we hope will be our first-born child. After 10 years that included four miscarriages, one ectopic pregnancy, and several consecutive years of not even conceiving, this is by far the longest I have carried a child. We are so grateful for the role CPT has played in my health and that they were willing to look outside the box to help heal women.

Stage II Endometriosis and Age 40

- Victoria's Story

After several futile years of trying to find the cause of my worsening pain and discomfort, I was diagnosed with stage II endometriosis in 2001. I had a pelvic laparoscopy during which the doctor removed the endometriosis (that he could see), adhesions, an ovarian cyst, and a uterine polyp.

I couldn't tolerate the oral contraceptives and was not willing to take medications that would put me into a pseudo-menopausal state.

I was then advised to go on oral contraceptives to control the pain and growth of the endometriosis. I was relieved to know the reason for my pain and was hopeful that I would soon feel good again and be able to live my life without fearing the return of the pain.

Unfortunately, I couldn't tolerate the oral contraceptives and was not willing to take medications that would put me into a pseudo-menopausal state. The doctors offered me no other solution or treatment, so I was left to deal with my pain on my own.

A few years later, at 39, my husband and I decided we wanted to try to have children and we'd better try now or it could be too late. We tried to conceive for six months. This was not easy with the pain I always experienced around the time of ovulation.

I entered the whole process at CPT with a lot of skepticism...I had no expectations whatsoever of the treatment having any effect on my ability to conceive.

When we were unsuccessful, we sought the advice of a reproductive endocrinologist. I was 40 years old by this time and the doctors were very straightforward about the declining possibility to become pregnant or carry a baby to term at my age.

Finally, after a lot of testing, we decided on the fertility clinic we wanted to use and went through a four-week cycle of in vitro fertilization. We were excited when we came out with four embryos to transfer.

I was disappointed to find out, a couple weeks later that I was not pregnant and the IVF procedure had failed. I was feeling pretty hopeless about my body's ability to conceive and decided just to try to find a way to relieve the physical pain from the endometriosis.

While researching endometriosis on the Internet, I found the Clear Passage Therapies (CPT) website and called them. They sent me a detailed form to fill out about my history and symptoms. After completing the preliminary review to determine if I was a good candidate for therapy, I scheduled a five day intensive treatment program.

I began the blood tests for IVF and found out I was pregnant, naturally!

I entered the whole process at CPT with a lot of skepticism about their ability to help me with my pain and a lot of anxiety about whether my insurance would cover any of it. I had no expectations whatsoever of the treatment having any effect on my ability to conceive, even though many of the therapists and staff there said that "it happens."

The treatment ended up being more intense (and painful at times) than I imagined it would be, but it also was extremely cathartic — something I expected.

After I went home I somewhat reluctantly decided to try one more cycle of in vitro fertilization. I began the blood tests for IVF and found out I was pregnant, naturally! This came as a complete surprise as I had no medical assistance and became pregnant "on my own." The only thing I could attribute my "success" to was my treatment at CPT. Despite my reluctance to believe it, it was the only variable in the equation. It had happened just like the therapists at CPT told me it "could."

Now, three years later, I have a lovely two year old daughter who has brought so much happiness to my husband and I and everyone in our family.

Suspected Endometriosis, but Hesitant to Undergo Laparoscopy

- Jasmine's Story

"I suspect you might have endometriosis," my doctor told me. For years I had experienced lower abdominal pain, cramping, and painful intercourse. I was relieved to know there was a cause for my pain, but also dismayed to learn that the only way to diagnose endometriosis was through laparoscopic surgery. My doctor informed me that endometriosis was a leading cause of infertility and that surgery could improve my chances for a successful pregnancy.

I researched online and learned that some patients were in more pain after surgery. Furthermore, my doctor wanted me to be on birth control after the surgery to prevent the re-growth of endometrial tissue. My husband and I were trying to get pregnant at the time, so I knew that option wouldn't work for us.

While researching about endometriosis, I read about Clear Passage Therapies (CPT). I learned they could help reduce the pain associated with endometriosis and prepare my body for a successful pregnancy. I asked my doctor and he said I should go ahead and try it if I wasn't comfortable with surgery.

> ***I researched and learned that some patients were in more pain after surgery.***

I scheduled an intensive week of treatment. My primary goal was to become pregnant and one week after treatment —

I was! My pregnancy went very well and I was also blessed to no longer experience painful intercourse or lower abdominal pain.

I am so thankful for the people at CPT. The therapists were wonderful and I will always remember the last day of treatment. As my husband and I drove off, she was sitting by the window and waving, just like an angel. And she was our angel who gave us hope, and the opportunity to conceive a baby.

My primary goal was to become pregnant and one week after treatment – I was!

As I look at my beautiful baby now, I am happy I took the initiative to research and find a treatment that was healthier and safer for my body. CPT was a true blessing for us.

Chapter Eight

Hormones and Fertility

We never imagined that we would be able to help women with hormonal conditions, such as PCOS or high FSH. Once again, it was our patients who spurred our inquiry in this area, when they kept calling us and reporting unexpected positive results after our treatment. After hearing reports of so many dramatic turnarounds in our patients, we realized that we had to investigate this phenomenon.

- Belinda Wurn

1997 - "There is no reason to believe that we can assist hormonal conditions with this therapy." - **Richard King, MD**

2000 – Patient One Chart Review: "This patient was diagnosed menopausal; she was refused IVF three times due to very high FSH, but had two natural full-term pregnancies after therapy."

Her reproductive endocrinologist told her she was "out of options."

2001 – Patient Two Chart Review: "This patient says she did not have a period for a year; then after therapy, she started ovulating again."

2003 – Patient Three Chart Review: "This patient reports she went six months or more without a period. Oral and injected hormones, several IUIs and three IVFs all failed to bring her dream child. After therapy, she had a full-term pregnancy without drugs or surgery."

2004 - "I may have been wrong about therapy not improving hormones; let's investigate this." - **Richard King, MD**

As we age, fertility declines; it's as simple as that. Medical literature is replete with references that indicate that a woman's 35th birthday marks the decline of her fertility as she moves toward menopause. However, the age of this "marker" can vary from woman to woman.

This statistic is especially daunting to highly motivated career women. Having completed college and often postgraduate degrees, these overachieving women enter the work force hoping to create a career and independent lifestyle for themselves. Whether married or not, they are proud to have rolled up their sleeves and set to work to create a professional self-sufficient way of life. All of this takes a tremendous amount of time and dedicated effort. Thus, by the time they are ready to think about a family, ten to fifteen years have passed since they left college.

When they have difficulty conceiving and consult their gynecologists, they are dismayed to find that their prime reproductive years have already passed them by. It is a cruel and unfair twist of fate, but it is also statistically accurate. Thus, any way a physician or a physical therapist can help turn back the clock for these women is a huge advantage, allowing them to look forward to functional reproductive years and to the family that they have worked so hard to create.

Measuring the Biological Clock

Reproductive endocrinologists and other infertility specialists have created specific criteria to measure declining reproductive ability as women age. There are several methods, but perhaps the most commonly accepted measure of age-related decline in fertility is to determine the level of FSH (follicle stimulating hormone) in the blood, early in the menstrual cycle.

As a woman ages, her eggs have a more difficult time maturing. Thus, the pituitary gland must create more and more FSH to stimulate follicle growth with each passing year. When physicians note this increase in FSH levels, they have a good indication that fertility is declining, and a measurement to quantify that decline.

In order to get reliable results, testing for FSH levels should be done on the second or third day of the menstrual cycle. Many physicians believe that a one-time increase in FSH levels above 10 IU/L (international units per liter) indicates that the woman will likely no longer be able to conceive her own child. Others feel that if FSH can be brought back down to below 10 (or sometimes 12), there remains an opportunity for conception to occur naturally, or by in vitro fertilization. To assist the reproductive process for women 35 or older, some physicians will administer FSH to help eggs mature.

Many physicians now acknowledge the importance of checking estradiol in addition to FSH levels, because a high estradiol level can suppress FSH, making the FSH level appear lower than it really is.

A procedure known as the Clomiphene Challenge Test enables a physician to check both FSH and estradiol levels. After obtaining blood tests on the third day for both hormones, women are instructed to take clomiphene on days five to nine of the menstrual cycle. Then, physicians check FSH levels again on day ten. Ideally, a Clomiphene Challenge Test would show a low FSH level on day three, a low estradiol level on day three, and a low FSH level on day ten.

FSH levels are a primary test for a woman's ability to conceive and carry a birth to term naturally, and by IVF if she plans to use her own eggs. Women with high FSH levels may be encouraged to adopt, or to use eggs from another woman (called donor eggs). If the body's endocrine system could be adjusted to turn back time and proper FSH levels could be restored, a woman would presumably have a better chance for a full-term pregnancy, whether naturally or through assisted reproductive techniques.

The Diagnosis of "Infertile Due to High FSH"

Early on, we were approached by women whose physicians had diagnosed them with hormonal problems, such as decreased ovarian reserve, advanced reproductive age, "old eggs" (a commonly used but insensitive phrase), or high FSH. These diagnoses generally indicate a hormonal condition in which the body is unable to produce eggs that will mature and grow.

Many of these women were in their mid-to-upper-30s or 40s, and frustrated that their fertile years were slipping away month by month. Our hearts went out to these women, and naturally we wanted to help if we could, but the idea of helping hormonal infertility seemed far-fetched.

While we had good evidence that we could improve "mechanical" issues, such as scarring, adhesions, pain and blocked fallopian tubes, there was little reason to believe that we could help "medical or hormonal" infertility which has always been considered to be in a totally different arena from mechanical problems.

When we consulted our gynecologist medical advisor, he discouraged us. "I can see where you can help the biomechanics of reproduction," Dr. King said. "It makes sense that you are able to decrease adhesions, help implantation, and help sperm meet egg. We have seen the evidence and met the children," he said. "But there is mechanical infertility and there is hormonal infertility. We just don't have any evidence to show that you can help that condition, and I don't think that you can."

Thus, not wanting to waste our patients' time or money, we routinely turned down women whose infertility was caused solely by a hormonal condition.

Advanced Age and "Old Eggs"

The diagnosis of "advanced age" and "old eggs" seemed somehow counterintuitive to us, once we actually met some of these applicants for therapy. Here were women who appeared to be in the prime of their lives, yet they were receiving diagnoses that made them seem like matrons. With the rest of their bodies so youthful, it was curious to us that they were diagnosed infertile due to advanced reproductive age. These feelings were strengthened in many cases when we heard from them that their mother, aunt or grandmother bore children well into their 40s.

While we had witnessed several dramatic successes with cases of mechanical infertility, we were not reproductive specialists. So we turned to the experts, and followed the established assumptions. In short, we continued to discourage women with these "age-related" diagnoses from attending therapy. Perhaps we should have been listening better to our intuitions.

Breaking the Biological Clock

One day a patient with severe hormonal dysfunction, and adhesions, came to see us for therapy. Her case forever changed our minds about our ability to help hormonal conditions.

Menopausal Hormone Levels (FSH of 28)

- Lisa's Story

After years of struggling with infertility, unsuccessful surgeries, and hormonal treatments, Lisa turned to her last option — in vitro fertilization.

She started the cycle of fertility drugs that would prompt her ovaries to release multiple eggs. However, her IVF cycle was canceled when she didn't produce any eggs. She was in shock and immediately returned to do the necessary blood work for a second IVF cycle.

The results showed that, at 19, her FSH level was much too high to undergo IVF. Her RE's cut-off point was 10, and Lisa was far beyond that number. Unwilling to accept "no" as an answer, Lisa waited a little while, then returned to test her FSH again. This time, the number had jumped to 28 — indicating she had become menopausal. Her reproductive endocrinologist told her she was "out of options" to carry her own biologic child; the only thing he could suggest was egg donation or adoption.

That was when Lisa hit rock bottom. IVF had always been her safety net — a choice she could turn to when nothing else worked. Lisa felt devastated and isolated from her friends, who were already celebrating the baptisms and birthdays of their children.

She told us that this constant sadness propelled her to search for other solutions. She kept looking at Internet bulletin boards and reading everything she could. She learned that acupuncture and herbs could help FSH. She started going to the acupuncturist once a week, and she drank a special herb tea twice a day.

She continued to research on the Internet and happened to stumble upon our website. Lisa became intrigued when she learned our treatment had been successful in relieving endometriosis and intercourse pain, two conditions she suffered in addition to infertility.

Constant sadness propelled her search for other solutions.

Lisa decided to complete the 20-hour treatment program in one week. At the time we did not treat patients with strictly hormone related infertility, and thus we told Lisa that we likely could not help that aspect of her infertility. We felt we could help her with her pain, however. Thus, we treated her as an endometriosis pain patient.

Lisa had been diagnosed with stage IV endometriosis during laparoscopic surgery, and when we palpated her pelvis, we felt she had developed adhesions throughout her reproductive tract. We felt with our hands for adhered areas and worked hour upon hour to free her organs from their adhesive straight-jackets.

By the end of treatment, Lisa was thrilled to find that intercourse no longer hurt. We had become used to seeing this positive result in patients who came to us with complaints of intercourse pain, but for Lisa, pain had been so severe that she was almost shocked to have pain-free sex after just a week of therapy. (See Chapter Seventeen for more information on endometriosis pain and Chapter Twelve for more information on sexual intercourse pain.)

These results made Lisa and her husband optimistic that the treatment might help her to become pregnant. A month after treatment, Lisa was disappointed when her period came. However, the next month, her hopes rose when her period was late. She rushed to the doctor's office for a blood test, which confirmed she was pregnant naturally. After all of her problems, the pain, the endometriosis and the failed medical treatments, Lisa and her husband were joyful but cautious. They called us to tell us the good news.

Lisa gave birth to her baby daughter in April 2003 and our hopes of helping other women like her were reinforced. Little did we know, our work would have lasting effects – Lisa had a subsequent natural pregnancy two years later and gave birth again, in 2005!

Frankly, we and Lisa's reproductive endocrinologist were stunned by her natural pregnancy. We were wondering if (and really assumed that) her pregnancy was a total fluke. But when Lisa had a second natural pregnancy and childbirth two years after her first "miracle baby," it really piqued our interest. Our hopes of helping other women like her were cautiously optimistic, and we decided to accept other women with high FSH levels. We told them that we had no scientific proof we could help high FSH, but we also shared Lisa's story with them. Several of these women chose to attend therapy. In all cases, we requested they test their hormone levels both before and after therapy.

We set to work to conduct clinical trials for these women, for whom no other option existed for a natural child of their own. We cautioned each of them again that we had no published science on possibly improving pregnancy rates for women diagnosed with hormone-related infertility, but also advised that we had seen some encouraging results.

Our initial study design to test and measure our chances for improving fertility in women with high FSH was very straightforward. Women with high FSH would be asked to have their FSH levels tested before therapy. Then after therapy, we would send them back for a re-test.

In essence, while we were following a basic scientific protocol, we realized that there would be holes in our data. In a full study (which we plan to conduct, based on results of this simple pilot study), we would have each woman attend the same laboratory for pre- and post-therapy tests.

But at this point, we just wanted to get a sense if we should look further into the question of whether or not we might improve fertility or hormone levels in women who came to us diagnosed infertile due to high FSH. While we were hopeful, we were neither optimistic nor pessimistic. How could we be either? We had no data, except one remarkable case.

Still, we remembered how our first surprise case of opening blocked fallopian tubes led to a remarkable discovery and two pioneering published studies to date. Thus, we felt it was necessary to ask the question, test the women, and let the data tell us whether there was reason to pursue this inquiry further.

We called our biostatistician, a Ph.D. professor of biostatistics at a respected medical school, to ask how many women we needed to test in order to get a good sense of whether or not we were helping them. This scholar-scientist had published over 200 studies in peer-reviewed journals. At the time we consulted him, he directed over $10 million in funded studies for the US National Institutes of Health (NIH).

He said, "It really depends on what kind of results you are seeing, along and along. The better the results, the less people you would have to test. I suggest you start with eight participants. That should give us a good start. We'll check your results then, and make a decision of whether you need more, or if it is even reasonable to continue."

We set up our protocol to check FSH levels "before and after" therapy on the first eight women who chose to attend therapy with us, and who reported an FSH level above 10 — which seemed to be the cutoff point for a reasonable opportunity to achieve pregnancy, as determined by reproductive endocrinologists across the country. We assigned a team to the task of gathering data on any women who attended therapy with FSH levels above 10.

As it happened, we got busy and by the time we got around to checking, we had 16 subjects for this "FSH pilot study." Since this was double the number our biostatistician suggested, we knew that the results would be highly indicative of our ability (or inability) to help these women. As we do with all of our studies, we included all women who qualified, which is the proper and most conservative way to gather scientific data.

When we compiled the data from these women, we were shocked to find that the results were not just promising — they were nothing short of astounding! Here's what we found:

My hormone level of FSH was 26.2, indicating that my body wasn't producing quality eggs. In fact, I was officially diagnosed as menopausal.

– Jen, former CPT patient, naturally pregnant one month after treatment

Of the 16 participants in the study, the average pre-therapy FSH level was 20.4 (low of 10.7, high of 37.6). While we were hoping to get pre- and post-therapy FSH levels on all of the women, six became pregnant naturally right after therapy, so we never got a chance to check their post-therapy FSH levels. Our physician advisor said that since they conceived naturally, we could assume that their hormone levels improved. In a population of women who should not be able to conceive with an FSH level above 10, the pre-therapy FSH levels for the women who became pregnant naturally after we treated them were: 11.3, 13.6, 18.0, 23.1, 28.0, and 33.1.

That left only 10 women whose FSH levels we could tabulate. Of these, FSH levels declined in 9 of them, in many cases precipitously. In one case, FSH levels climbed — one point. There were some dramatic turnarounds that don't show on the chart; for example, one woman with pre-therapy scores of 37.2 became pregnant through IVF after therapy. The woman who had an FSH of 37.6 before therapy reported that her FSH decreased to 21.7 after therapy. One woman who had a pre-therapy FSH of 28 has now had two natural pregnancies and births since therapy.

Age is another consideration for women who are concerned about hormone levels, and the age of women in this pilot study averaged 39.3 years at the time of their therapy. The oldest woman to become pregnant naturally in our pilot study was 44.9 (45) years old when she completed her therapy. Her pre-therapy FSH level was 33.1.

One woman aged 42.3 (42) had a natural full-term pregnancy after therapy (which also opened her fallopian tubes). Another woman aged 41.8 (42) had two natural pregnancies after therapy. Although she miscarried the first, she was 8-weeks pregnant with her second natural post-therapy pregnancy the last time we spoke with her. The oldest woman in the study was 45.8 when she completed her therapy. We opened her blocked fallopian tube and her FSH decreased from 18 to 13.2. We were testing for FSH levels, not pregnancy, and we were surprised to have so many unexpected pregnancies so quickly. We do not have pregnancy data on most of the other women in the study whose FSH improved.

In total, 15 of the 16 women in our FSH/hormonal pilot study had improvements, many of them quite significant. The full results of this pilot study are shown in the table on the next page.

We hope to conduct a two-year post-therapy follow-up with all of the women, but as we saw, the data was both surprising and telling. Thus, we now encourage women with high FSH to consider attending therapy.

FSH Pilot Study - Detailed Results

Patient Number	Age at Therapy	FSH Before Therapy	FSH After Therapy	Change After Therapy
1	41.8	18.0	Two natural pregnancies	
2	34.8	28.0	Two natural full-term pregnancies	
3	39.7	12.5	8.1	4.4
4	45.8	18.0	13.2	4.8
5	39.9	14.0	9.5	4.5
6	39.2	15.6	6.0	9.6
7	39.4	10.7	5.3	5.4
8	39.8	15.0	16.0	-1.0
9	42.3	13.6	Natural full-term pregnancy	
10	31.3	37.2	18.0	19.2
11	37.7	27.1	14.4	12.7
12	29.9	37.6	21.7	15.9
13	39.6	12.0	4.1	7.9
14	41.4	23.1	Natural pregnancy	
15	42.0	11.3	Natural pregnancy	
16	44.9	33.1	Natural pregnancy	
Average	39.3	20.4	11.6	8.3

Three years after Lisa's case, it became clear to us that a high FSH test reading signified merely a "snapshot in time" for these women. Their doctors' warnings of "premature ovarian failure" ended up being inaccurate for Lisa – and ultimately for a number of other women we were treating.

Because our work had been shown to improve the function of blocked fallopian tubes (which are significantly smaller than ovaries), we wondered if the same process of freeing adhesions might be improving the function of the neighboring ovaries. In other words, is there a mechanical process involved in the hormonal changes that we see in the body as we age? Simple logic appears to say "yes." The rest of the body demonstrates aging in mechanical ways over time. Thus, why wouldn't the same be true for the endocrine glands, and the communication processes among them?

Truth be told, we do not know exactly how we were helping in this instance – whether we were increasing blood flow, nerve conduction, improving the ovary's motility (the natural movement inherent within any organ), or reducing the biomechanical stressors on the pituitary and hypothalamus, which we discuss more extensively later in this chapter. We can only surmise, but this preliminary clinical study shows that something positive happened for nearly every one of these subjects. Furthermore, the mechanism of the improvement may be different for each woman, depending on her specific pathology. We may never know the answer to why this manual physical therapy was so successful in treating so many cases of high FSH, but we are inspired to continue this investigation.

A New Key to Treating Hormonal Infertility

We speculate that one reason our treatment was successful for these women was that (as well as treating the ovaries) we felt it incumbent on us to address and treat any adhesive processes that might affect the dura and fascia which surround the spinal cord and brain. These are very important structures in life, and in reproduction, so it is important to understand a bit of their location, and the areas they affect.

The dura starts at the tailbone (coccyx), then surrounds the spinal cord to the base of the skull. It has strong attachments at the sacrum, the vertebrae at the top of the neck, and at the base of the skull.

The dura and its fascias then enter the cranium via a large opening in the base of the skull. From there, they rise into the cranial cavity and surround the entire brain and all of its structures.

A strong collagenous sheath of the dura (the falx cerebri) divides the left and right brain; a paired sheath (the tentorium cerebelli) divides from it and creates the floor of the brain at the level of the eyes and ears. Strong collagenous fascias spread like a tree, to surround and separate literally every structure within the brain – including the hypothalamus and the pituitary, which is considered the master gland of female reproduction.

There is a recognized feedback communication loop between the ovaries and the pituitary-hypothalamus region of the brain. The positive responses in 15 of the first 16 women we tested and treated with high FSH indicated to us that a large part of this feedback loop is mechanical in nature, and subject to the same improvements we observed when we treated adhered tissues in other parts of the body.

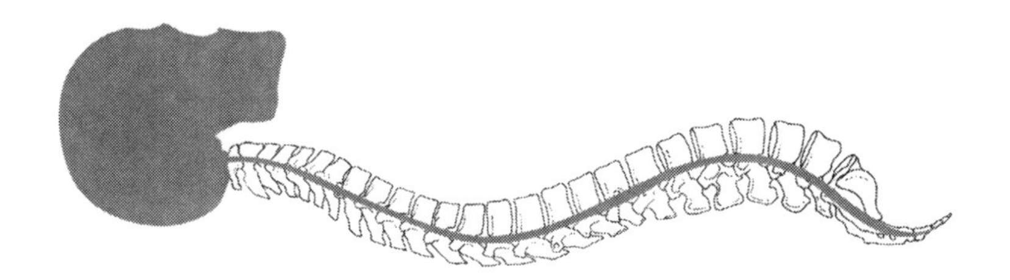

Keys to good communication between ovaries and pituitary may include structural elements such as fascia that surrounds those structures, and the dura which covers the spinal cord and brain.

The hypothalamus, which closely neighbors the pituitary gland, constantly monitors female hormone levels in the bloodstream through its sensory receptors. It responds to the information it receives by regulating the release of "messenger hormones," such as Gonadotropin Release Hormones (GnRH), to the pituitary gland.

In response to the "messenger hormones," the pituitary gland determines the exact amount of hormones that it will then release to stimulate the ovaries. These hormones, or gonadotropins, are called follicle stimulating hormones (FSH) and luteinizing hormones (LH).

The hypothalamus closes the feedback circle by measuring the level of hormones produced by the ovaries while at the same time monitoring the release of LH and FSH by the pituitary gland. This "push-pull" interplay of messages and responses produces the cyclical hormonal environment in women that is designed to promote a successful pregnancy.

In short, there must be good communication among all of these structures in order for reproduction to take place, and (especially) in order for a new follicle to mature during the first phase of the menstrual cycle. If one or more of these structures is restricted by adhesions or other biomechanical forces, it will not be able to perform its function properly or with full efficiency.

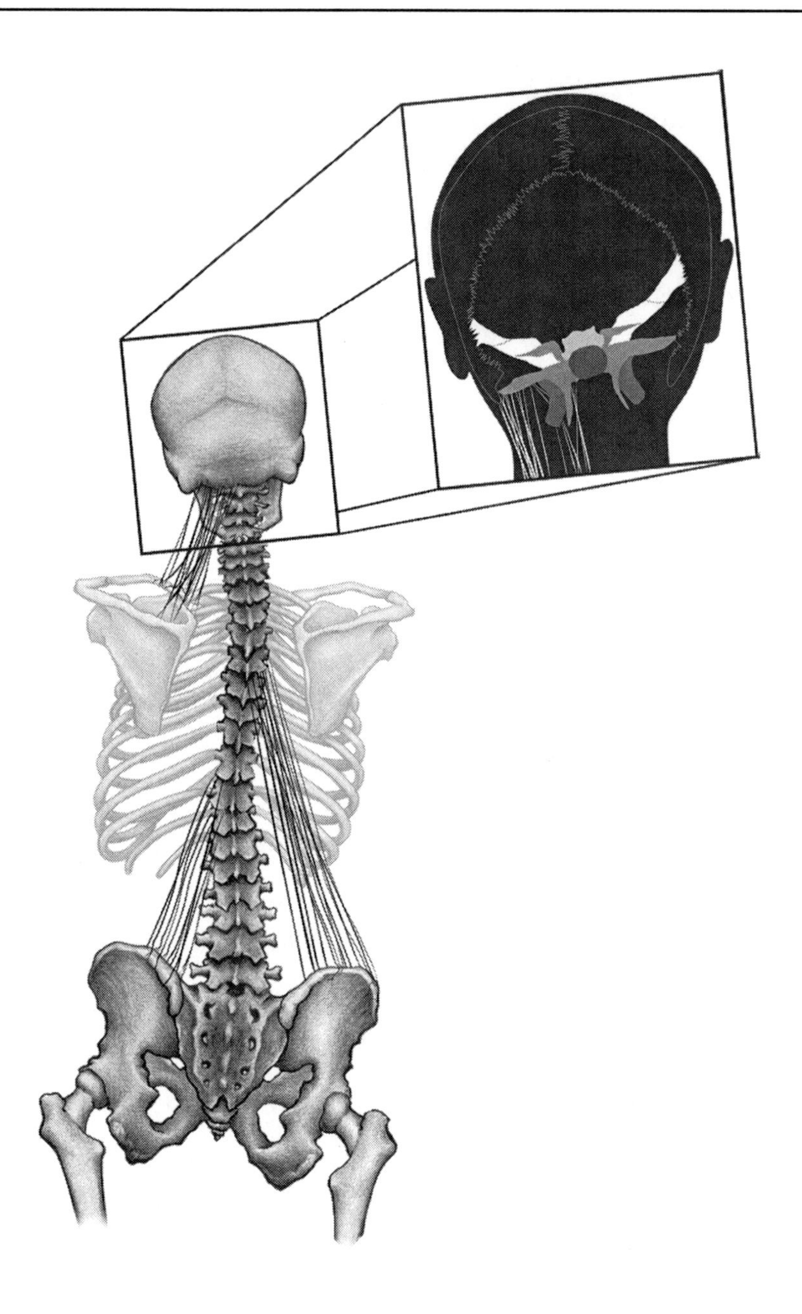

Cranial bones may be pulled out of alignment due to adhesions or spasm further down the body.

Fascia surrounds the brain, and all the structures in the cranium; these include the pituitary gland, the hypothalamus, and attachments to the 28 bones of the cranium.

During life, the fascia in our bodies is constantly being pulled down toward our feet by gravity. In addition, trauma and compensatory adhesions in the upper back, neck, and chest create a pull at the fascial attachments of the dura, which surround the spinal cord at the base of the skull. From there, this highly structural fascial sweater climbs into the cranium where it surrounds the pituitary gland — and virtually every other structure in the brain! (See Chapter Two for more on the structure of fascia.)

Because of our unexpected positive results treating women with high FSH, we began examining the anatomy and biomechanics of the pituitary and its surrounding fascia. Our investigation brought to light a few important discoveries. Most of our women with high FSH had one or more of the following mechanical anomalies or asymmetries:

1) One of their mastoids (the bony protuberance below the ear) was notably lower than the other side,

2) One of their zygomatic arches (the bone at the front of the cheek, on their face) was lower than the other side,

3) They had tightness, tenderness or jamming at the cranial base (the place where the back of the skull meets the top of the neck),

4) Their tailbone was pushed forward, or to one side, or

5) Some cranial bones appeared totally immobile, and adhered to their neighbor. (While cranial bones do not 'move' in the sense of other joints, they do not become totally fixed until very late in life, if at all.)

The first three of these all related to the direct pull of cranial fascias on the pituitary and hypothalamus gland. When these bones were out of their relaxed, midline alignment, the sphenoid bone that contains the pituitary gland will be pulled out of alignment as well. Consequently, we surmised that the tiny and delicate pituitary gland was subject to being compressed or otherwise restricted by the (relatively) large sphenoid bone which surrounds it.

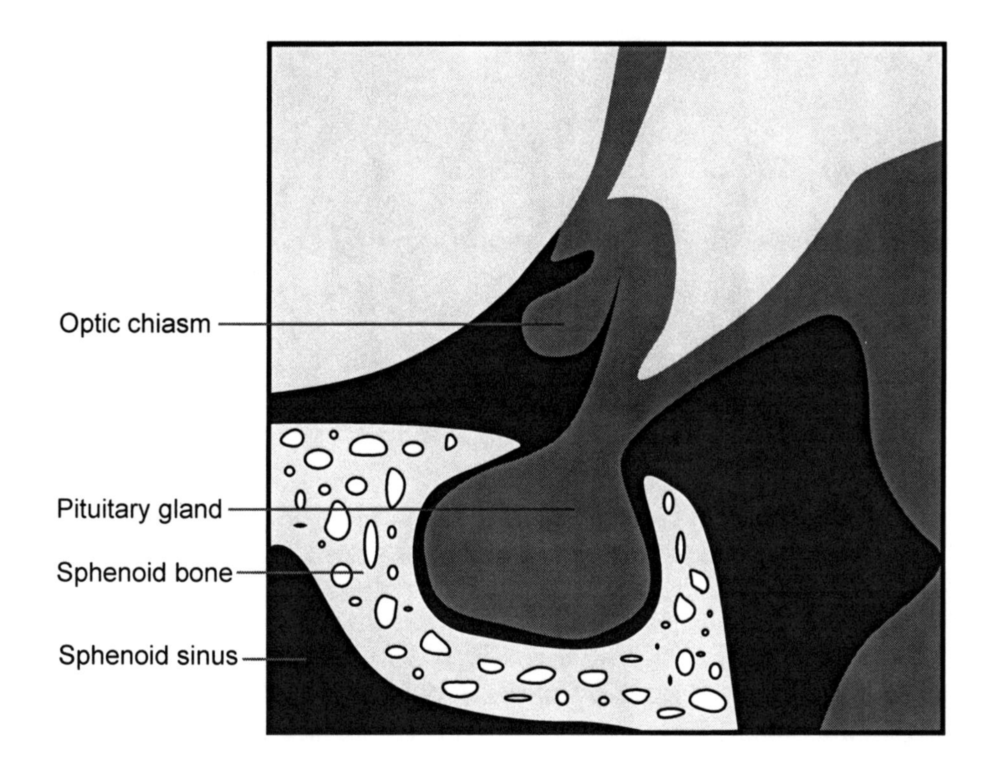

In its normal state, the pituitary can function with normal mobility

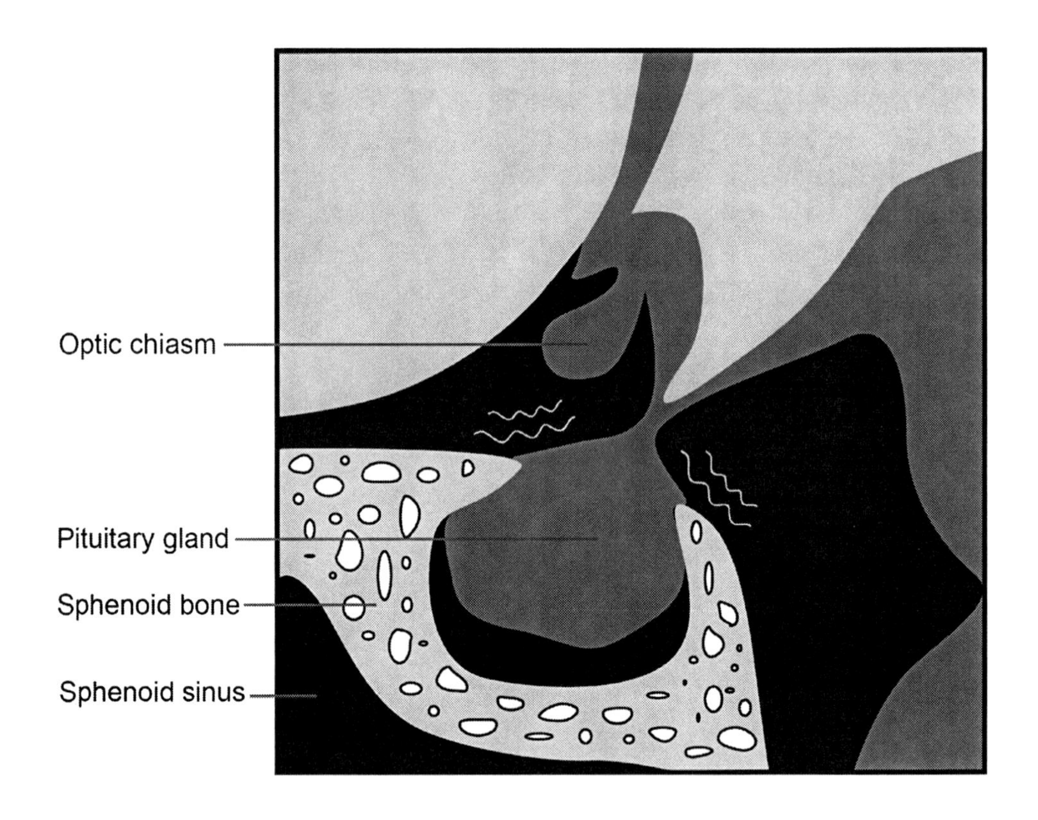

We speculate that a poorly aligned sphenoid can pull on the pituitary gland, restricting its mobility and decreasing its function

In the fourth case (coccyx pulled forward or to one side), we wondered if the forward position of the coccyx was pulling down on the dura – that strong fascial sheath that totally surrounds the spinal cord, brain, and pituitary gland. If that were true, might it be that pulling that coccyx back and restoring its normal mobility would relieve the pressures all the way up the dura and into the brain?

Certainly, we knew we would do no harm by treating either of these areas, both of which we had treated for many years in patients with headaches (for the cranial area) or with constipation, tailbone, or intercourse pain. Thus we treated these areas in women with high FSH, along with other adhered areas that were pulling on structures that could affect hormones (ovaries and neighboring structures).

The results of treating adhered tissues affecting all of these structures are shown in the table earlier in this chapter. By treating these and other adhered structures throughout the body, we found we were able to improve the function of the entire system, including structures with fascial attachments deep within the brain. As we found in our clinical review of women with high FSH, we witnessed some remarkable improvements when we expanded treatment into these areas for women diagnosed with premature ovarian failure, "old eggs," and high FSH.

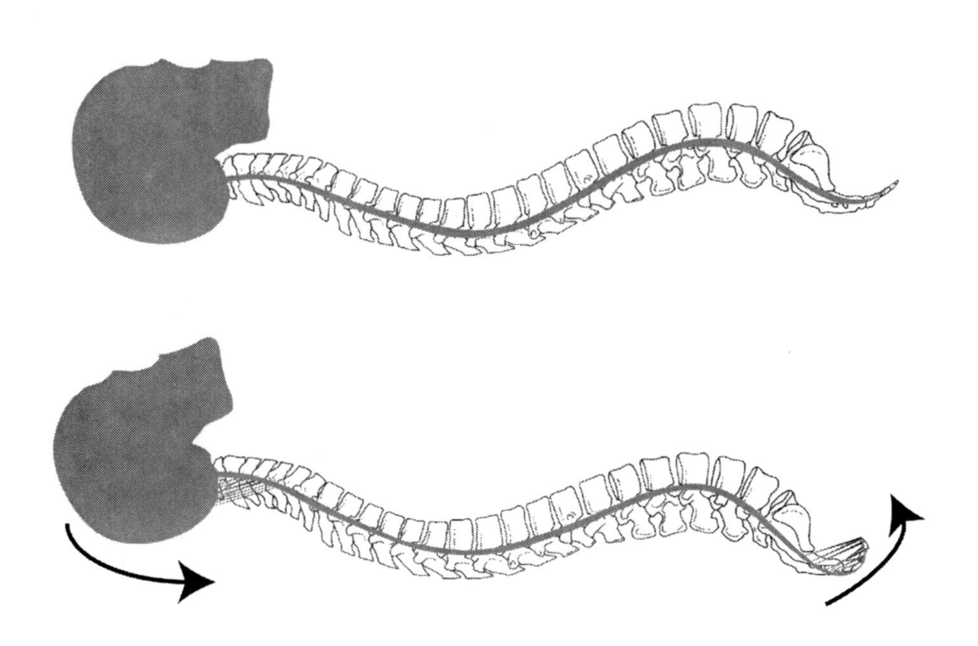

When the tailbone is pushed forward after a fall, it can pull down the fascias that surround the spinal cord and brain, causing dysfunction

Two Prior Miscarriages and Hormonally Infertile

- Paty's Story

When Paty came to us for treatment, she had struggled with hormonal infertility for four years. "At first, I didn't realize I had these problems," she told us. "I became pregnant with no problem four years ago." But then she miscarried and her doctors could not find the cause.

When Paty and her husband tried again, she again became pregnant easily. "But then I miscarried again," she said. Her doctor felt she should consult a reproductive endocrinologist, which she did. The specialist immediately tested her hormone levels.

"They found I had serious hormone problems," Paty told us. "They told me I could never carry a baby to a full-term birth unless I underwent hormone therapy."

They told me I could never carry a baby to full-term birth unless I underwent hormone therapy.

Paty immediately changed her eating habits. She added more natural foods to her diet and began researching for other natural ways to improve her infertility. Her research led her to our website, where she learned about the physical therapy protocols we had developed to treat infertility.

"I was skeptical at first," Paty told us. "But the more I learned about it, the more I felt that the treatment could help improve my hormones — and hopefully prevent another miscarriage." She decided to attend an intensive week of treatment.

Because we knew Paty's hormones were one of the key factors preventing pregnancy, we first examined the structures along her hypothalamus-pituitary-ovarian axis. This included her pelvis, spine, neck, and cranial bones. Using our hands and feedback from Paty, we found several areas of tightness along that route. Then we gently broke down the adhesions that were restricting those areas. Before treatment, Paty had experienced low back and neck pain. After we treated those areas, she found that her pain was gone.

We then focused on the soft tissues of her reproductive organs to help restore proper mobility and motility (the inner inherent movement of all organs). We paid special attention to her uterus to address any micro-adhesions (tiny strands of collagen that can change the uterine surface, prevent successful implantation of an embryo, and restrict the mobility of uterine ligaments). We also addressed any restricted mobility in the ligamentous support structures of her uterus.

"Treatment was very nice," Paty reported. "As well as the physical changes, it also helped me calm my mind and emotions. The therapists ensured that both my body and mind were ready for pregnancy."

One week after her treatment, Paty became pregnant naturally. Although she was excited, Paty knew she had to be cautious with her hopes.

After the first trimester passed with no complications, Paty breathed a sigh of relief. "The rest of my pregnancy went

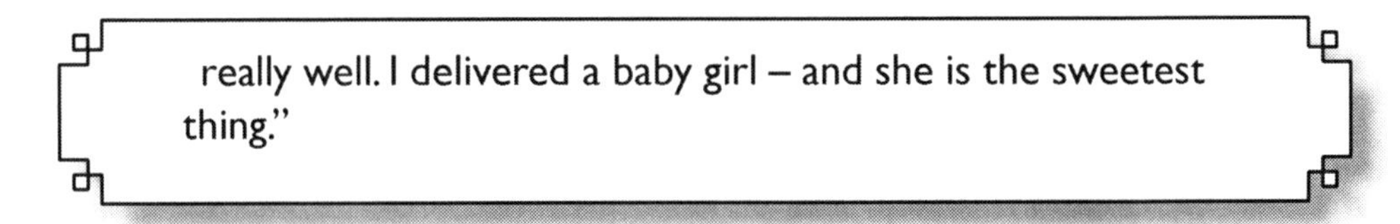

really well. I delivered a baby girl – and she is the sweetest thing."

Restoring Fertility

We became so fascinated with all of these women's hormonal success stories that we decided to "open the gates" and encourage women with high FSH, advanced age and decreased ovarian reserve to attend therapy. Always conservative on our patients' behalf, we told them all that we had not yet published scientific results on this aspect of therapy. Still, we were encouraged and excited with our results to date.

As noted earlier in this chapter, 15 of the 16 women who tested with high FSH showed improvement after therapy. Said another way, 94% of the women in this early study showed improved FSH levels, or became pregnant naturally before we had a chance to conduct their post-therapy test. These results were particularly interesting to us and to our physician advisors because before this clinical study, hormonal infertility was thought to be treatable only with pharmaceuticals, such as hormone injections.

As one researcher at a local medical school, a gynecology nurse-researcher with two decades of experience, told us, "This is really remarkable; in medicine the best we can do is to give injections or medications to improve hormone levels. Here you have apparently improved hormone levels in the blood with

The infertility specialist told me that the grade of my eggs was low because of my age, and encouraged me to pursue donor eggs.

– Nicole, former CPT patient, became naturally pregnant and delivered a healthy baby girl after treatment

a non-surgical, non-pharmaceutical physical manipulation. It really stretches the bounds of our present understanding of the cause of hormonal conditions. We always thought that hormone levels were strictly ruled by endocrine function. With your clinical trials and several pregnancies, it appears that there may be a strong mechanical aspect to hormone levels as well."

Unable to Ovulate

- Sophia's Story

My husband and I started trying to conceive a child in January 2003. After several years of being on birth control, my cycles were not returning. I spoke with my doctor and after being tested, he told me there was nothing "wrong" with me or my husband that should have prevented conception.

We then tried Clomid for three months and that did not work. My doctor was unable to determine why I was not ovulating and wanted to put me on experimental medication. We were dissatisfied with this diagnosis and did not want to pursue this type of treatment.

Around that time, I learned of Clear Passage Therapies (CPT) through a friend who had heard of them on the Internet. Their treatment appealed to me because it was natural.

In fall 2003 I went for treatment at CPT. It was soothing and uplifting and I felt very good about the process.

After the first month of beginning treatment, I ovulated and conceived, but unfortunately suffered a very early miscarriage.

The next month, I returned to CPT to complete my treatment. Again, I felt very positive about the treatment. The therapists listened to me and provided very positive assurances. That month, I ovulated and conceived. I delivered my son in August 2004. I nursed my son for 13 months and did not have a period during that time. After stopping breastfeeding, I immediately got pregnant again. I lost that baby but got pregnant a couple of months later and had a little girl in October 2006.

I definitely attribute the treatment to the return of my ovulation.

History repeated itself when I nursed my daughter for 13 months and did not have a period during that time. After stopping breastfeeding, I immediately got pregnant (again). I miscarried but then got pregnant a couple of months later and am due in one month with my third child.

I definitely attribute the treatment at CPT to the return of my ovulation and putting me in a positive frame of mind which ultimately enabled conception. I highly recommend CPT to those experiencing any infertility issues. The atmosphere, hands-on therapy, and natural healing of CPT are a great benefit to many women trying to conceive. It certainly helped me!

High FSH and Secondary Infertility

- Jocelyn's Story

"My FSH is 14.2," Jocelyn told us. "Do you think you can help?"

Four years earlier, Jocelyn had become pregnant and given birth without any problems. But when she and her husband wanted to conceive again, it didn't happen as quickly as before.

Jocelyn told us, "I wasn't fully aware it was a problem until a year went by. That was about the time I had my yearly visit with the Ob/Gyn, so I asked her what she thought." Her doctor performed a battery of tests and found Jocelyn had high FSH.

"She immediately referred me to a reproductive endocrinologist," Jocelyn explained. Her RE completed more tests and confirmed that she had high FSH. He recommended IVF or hormonal shots to try to lower her FSH.

"I'm a naturalist," Jocelyn told us. "I wasn't excited with his options. I didn't want to take any form of drugs for the purpose of getting pregnant."

She then researched on the Internet to find natural treatment forms. Jocelyn explained, "I knew I could very easily get stressed and emotional about my infertility, but I refused to let myself go there. I didn't let my infertility become me. I saw this as an opportunity to make myself better — to really get my mind and body in a healthy state."

During her research, Jocelyn found the Clear Passage Therapies (CPT) website. "I was totally blown away," she told us. "I couldn't believe the clinic was only an hour from my home."

Jocelyn asked her RE what he thought of CPT, and she was dismayed to hear him sternly recommend she not waste her time or money because there was "no published evidence yet to support that the treatment could lower FSH."

Jocelyn scheduled a consultation with our head therapist to discuss treatment further. Our therapist explained how treatment generally works and the philosophy of how we believed it may be helpful in improving hormone levels. Admittedly, we had no clinical studies addressing FSH yet, but we shared with her the numerous cases of patients who had come to our clinic and experienced success despite a diagnosis of high FSH.

"My husband and I decided it was the right treatment for us," Jocelyn said.

All of my aches and pains are gone. I feel much more flexible and better overall.

When she came for treatment, her therapists noted different areas of stiffness in her body and evaluated areas where she felt pain. They worked to release the tension in those areas and restore mobility to her pituitary-hypothalamus-ovarian feedback loop.

After treatment, Jocelyn told us, "All of my aches and pains are gone. I feel much more flexible and better overall. People tell me I look younger, but it's hard to tell if it will help my fertility."

Jocelyn didn't have to wait long. She became pregnant just one week after she returned home.

Jocelyn is now four months into her pregnancy. "It's pretty exciting," she tells us. "The ultrasound shows a big, healthy baby."

42 and Denied IVF Due to Hormonal Factors

- Chloe's Story

I met my husband at a sailing club in downtown Manhattan in July of 2000. I was 39 years old. We got engaged when I was 42 and since we both wanted to have a child, we didn't waste any time.

I had taken an HSG dye test at an earlier age and the test had indicated that both of my fallopian tubes were totally blocked. At that time, the doctor thought that it might be due to just mucus so I was eager to find out if the HSG would be successful this time around.

Despite the technician's attempt to force the dye through my tubes, they both remained completely occluded. My fertility specialist felt that surgery to unblock the tubes would be fruitless.

I did not get too discouraged, thinking that I could always do IVF. But I was wrong. My hormone levels were too high to be accepted into the program.

Eventually I stumbled across Clear Passage Therapies (CPT). At the time, they had no published data about their success with hormonal dysfunction, but they had shown success with opening blocked fallopian tubes. I showed their literature to my fertility specialist, who shook her head and said, "I don't think this will work, but if you are going to try it, do it soon so we can move onto other options."

The following month, I spent a week at CPT. Everything about the place seemed comforting. The therapists were highly trained in several physical therapy modalities. They were medically competent and emotionally intelligent. I felt as if they had a personal vested interest in helping me get pregnant.

I left CPT and flew immediately to San Francisco to meet with a doctor who specialized in Chinese medicine. I worked with her for a week in different modalities and began taking her prescribed herbs and supplements to help with my hormone levels.

I know they helped improve my hormones… because after just a few days of their therapy, my period has returned!

When I returned to my doctor the next month, I learned that my hormone levels had skyrocketed. I discussed the supplements and herbs I was taking and my doctor was shocked at the amounts of Chinese supplements and herbs I was prescribed. He advised me to immediately stop taking them and sure enough, the next month my hormonal levels dropped to a normal level. I knew that my hormone levels had peaked and then dropped because of the Chinese supplements, but I wondered if CPT helped bring my levels to a normal level.

It didn't matter what did it - if my hormonal levels were in range, all I needed was an open tube to become pregnant! I asked my doctor to take a look with a sonogram. I saw him shake his head. "You see that black spot on the screen? That is your left ovary stuck against your uterus. Your tubes are probably so damaged that the only hope for you is a donor egg." After my appointment I walked through Central Park to home — and cried all the way.

That week I missed my period. Five days after my visit with the fertility specialist I took a pregnancy test. I was pregnant! That black spot on the screen was my baby.

It was then I knew that CPT must have opened at least one of my tubes. Nine months later, I gave birth to my beautiful daughter, Natalie.

I was so happy with my time at CPT that I recently returned for a bit more treatment. I hoped they could help me relieve pain I experienced after the C-section with my daughter. Due to stress in my life, I had also stopped menstruating eight (or so) months earlier.

While I suspected that CPT helped my hormones before I conceived Natalie, I did not have hard evidence to say they helped that aspect. That changed with this visit. I know they helped improve my hormones this time because after just a few days of their therapy, my period has returned! In fact, my overall function is noticeably better.

Three Unsuccessful IVFs

- Faith's Story

After trying to conceive for over a year, I started down the path of infertility treatments. I was 35 years old and the doctors reminded me that I was getting "old." I started with IUI treatments (two), but when both failed the doctors told me I should start IVF treatments.

I had my first IVF in September 2005 and had three embryos transferred. Then in October, I started experiencing a lot of pain. I went to the hospital and the doctor discovered one of the embryos had implanted in my right tube causing an ectopic pregnancy. He immediately scheduled me for surgery to remove the tube. After the surgery, the doctor told me I had a lot of scar tissue at my right tube and that I probably had scar tissue surrounding my left tube, as well.

Remarkably, the other two embryos were still alive inside my uterus. However, on a business trip to California in November, I started getting sick. When they diagnosed that pain, the physicians said that my gallbladder had to be removed. When they then checked on the embryos, we found that they didn't make it. Crushed, I had to have a D&C as well.

After the last round, my doctor again reminded me that I was getting "old" and the only way to get pregnant was to go through another (fourth) round of IVF.

When I returned home, my doctor tried to be positive and said that we should start right away on another round of IVF, but when they checked my uterus, they found that I had remaining tissue and I had to have another D&C before we could start .

I could feel the changes occurring in my body . . .

My second round of IVF began in May 2006 and they transferred two embryos, but with no success.

My third round of IVF treatments started in August 2006. Unfortunately, the doctors discovered that my uterus lining was not thick enough, so they had to freeze those embryos until my uterus was "ready." The third transfer finally occurred in November 2006; it was also unsuccessful.

After the last round my doctor again reminded me that I was getting "old" and the only way to get pregnant was to go through another (fourth) round of IVF.

Even though the IVF doctors told me it would not happen (and I was too old) I have proved them wrong!

I felt that my body had been beat up and I was sick of all the shots. I wanted to try to heal my body and think about next steps, which is when I found Clear Passage Therapies (CPT). I found their clinic online and thought it might be the right path for me after what I had experienced. It made sense to me that my body needed to heal and that the therapy was something I needed.

I spent one week (20 hours of therapy) in the Florida location in February 2007. All of the therapists were wonderful and I could feel the changes occurring in my body. I left feeling that my body was in a much better state than when I arrived.

When I returned home, I thought about other natural treatments to help heal my body. I started to see a homeopath and began yoga to get my body in shape. I realized that I needed time to heal from all the treatments and surgeries and I wanted to feel stronger.

In January 2008, I added acupuncture to my other holistic therapies and found that I could feel changes after each session.

Then in March 2008, I found out that I was pregnant – naturally! I am still a little shocked because I feel great. I think the reason why this worked for me is a combination of everything, but it started at CPT. I know that I will have a healthy baby and even though the IVF doctors told me it would not happen (and that I was too "old") I have proved them wrong!

Age 40 with High FSH

- Janell's Story

Since you are reading this, you probably know that life doesn't always go according to plan. In my perfect world, I would have been married in my mid to late 20's and started my family before I was 30.

Instead, I didn't get married until my mid 30's or start trying to conceive until my late 30's. I had a miscarriage, then couldn't get pregnant again, despite religiously taking my temperature, banning alcohol from the house, and making my husband wear different underwear.

As time passed, we became more anxious. My biological clock was ticking so loud that my husband could hear it.

My husband and I began to struggle with some of the most emotionally difficult decisions of our marriage. "Do we try IVF? Do we choose adoption? What about the finances? Is it unwise to spend that much money on a 15% or less probability? Wouldn't the money be better spent on adopting a child in need? Could we be happy and fulfilled without children?"

We felt adoption was an excellent option. We still do. However, as we considered how we would feel at the end of our lives, we wanted to be able to look back and say, "Yes, we did everything in our power to conceive a child. No doubts. No regrets."

It was time to get serious and see if there was anything wrong physically that was preventing me from getting pregnant. As luck would have it, my HSG test was scheduled on the day of my 39th birthday. Not good. The technician blurted out, against medical protocol, that I had a blocked fallopian tube. This birthday turned out to be the worst birthday in the history of birthdays!

My doctor gave me the option of surgery but she didn't really push for it, probably due to my age and the fact that I would need to take medication to increase egg production for the ovary beside my only clear fallopian tube. I was also not keen on the idea of surgery because I knew that it could cause more scar tissue. My husband and I then pursued intrauterine inseminations (IUI), but learned that my FSH levels were fluctuating on the borderline between normal and high. This made me ineligible for IUI during cycles when my FSH level was too high.

It was time to get even more serious! I started researching hormone levels and looking into IVF.

During this time, I discovered Clear Passage Therapies (CPT) in one of my Internet searches. My husband and I decided that I should do the therapy because it could help my two problems — the blocked fallopian tube and my FSH level. Since we'd decided that we were going to pursue IVF, we also wanted to do everything possible to make that a success. I did the 20 hours of therapy over several weeks because I live close to one of the clinics.

The odds of my conceiving with an FSH level of 17 is about 1% . Couple that statistic with the fact that I had a blocked fallopian tube, and the odds drop further.

After CPT, I tried one more IUI. While the IUI failed, I learned that my FSH level had dropped from 11 to 6! I attribute this to CPT. The following cycle, I started the process for IVF, only to be told that my FSH was too high (17) for a possible pregnancy with IVF. That was a real emotional blow.

Later that same cycle, my husband and I did our thing and said our prayers. Incredibly, I got pregnant. God answered!

After I became pregnant, my husband learned that the odds of my conceiving with an FSH level of 17 is about 1%. Couple that statistic with the fact that I had a blocked fallopian tube, and the odds drop further. CPT could have opened my fallopian tube, but I did not have that tested before I became pregnant.

I was 7 months pregnant at my 40th birthday party. It turned out to be the best birthday in the history of birthdays!

I truly believe that God used CPT to provide us our miracle baby. He saw our circumstances and led us in our decisions, to bring us a child.

Treating Polycystic Ovarian Syndrome (PCOS)

Polycystic Ovarian Syndrome (PCOS) refers to an endocrine disorder that affects approximately 5% of all pre-menopausal women. PCOS occurs among all races and nationalities, is the most common hormonal disorder in women of reproductive age, and is a leading cause of infertility. The principal symptoms of PCOS include lack of regular ovulation or menstruation, multiple ovarian cysts, and excessive amounts or effects of androgenic (masculine) hormones.

Symptoms may include acne and male pattern hair growth (hirsutism). Insulin resistance, diabetes, and obesity are all strongly correlated with PCOS. Symptoms and their severity vary greatly among women, and PCOS may occur without outward symptoms.

The proposed causes of PCOS include excess androgen production by the adrenal glands during puberty or stress, or disturbances in the cyclic pattern of GnRH release by the hypothalamus. Polycystic ovaries are not the primary cause of amenorrhea or hirsutism in this condition. Rather, they are one sign of an underlying endocrine disorder that ultimately results in these symptoms.

In some cases of PCOS, adhesions will partially or totally envelop the ovary like a thick sock, preventing the ovum from escaping. Surgical treatment can involve drilling several holes in the adhesive envelope to allow the egg to escape. Other treatments for this condition consist of birth control pills and fertility medication.

The Wurn Technique® has shown good results clinically in some women who presented for therapy with PCOS. As happened with FSH, we initially discouraged women with PCOS from attending therapy. But as also happened with FSH, some women with PCOS chose to attend despite our lack of data. As a result, we are just beginning to compile data on the results of therapy for women with PCOS. We have been able to help several PCOS patients that have come to us.

Three Prior IVFs and Two Surgeries for PCOS

- Tamás and Bianka's Story

My name is Tamás (Architect) and my wife's is Bianka (Pharmacist). We are from Hungary, a country where the level of medical science and service is as high as the USA — and is theoretically free.

My wife and I endured incredible highs and lows as our journey unfolded. We hope it may inspire you to persist, and not give up your dreams. We never gave up though it was not easy, and now we have beautiful twins — a boy, Gábor, and a girl, Nikolett. We are sure that we have Clear Passage to thank for them.

Bianka and I married in 1999 after a fairly short dating period and ever since, our love for each other has made our time together wonderful and peaceful. Bianka had been very sick as a child, and we knew we would have some problems conceiving because Bianka had irregular periods. In fact, her hormones were so "off" that she would sometimes go six months without a period at all. Despite this, we had faith; we decided to try to have a child from the very first day of our married life.

When doctors learned of her severe hormonal problems, most of them wanted her to take contraceptive (hormone) pills to help regulate her period. We felt that would just be a "patch;" it would not solve the root of the problem. Besides, you can't get pregnant taking contraceptives. Before we were married, they told Bianka, "Please come back when you think you are ready to have a child and we will look at the problem again."

Like many women, Bianka felt uncomfortable being so exposed at her gynecology visits. Besides, she often felt rushed through her appointments, more of a burden than a special client. Thus, we did not spend much time seeking second opinions from other doctors at that time. Little did we know how much that aspect of our life was about to change!

We were both heartbroken when Bianka was officially diagnosed with Polycystic Ovarian Syndrome (PCOS). At last, we realized that we had to take whatever steps were necessary to solve the problem. In order to achieve our aim we agreed to see several doctors and to hear different opinions. Each physician seemed to have his or her own ideas of what she needed. Bianka began to feel like an experimental doll in the examination rooms.

In my society, we were already relatively old to have children; Bianka was 29 and I was 26. For us, it was not about the age — it was about being able to care for a child financially. We wanted to have a secure foundation under us to be able to support our children until they were able to start their lives. We did not have that.

Even though healthcare is theoretically free for everybody in Hungary, it can be costly to get the kind of medical attention and physician time that special cases such as Bianka required. The continuous traveling, the prescribed medication and the extra costs added up to a lot of money in the end, and we still had no results — no baby!

Bianka had to take Clomid treatments to help regulate her hormones and also had to inject herself daily (under her skin) with medications for seven rounds of hormone treatment to help with the PCOS. Then she went to the doctor later each day for more hormone injections into her muscles. The adventure to become parents that started out so positively was becoming exhausting, depressing and terribly difficult. The strong hormones Bianka had to take only made a deeply emotional experience even more difficult — really, for both of us.

The PCOS also caused "tentacle-like" adhesions to form on and over her ovaries. They told us that surgery would help, but that would be a temporary measure. The PCOS adhesion surgeries might have to be repeated as often as every year. We visited even more physicians, some of the best in the world, from our investigation. Bianka underwent surgery for PCOS. So many of these doctors and their staffs were great, but the doctors said she would eventually need another surgery to conceive.

People who have never experienced the deep and powerful yearning for a child, followed by the recurring disappointments, will never understand what it feels like.

After her first surgery, she continued with Clomid and intrauterine inseminations (IUIs). By Hungarian law, we first had to undergo five intra-uterine inseminations before our insurance would pay for IVF. Bianka underwent five separate IUIs without success. Well, she did get pregnant once, and we were thrilled. That elation lasted just a short time, as we faced the trauma and further heartbreak of a miscarriage. It was like a funeral shroud landing on a ray of hope. It was just terrible.

After that first PCOS operation, 25 rounds of Clomid, 5 IUIs, and that miscarriage, we had spent most of our funds. Instead of months, we were starting to measure our quest for a baby in years. Frustrated but determined, we decided not to waste any more time and money on IUI procedures. After our fifth failed IUI, we finally made it to the IVF program, and decided to go straight into that.

By this time, we had consulted several physicians. We settled on a Hungarian institute founded by a Hungarian American doctor. The doctors and the atmosphere were great, and their success rates were among the highest in the world.

We had to go through all the examinations again and the doctors started a new experiment on her. I use the word "experiment" since the doctors add hormones and other elements so they can create the best environment in each patient to help create a pregnancy.

The doctors and the nurses were really great and they did their best. The first IVF resulted in a pregnancy, but after five weeks, we endured another miscarriage — another funeral.

Her doctors decided she needed another PCOS surgery, so we did that. Directly after this (her 2nd PCOS surgery), we had another IVF. This time, there was no pregnancy at all. Every time a procedure failed, it was an enormous heartbreak and it was worse each time. But in order to persevere, we found we needed to try it over and over again. And we did. The third IVF did not even bring a pregnancy.

By this time, we started losing faith. People who have never experienced the deep and powerful yearning for a child, followed by the recurring disappointments, will never understand what it feels like. As a man and husband, I knew that I had to support my wife more than ever in this situation. I think the pressure on a woman is much higher than on the man. Even though I suffered deeply, I had to act as if everything was all right.

Other circumstances in our life began to change. At the same time nothing seemed to work for our family plans, I lost my job; now, it was only my wife who made money. To pursue our dream of a family, we sold everything we could to have enough money for the treatments. Finally, we got to the point where there was nothing else left for us. Something had to change.

I had no other choice but to come back to the States and get a job in 2005. Slowly, change began to come into our life. My friend Chris gave me a place to stay and helped me with everything. Every night I was hopelessly searching the Internet and sending every IVF institute a letter in which I asked for information or for help. Nothing happened from all of those efforts.

At this point the doctors said that she should have a third surgery for the PCOS. Thus, no closer to our goal, we found we would have to start the entire process all over again. Then, a small light emerged into our dark night.

She spoke in a manner that was scientific, but she phrased her message into sentences that anybody could comprehend.

One night I came across the website of Clear Passage Therapies (CPT). To be honest, I was not expecting anything special from this company either. But I read through its profile because I did not want to miss anything. What can I say? The numbers were gorgeous and we seemed to fit in the program. But there came the haunting question: Could this work for us?

We really had no other options, so I forwarded the site to my wife in Hungary, and also to our doctor. Bianka was very excited, but the doctor was cautious. We made up our minds and I called them. They told me everything I needed to know and they sent me all their information in printed form.

I remember that summer very well. I lived in the New York area trying to make some extra money, and Bianka was still in Hungary. There were only two Clear Passage offices and none were within a few thousand miles of me. Originally, Bianka was going to visit me early September and we were to go home together a few weeks later.

As it happened, the company was due to open a New York office in August. We had difficulties collecting the necessary doctors' forms and papers we needed, but finally Bianka managed to put everything together.

It took about a week after she applied before we got the word that she had been accepted in the program. The secretary was unbelievably helpful and understanding. She managed to set up an appointment in the New York office for us in September

The timing and everything seemed to be just perfect for us. Bianka's first appointment was on Labor Day and I had the chance to go in with her for her first appointment. I spoke with the therapist and asked her all kinds of questions. She was nice and funny, but was very scholarly. She explained everything to us and answered all our questions while creating a very calm and friendly atmosphere. She spoke in a manner that was scientific, but she phrased her message into sentences that anybody could comprehend. Once she had answered all of our questions, she started the treatment right away.

This physical therapy consisted of two sessions every day for five days: one in the morning from 10 to 12 and one in the afternoon from 1 to 3. Even though some people liken this work to massage, it is really nothing like you can imagine. The therapist worked on every part of her body, and I mean everywhere! There were some situations where I thought I should leave and come back a little later because it was so intimate and I did not want to discomfort anybody.

But the therapist said I could stay. She wanted to make sure I understood everything she did, and she wanted to do whatever Bianka needed to give us our best chance at success.

The therapy gave us new direction; we did whatever, whenever we wanted it. We felt more natural and free, so our sexual life became fun again.

After we explained Bianka's history of PCOS and the surgeries she had for that, the therapist paid special attention to Bianka's ovaries. Most women with PCOS experience a constant discomfort around the ovaries. This can be very painful, especially around the ovulation. Another problem with PCOS is that the woman can develop adhesive "tentacles" that glue it in place so the natural fluid movement of the ovary in the body does not happen. Physicians cut these "tentacles" during the surgery because it is very important that the ovaries can float freely. Unfortunately they don't stay free for long, for most women. With luck, after the surgery you can have better mobility about a year. After that, doctors are almost 100% sure that they will glue down again. Our doctors wanted Bianka to have a third PCOS surgery to clean up her adhesions, but we went to CPT instead.

To Bianka's and my big surprise, our therapist determined the exact location of her ovaries. She placed pressure on the right spot until Bianka felt something similar to when a fishing-line splits. The best part was that all the pain she was feeling around her ovaries disappeared right away. This was an unbelievable experience. Our therapist had enabled the "tentacles" to detach from the ovaries.

I was happy I could be there at least one day with her. After that, I had to go back to work and Bianka had to commute alone to New York for four more days. I was very proud of her and I still am because she never gave up, even when we almost thought that there was no hope left.

Once treatment was finished, our therapist told us that the treatment helps increase a woman's sexual function as well. Well, all I have to say about this is that she was right on that! The treatment helped change both our lifestyle and our relationship with infertility. We did not care about timing, temperature and things like that any more. The therapy gave us new direction and we did whatever, whenever we wanted it. We just felt more natural and free afterwards, so our sexual life became fun again.

Even though we were done with the treatment after five days, it did not mean that the therapy was over. For Bianka, the real work started from then on. With the help of therapy, all her body parts, muscles, joints etc. were loosened and she had to maintain this state. She was given a detailed description, illustrated with pictures of special stretching exercises which she had to practice twice a day. Thank God Bianka was very, very dedicated.

When we returned home to the infertility clinic in Hungary, we asked if we could do the regular insemination, instead of IVF. We were feeling really good; we just wanted to make sure that the sperm got where it needed to be. We didn't do anything else. No special medications, just the usual folic acid and our regular vitamins.

We had two inseminations. The first one had no result, but that was right after the therapy and the therapist said it might take a few weeks for Bianka's internal organs to return to normal, after therapy. We did the second post-therapy IUI a little later, so Bianka had time to practice her exercises.

I remember the day so well. I could not believe my eyes when the nurse took me into the examining room that day to show me the pictures of Bianka's pregnancy on the monitor. The doctor explained the image to me. He was careful to mention that he only saw one embryo. But you know after a while all husbands become "experts" on this topic and so did I. So when we left the room I told Bianka that I was almost 100% sure that there were two embryos. Turns out, I was right. I guess the doctor was trying to protect us from another shock in case something happened to one of them.

It is amazing to both of us that after all the drugs, all the surgeries, all the failed medical attempts, these two beautiful children came to us without surgery or drugs.

Even though the babies came on week 33, until that moment we had no complications. Everything went smooth and by the book. By then we were in a regular hospital with a doctor we chose, who was supposed to be very good. In fact, he made a big mistake and our story almost ended up in a catastrophe but thanks to God and the nurses, our two angels came out fine. For us they are the most perfect children in the world.

Over all I have to say we thank God and CPT for our children. It is amazing to both of us that after all the drugs, all the surgeries, all the failed medical attempts, these two beautiful children came to us without surgery or drugs. I wish others who are searching could know about this therapy. I hope our story may give someone a bit of inspiration and extra strength to go on, and never give up.

22 Negative Pregnancy Tests and PCOS

- Alyssa's Story

I was diagnosed with PCOS when I was 21. My doctors informed me that when I was ready to get pregnant, I would need fertility drugs.

In 2001 when I was ready, I spoke with an infertility specialist immediately. I was placed on Clomid and another medication to help me menstruate.

After six months of Clomid, I was switched to Gonal-F. For the next year and a half, my doctor slowly increased my dosage to 4 ampules a day. I tried multiple intra-uterine inseminations as well, but I still could not become pregnant.

After 22 negative pregnancy tests, I didn't know where to turn for help and I was considering pursuing IVF. Around that time, my cousin called me and told me about a new fertility treatment she had heard about on the news. I didn't think much of it until she called me again and urged me to research it. I looked at the clinic online and learned about Clear Passage Therapies (CPT).

I decided I wanted to go, but my husband was completely against the idea. I was determined to come up with the money. I am a real estate agent, so I worked hard and put in the extra time to make the extra sale I needed to have the money.

In 2003 I attended an intensive week of treatment at CPT. As they made adjustments to my body and tissues, I could feel slight changes. The pain I regularly experienced in my pelvis and lower back also decreased.

Shortly after treatment, I became pregnant. I was still on the Gonal-F, but I had been on the same dosage for almost a year. I think my body was out of alignment before and the techniques at CPT fixed my body and enabled me to become pregnant.

I now have an incredible four year old. It took me almost three years to get to CPT, but I'm glad I went.

Extensive Adhesions and PCOS

- Elyse's Story

In early 2004, my husband and I married. We were ready to start a family right away and I stopped taking oral contraceptives. I had been on the pill for twelve years in order to regulate my periods and never had any problems. But when I went off of it, my period did not return for five months.

I went to my doctor and he immediately referred me to an infertility specialist. My specialist examined my medical history and did some blood work. He discovered that I had poly-cystic ovarian syndrome (PCOS), a condition in which you do not ovulate regularly. My doctor explained, "You have a lot of immature follicles in your ovaries, which causes an imbalance in your hormones."

He placed me on Clomid, a drug designed to regulate ovulation, but nothing happened. He then recommended I start IVF. I was uncomfortable with this option as I had always wanted to pursue the least invasive option first, but he continued to push it hard.

As a result, I decided to meet with another specialist who would respect my wishes with regard to treatment. My new doctor, husband, and I decided I should try Clomid again, but after a few unsuccessful cycles, it was obvious the medication was not helping. He told me, "Elyse, your only option is IVF." He understood I was upset and explained that because my hormones were not regular, IVF was my best chance to produce mature follicles and carry a viable pregnancy.

One of the specialists even cried as she viewed the screen during my ultrasound.

Since both doctors had suggested IVF, I agreed and began IVF in December of 2004. It was a painful process both mentally and physically. I had always been terrified of needles. However, in January, when I learned I was pregnant with twins I rationalized it was worth all the pain. My joy was short lived. At the 8 week ultrasound to hear/view the heartbeats we learned they were conjoined. Moreover, one of the fetuses was not developing at the expected rate and was already much smaller than the other. The doctor appeared disappointed and doubtful they would make it. However, he encouraged us to get a second opinion. We obtained opinions from three other specialists, who all reported poor prognoses. One of the specialists even cried as she viewed the screen during my ultrasound. My husband and I made the difficult decision to terminate the pregnancy. It was one of the most difficult decisions of my life.

On March 9, I had a D&C. I was hysterical while being put under anesthesia even though I knew it was for the best. I awoke with a terrible emptiness and cried endlessly for weeks.

I felt absolutely miserable, but certainly was not ready to give up.

I felt absolutely miserable, but certainly was not ready to give up. Our doctor explained our options. He had retrieved 28 of my eggs for the initial IVF procedure which resulted in "plenty" of frozen embryos for transfers. The doctor joked I could have a "football team" if I wanted. Our embryos, he explained, were all in great shape. We confirmed this through pre-genetic implantation diagnosis just to be sure. I began frozen transfers in May and continued through July — but none of them took.

During this process I tried all kinds of treatments, including Viagra® suppositories. A study had found that it increased blood flow to the uterus, thereby aiding implantation.

In August, my doctor decided to perform a hysteroscopy to see if there was scar tissue in my uterus that was preventing the embryos from implanting. His suspicion was correct, and he found extensive scar tissue that had formed as a result of the D&C. He removed everything he could and was optimistic that I would then be able to become pregnant.

He did another embryo transfer two weeks later, but it didn't take either. My doctor was concerned that more scar tissue had formed and used a hydrosonogram to check my uterus. He found that scar tissue had grown again in my uterus.

I was extremely upset, but we decided to try one last embryo transfer. When it didn't take, my doctor wanted to perform another surgery to remove the scar tissue.

My doctor had given up on me. However, I didn't give up on me.

"Absolutely not," I told him. It was obvious to me that my body was feeling like it was under attack and it was overproducing scar tissue to compensate. I felt like I was ruining my body with the surgeries and medications. My body was becoming a "toxic waste dump," and I was mentally exhausted. I wanted a break.

In November, I began seeing an acupuncturist, to see if she could help regulate my hormones naturally. While I saw the acupuncturist, I continued visits with my doctor. In February, he told me that I "didn't have the right uterus" and needed a surrogate. My doctor had given up on me. However, I didn't give up on me. I decided I needed to find a way to eliminate the scar tissue that had formed without using an invasive surgical procedure.

I decided I needed to find a way to eliminate the scar tissue that had formed without using an invasive surgical procedure.

I decided to research online whether anything like this existed. Although I had always had a hard time using the computer, I was determined to find something. Not knowing how to refine searches on the Internet, I typed in an extremely long phrase "non-surgical removal of scar tissue" and the Clear Passage Therapies (CPT) website was one of the first that showed-up. I printed all of their pages and when my husband came home that day, he couldn't believe I had found a website that described the type of treatment we were looking for. We were both genuinely excited.

After reading their literature, we knew their focus on reducing adhesions and scar tissue would be helpful to me. I scheduled myself for an intensive week of treatment. Because I was going to their clinic in California, I had to receive an authorization form from my doctor. When I told him about the treatment, he was doubtful about whether it would work. He had never heard of anything like this. He cautioned me about spending too much time trying alternative treatments such as physical therapy, nutritional detoxification, acupuncture, and herbs. If I waited too long before trying another transfer, I would risk more growth of scar tissue. I silently reminded myself of the two week period it took for scar tissue to form and did my best to ignore his comments. The doctor reluctantly signed my forms, which allowed me to begin treatment with CPT.

I attended therapy in March and I found it was very intensive. I could feel my therapists breaking apart scar tissue. After the first day of treatment I went to the bathroom and I actually saw scar tissue in the toilet. I couldn't believe it. My therapists explained to me that scar tissue had probably formed within my uterus and that they helped it detach from the walls. I was filled with hope that they would be able to remove the remaining scar tissue in my body.

After treatment, I knew I still needed to address my hormone imbalance, which was the original reason for seeking assistance with fertility. I saw a new fertility specialist, who respected my decision to start at the beginning once again. The doctor placed me on Clomid for two cycles. The first time, I did produce one egg, but it wasn't fully developed. During the second cycle, the doctor did not find evidence of ovulation until well past the time Clomid would have produced an egg. He did an ultrasound and saw a "big beautiful egg" just waiting to be released from my right ovary. He exclaimed, "How in the world did you do that?"

As I look at my twins, I am glad I trusted my instincts and found treatments that coincided with what was the best for me.

I knew that the acupuncture, herbs, and nutritional counseling had helped regulate my hormones and CPT had enabled my uterus to prepare for a successful implantation. I took all of the information I had to my previous doctor and my growing belly as proof!

To our delight, we soon learned that I was pregnant with twins! My twin girls were born March 8, 2007 — two years after my heartbreaking D&C and almost one year to the day of completing my treatment at CPT. As I look at them today, I am glad I trusted my instincts and found treatments that coincided with what was the best for me.

Three Prior IVFs, PCOS, No Natural Menstrual Cycle

- Sydney's Story

"You have Poly-Cystic Ovarian Syndrome, also known as PCOS," my doctor told me. "PCOS prevents you from ovulating, which explains why you and your husband have not been able to conceive." My husband and I had wed just six months prior and we knew we wanted children right away. Before getting married, I was on oral contraceptives, so I had no idea there was anything wrong with my ovulation.

My doctor recommended I try medications to help me start ovulating and have a normal menstrual cycle, but none of it seemed to do anything.

After six months, my doctor referred me to a fertility clinic. That clinic agreed that I had PCOS. The specialist said "PCOS often causes adhesions to form around the ovaries, preventing an egg from being released. Although your HSG report shows your fallopian tubes are clear, it is still possible you have adhesions around your ovaries. We can perform laparoscopic surgery to visualize this area. If there are adhesions, we can drill holes through the adhesions to access your ovaries. That will create areas for your eggs to be released."

My husband and I were uncomfortable with surgery, so we proceeded with medication. The physicians put me on stronger medication, which sometimes included daily shots in my hip.

In my fifth month of taking these new medications, I hyperstimulated. Because I had produced a large quantity of eggs, my doctors felt I should go ahead with IVF. I had not expected to jump to IVF so soon, but I was extremely hopeful it would work. They retrieved 28 eggs during the procedure.

We did two transfers, but nothing worked. My doctors wanted me to have another IVF, but we just needed a break.

They placed two fertilized embryos in my uterus and froze the other eggs for future transfer. When the two embryos did not take, I was devastated. My nurse told me, "I knew you had too much hope."

That was such an insensitive thing to say; I became really upset, and wondered "Why am I here?"

But after a while, my husband and I decided to continue transferring the frozen embryos. We did two transfers, transferring three each time, but nothing worked. My doctors wanted me to have another IVF, but we just needed a break.

My husband and I started to research our options online. While looking for information on our infertility clinic's website, we saw a page for alternative medicine. There, we read about a manual physical therapy that had some scientific success in helping women become pregnant. After reading through the website, we decided to attend treatment at Clear Passage Therapies (CPT).

I spread my treatment out over two weeks and it was absolutely great. CPT changed my way of thinking about infertility. Instead of thinking, "This one part of my body isn't working — and I hate it," they helped show me that the whole body works together. While treating my entire body, they also resolved back pain I had for years. I had even seen several physical therapists before and one of them told me, "You will need surgery by the time you are 40." But after CPT, I had no pain. I also experienced a great reduction in intercourse pain. I had always thought the pain I experienced with intercourse was normal.

The most astounding result from my treatment was that my menstrual cycle returned! Although the exact cause of PCOS is unknown, one of the main symptoms is an irregular or missed cycle – yet here I was, finally having a regular menstrual cycle!

The most astounding result from my treatment was that my menstrual cycle returned!

My husband and I decided to find a new infertility doctor who was more alternative. When he heard I had PCOS, yet now had a regular menstrual cycle, he asked, "What have you been doing?" He was thrilled my treatment at CPT helped, but he still felt I should go back on fertility medication to further increase my chances of ovulating successfully. Because the doses were so high, I had to have ultrasounds daily. After six months, nothing seemed to be working, and he suggested laparoscopic surgery to drill holes into my ovaries.

I knew from my time at CPT that surgery might help, but could also have numerous detrimental affects on the body. Furthermore, I knew from my own personal research that the surgery would only provide a small window for success. After that, the holes would close again.

So instead of the surgery, we decided to return to CPT for an additional 20 hours of treatment. Once again, my treatment was outstanding. Prior to my treatment, I had a lot of infections and inflammation in my vagina and my doctors and I couldn't understand why. After my treatment at CPT, I stopped having those problems, completely.

> ***We went through with this, our fourth IVF cycle, and the first one after CPT. This time, things were different… in fact, everything went fine.***

When we returned home from the clinic, we decided our lives would not be dictated by infertility, so we started the adoption process. A few months later, we were surprised to hear we received a grant for IVF. We had applied for the grant many months prior, and we had just assumed we didn't receive it.

We went through with this, our fourth IVF cycle, and the first one after CPT. This time, things were different. In fact, everything went fine. They implanted two embryos and both took well. I had no problems through my pregnancy. I was able to work until the day of my C-section. I really felt it was because of the treatment I received at CPT – I just felt so good.

My boys were born in October, and today they are doing great. I am thankful I had treatment with CPT, I just wish someone would have told me about them earlier. They educated me about my body so I could figure out what was right for me, and their therapy helped my body heal naturally. If I'd

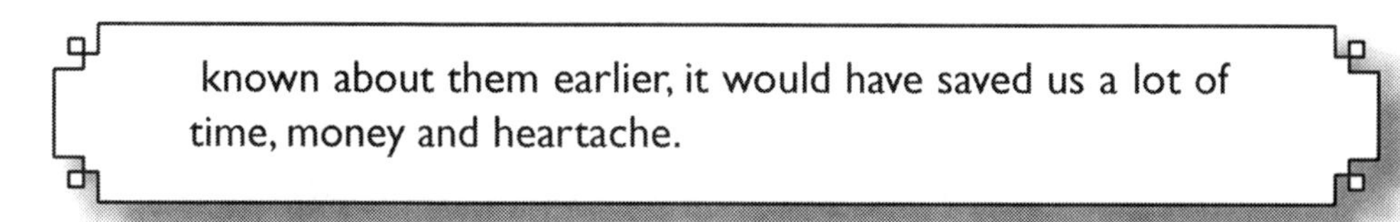
known about them earlier, it would have saved us a lot of time, money and heartache.

Unexpected Patient Successes

If high FSH and hormonal dysfunction are a natural byproduct of aging, then why are we seeing such dramatic improvements in FSH levels, natural pregnancies, full term births, and even subsequent births among women that have been diagnosed hormonally menopausal? We have asked ourselves this question, and the only thing that makes sense to us is that there is a strong mechanical component to the processes that dictate hormone release (whether in the brain, ovaries, endocrine glands or their "communication loop"). Knowing what we do about adhesions, it does not take a far stretch of the imagination to see that a large component of aging itself is a result of the mechanical actions of adhesions that form in all of us, as the years pass.

Over the course of life, adhesions develop throughout the body. They form whenever and wherever healing occurs from an accident, infection, surgery, or trauma. Once the injury has healed, the adhesions remain in the body as a permanent record of the physical insult to the tissues. This is a very real part of the aging process.

> ***We were told I should consider donor eggs since my FSH level was beginning to get high and I was not a good candidate to retry IVF.***
>
> *–Amania, who later became pregnant naturally and delivered a healthy baby girl after treatment.*

We have lost count of the number of times that, explaining remarkable turnarounds in our patients' symptoms, we have said, "It's almost like you are getting younger in that part of your body."

We are not being cavalier with such a statement. Adhesions form from healing events as we age. When we decrease adhesions and detach the cross-links that have bound our tissues over the years, mobility and function tends to return to those areas. In a very real sense, those organs and previously adhered tissues appear to "go back in time" to an earlier time in the healing process, or to a time before healing events occurred.

We have seen this happen time and again in the musculoskeletal system in patients who came to us with chronic pain. In a mechanical sense, the healing (and adhesive) process that occurs in the tissues of the reproductive system is not much different from those of our muscles or joints. As adhesions form, they bind tissues and structures together. As adhesions decrease, structures are freed from their prior bonds. When this happens, the structures are free to move with greater ease and mobility, as they did earlier in life.

We feel something similar is happening with these patients who come to us with high, even menopausal hormone levels. The vast majority of them either become pregnant naturally after we treat them, or their hormonal levels greatly improve. Decreasing adhesions that affect the reproductive organs and glands appears to turn back time to an earlier state of function.

Infertile for Eight Years and FSH of 18

- Mary's Story

After being married for 11 years, we were ready to start a family. Within a month, I was pregnant and we began to dream about life with our child. Seven weeks later, I was having cramps and began to bleed, hoping the baby would live. On Easter morning, I went to the hospital because I was having a miscarriage. Later that week, I visited my doctor, and because my HCG levels continued to rise, and there were no signs of a uterine pregnancy, they diagnosed an ectopic pregnancy. I was given methotrexate to end the pregnancy and to help preserve the tube.

The pregnancy was another ectopic.

A few months later, we tried again and I became pregnant right away. The pregnancy was another ectopic. An HSG was performed — a test where they use dye to show whether or not my fallopian tubes were open. It confirmed that my left fallopian tube was completely blocked. Nonetheless, my doctor was encouraging and assured me that I could still become pregnant with one working tube. I felt betrayed by my body and wondered why did I wait so long to start having children?

While I began graduate school, we decided to keep trying. Three more pregnancies later, and three more disappointing miscarriages, I felt like a battle worn soldier and began to see myself differently from my friends and family: childless. I hated to hear about my friends' pregnancies and couldn't bear to attend baby showers or even look at babies. I wanted to "move on" but couldn't.

After extensive research into fertility options, I came across Clear Passage Therapies (CPT) and contacted them for more information. They put me in touch with a former patient who had also experienced several ectopics. I asked her, "Do you really think the treatment works?" She responded, "Absolutely, they opened my blocked fallopian tubes." I was stunned. Was it really possible that they could open up her tubes without surgery?

That night I prayed about CPT. Every night I spent time with God and that night I asked for help in making a decision about what to do. What I heard was clear: to pursue CPT and let God heal me completely: body, mind and spirit.

The next day I looked at the Clear Passage website again and also looked at the option of IVF. My doctors and friends strongly suggested that I pursue IVF. I felt a range of emotions all coming from a place of fear. My mind kept repeating, "You're getting older." I was only 35 but felt like I was turning 50.

Ultimately my husband and I pursued IVF, with my leading. While the Lord was cautioning me on this path, I charged ahead and one month after graduation completed IVF. My FSH was on the high side, (12) but the procedure was successful and I became pregnant with identical twins! Within a few weeks, one of the twins died. Afterwards I continued to experience a lot of pain and kept returning to my doctor to see if something was wrong. My intuition kept telling me that something was very wrong. He dismissed my symptoms, even though the other "vanishing" twin was continuing to grow larger.

My intuition kept telling me that something was very wrong.

Throughout this time I continued my nightly prayers. Each night I prayed with my baby and God. I felt a strong connection among the three of us. At 19 weeks I was up one night having so much pain that I was unable to sleep. As I began to pray, I no longer felt a connection to the baby, and knew something had gone wrong.

The next morning when I rose, my water broke. I was terrified that the baby had died. I rushed to the hospital and with my husband by my side, the ultrasound showed a baby with no heartbeat. Our screams and cries echoed. It was a crushing blow for us. The doctor who had been treating me said I would never know what the cause was, but hours later we did know the cause. The babies were connected to each other through a vein. When one died, the other, healthy baby continued to pump blood into the body of the other twin. Eventually the healthy twin went into heart failure and died. That night I delivered my twin boys with much anguish and grief. I held our baby boy in my hands, marveling at his perfectly shaped mouth, and tiny hands and feet all in the palm of my hand. He was perfect. I felt as though I had let this child down, taken his very life away from him. When we left the hospital late that night I wished I could die too. I was broken and very angry.

The grief that followed me lasted for many dark months and left me feeling isolated from all normal life. So many things had gone wrong. I was angry at the doctor for not "noticing" the growth of the dead twin, I was angry at myself for not having pursued a specialist who could have saved the healthy twin's life, and I was alienated by many of the comments of doctors and friends who said things meant to bring comfort but which only brought me pain. I thought about writing a pamphlet entitled, "What not to say to those who have just had a miscarriage or stillbirth." Two weeks later we had a funeral under our large 100 year old oak tree outside our home, and shared our grief with our close friends and family.

The therapist recognized that I was in a fragile broken place. The week was more healing than I had expected, physically, mentally and spiritually.

Eventually I reached a point where I was ready to move forward. I was still hopeful that in some way our twins had forged the way for another life to take root. A few months later I tried IVF, but my body did not respond to the medication, even though they used the most aggressive protocol. My FSH was now 18, which in itself sent waves of fear over me, and my doctors said that I could not continue with IVF.

I thought about CPT again. I prayed and once again felt like it was the right thing to do. I scheduled myself for an intensive week of treatment. The therapist was a gentle compassionate person who recognized that I was in a fragile broken place. The week was more healing than I had expected, not only physically but mentally and spiritually. The therapist taught me to listen to my body, and I began to practice visualization. This allowed me to go deep into my emotions and thinking and see the patterns of thinking I had developed around pregnancy and my body. For the first time I began to imagine new possibilities for my body, my life, and what it would look like to be healed and whole again.

One month after treatment I retested my hormone levels to see if I could attempt another IVF treatment, but my FSH was still too high. My therapist at CPT told me that the human body sometimes needs six months to adjust after treatment and function properly.

After everything we had been through, my husband and I decided to go to Australia for some rejuvenation. We did a ten-day intensive no-frills health retreat where my husband and I spent time fasting, praying, taking long walks and getting plenty of rest. No phones. No TV. No town within 20 miles. During one of my long walks alone, I resumed a conversation with God and once again felt alive, really alive. It had been a long time away from truly living for me. I let go of my expectations, and let go of needing to have a child. Essentially I surrendered my desire — trusting and hoping that life was good with or without children in it. When it was time to go back home, one of the other participants asked us to stay and dog sit for a few months. The dog was a sprightly terrier living in the most beautiful beach house overlooking the ocean and the National Park of the Sunshine coast of Australia. This was another gift of healing. When we returned home, I became pregnant with Genevieve, who today is a bright, beautiful 2.5 year old, a daily reminder of the manifestation of hope and a source of eternal joy.

Almost 2 years after her birth, we looked forward to having another child. I became pregnant right away, but 7 weeks later miscarried. Afterwards, I experienced a lot of pain leading up to and during ovulation, and suspected something was wrong. After trying for nearly a year to get pregnant, I began to feel like I needed some outside help. I tried some medications, but nothing. Then I began thinking about IVF again. My

FSH was again 18 and my doctor did not think IVF would work. When we began to pursue other options like adoption and donor eggs, the doors didn't open. But, unlike other times, I did not feel desperate or fearful. Yes, I still had doubts, but I was beginning to trust and I believed there was another baby waiting for our family and that God was making a way once again. I knew then that I needed to go back to CPT. Always the planner, I made sure that when I returned home, my medications and fertility drugs would be waiting for me in the refrigerator, so I'd be ready to try another intensive protocol.

> ***Looking back, I know the road that I initially chose was one generated from fear. This fear pigeon-holed me and prevented me from following my instinct and divine guidance.***

At CPT I did a week of intensive treatment, with five hours of treatment each day for four days. On the third day of treatment, I ovulated and immediately noticed that I didn't experience any pain. When I returned home, I learned I was pregnant. I fell to the floor crying and praising God with deep humility and wonder. I didn't have to take any medication. I didn't have to go through years of waiting on adoption lists; I didn't have to use a donor egg. I didn't have to do more drugs, and wait any longer. As of this writing I am 17 weeks pregnant.

Looking back on my past, I know the road that I initially chose was one generated from fear. This fear pigeonholed me and prevented me from following my instinct and divine guidance.

Although I felt led to try a natural treatment option, I chose IVF because I thought it would work — quick and easy! It was only after experiencing the devastating loss of our baby boy that I turned to natural treatment — and it worked. Just before I attended my second round of treatment with CPT, my infertility doctor said I had less than a 2% chance of conceiving. Here I am, marveling at what has taken place.

Infertility has been the greatest source of my spiritual growth over the past 8 years. It has given me awe for what God is doing through the hands and hearts of people who are willing to serve others. I am the recipient of this love, compassion and dedication. This journey has given me a boldness to hold onto faith and hope. Hope never gives up, and there is always hope.

This journey has given me a boldness to hold onto faith and hope.

Chapter Nine

Pre-IVF Therapy

In vitro fertilization (IVF) is the gold standard for treating infertility diagnoses. It is usually conducted by gynecologists and reproductive endocrinologists (REs), often assisted by a PhD embryologist and other professional clinical staff. By the time a patient has been referred to IVF, she has usually exhausted all medical and surgical therapies, including intrauterine insemination (IUI) with her partner's sperm.

What Happens During an IVF?

IVF protocols vary by physician. The procedures any physician may choose are based on a combination of the doctor's training, skills, focus, and the specifics of each case. Notwithstanding individual physician approaches and philosophies, the course of IVF generally follows some variation of this protocol:

- Most physicians who perform IVF want to have as much control over the menstrual cycle as possible. Thus, many REs first choose to give a woman pharmaceuticals to stop her menstrual cycle. Now starting with a blank canvas, the specialist usually administers ovarian stimulating drugs to increase the egg production. This generally marks the beginning of the IVF cycle.
- Once they reach the desired size and number, the eggs are surgically removed from the ovaries. One or more of the best eggs are joined with the partner's sperm in a laboratory setting. Finally, these fertilized eggs are placed back inside the woman's reproductive tract — either into the uterus or the fallopian tube.

As precise and controlled as the process is, in vitro fertilization has one chance to work each menstrual cycle. If there is no clinical pregnancy or implantation, part or all of the process has to be repeated.

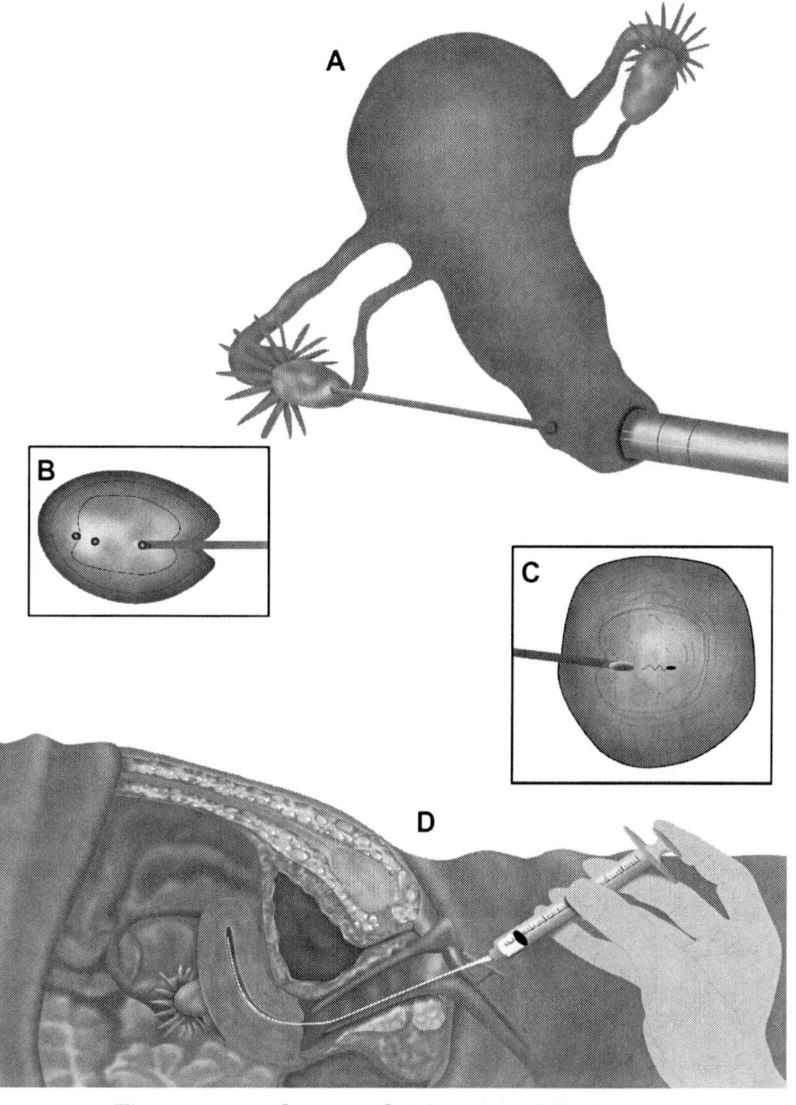

The process of in vitro fertilization (IVF) involves
A: Stimulating the ovaries to produce eggs
B: Extracting one or more mature eggs from the ovary
C: Introducing sperm into the egg or its close environment
D: Inserting the fertilized egg into the reproductive tract (uterus or fallopian tube)

Two major organizations, one governmental and one professional, have united to help the consumer better understand the process of IVF and the success rate of various clinics throughout the United States of America. The US Centers for Disease Control (CDC) and the American Society for Reproductive Medicine (ASRM) have developed a system for monitoring and measuring assisted reproductive techniques (ART). They publish their results each year in a report entitled Assisted Reproductive Technology Success Rates. This report is designed to inform the public each year of the number of procedures performed in every reporting IVF clinic in the US, the ages of the participants, the procedures performed, and the success rates of those procedures based by age of the mothers at the time ovary stimulating medications began.

CDC-ASRM gives success rates of pregnancies and number of live births per cycle rather than pregnancies and live births per transfer. A cycle begins when a woman begins taking ovarian stimulating medications. Only a certain percentage of these go onto the transfer stage in which a fertilized embryo is transferred into the female reproductive tract.

In short, the CDC and ASRM put forth a tremendous effort to create statistical data by which physicians can judge their successes and failures, and patients can be better informed about the success of the physician they are considering. CDC/ASRM gives copious amounts of great information at their "National Success Rates" website, including success rates for different age groups. According to their published data, the all-around live birth rate per cycle of live non-donor eggs (using the recipient's own eggs) was 28%.[19] The same citation notes the average cost per IVF cycle was $12,400; the book does not say whether this cost includes the medications.

You can print and view this data yourself, and print the entire book with success rates separated for every state and reporting clinic in the US at this web page: http://www.cdc.gov/ART/index.htm

Increasing IVF Pregnancy Rates with Therapy

In our early years when we were first investigating therapy for infertility, we had only seen about 20 natural pregnancies and births in women diagnosed infertile. Then a woman approached us and said, "I am scheduled for IVF. Do you think your work can help me?" We told her that we did not know, and in fact had never tested it.

Although we had never treated a woman preparing for an IVF transfer, it seemed reasonable to us that if we could help improve the function of reproductive organs of infertile women who became pregnant naturally, we might be able to improve the function of reproductive organs in women preparing for IVF transfer, as well.

We treated the woman, and she became pregnant with her first IVF transfer after therapy, although she had failed to become pregnant in two prior attempts by the same physician. Soon, other women in similar situations approached us.

In fact, six of the first seven women we treated prior to IVF transfers reported clinical pregnancies in their first IVF after therapy. Unless we and our patients were incredibly lucky, something of clinical interest was happening for these women.

When we began to track the success of the patients who came to our clinic to prepare their reproductive tracts for a more successful in vitro fertilization, the CDC-ASRM data proved invaluable. First, we knew that the national success rate of 28% per pregnancy after starting a cycle extrapolated into a 41% clinical pregnancy after transfer for women who made it to the transfer stage.[19] That data provided a comparison to our own success rate for women we treated before IVF transfer. The large database also provided a reasonable control we could use to compare our own patients' success rates with IVF vs. the norm (no therapy).

We studied the CDC-ASRM data measurement methods extensively in order to create a meaningful comparison suitable for publication.

After review by independent scientists and physicians, our research methodology was deemed valid.

We began to create a database of women who came to us for therapy and then went on for one (or more) IVF cycles within 15 months after therapy. Better understanding the scientific method now, we followed guidelines of the CDC and ASRM in tracking our success with these women, their cycles, and their transfers.

We gathered copious amounts of data, combed through every chart in the clinic, then called and recalled patients in order to create an accurate database of pregnancies, births, miscarriages, and successful and unsuccessful IVF transfers.

Twenty-five women were available for this study, which the biostatistician said was sufficient for statistical analysis. All of the participants received therapy, then underwent an IVF cycle after therapy using the mother's own fresh eggs.

This was a challenging group. Before treatment, 14 of the women reported a total of 21 prior natural pregnancies, but only 4 of the 21 pregnancies (19%) resulted in a birth.

Many of these women had also undergone earlier medically-assisted reproductive techniques (ART) such as IUI and IVF. Before therapy, the participants reported undergoing 78 prior ART attempts, including 54 intrauterine inseminations (IUIs). These 78 medical attempts resulted in only 3 pregnancies, and one full-term birth. This was a challenging population to treat, indeed!

After therapy, each of the 25 returned for follow-up IVF. Some chose to have more than one, so we limited the time frame to 15 months after therapy. We tracked the 33 IVF transfers completed within that time.

Results were fairly staggering, in that 22 of the 33 transfers (67%) after therapy resulted in clinical pregnancies and 15 of those (68% of pregnancies) resulted in live births. Such numbers would have been good, even for a less-challenging population.

Finally, we submitted our numbers to our biostatistician for statistical analysis and comparison to IVF without therapy. That analysis showed that IVF clinical pregnancy rates after therapy were 67%, compared to the control group's 41% success rate, which was an excellent result.

We then had to consider the significance of the numbers, i.e., did we have enough people in the study to provide meaningful results? In fact, we scored very high in statistical significance, with a probability score of ($P<.001$). This score indicates a very high degree of reliability, despite the fact that it was a relatively small study.

Several physicians and PhD scientists collaborated and created this study, which we submitted to *Medscape General Medicine*, likely the largest peer-reviewed medical journal in the world. *Medscape* is owned by WebMD, and had a readership of 2.5 million physician subscribers in 249 countries when they accepted our study. That study is available today at the US Library of Medicine or on the Internet via Medline search.

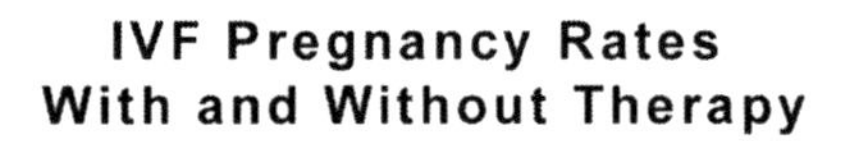

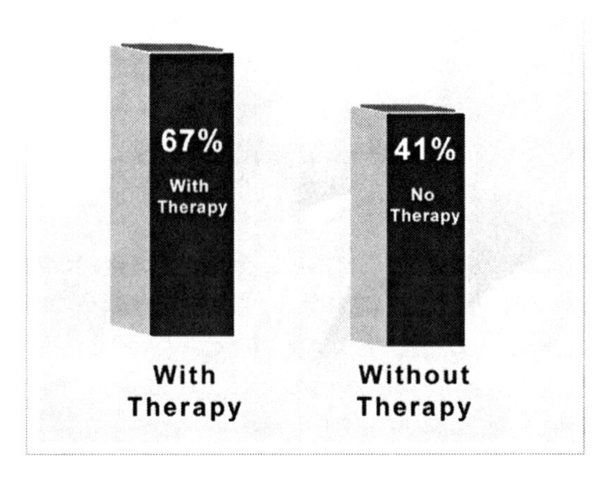

Six Keys to Boosting IVF Success

Why does our work increase IVF success rates? We can only surmise, but after assessing and treating these women, then reassessing them after therapy, we feel there are several areas in which therapy may have helped these women.

How Therapy Helps IVF

- Increases blood flow to ovaries and uterus
- Improves cervical mobility and ease of transfer
- Improves receptivity of uterine wall
- Decreases adhesions and spasm in the
- reproductive tract
- Improves hormonal function
- Improves whole body function, including pituitary-hypothalamus-ovarian communication

Increase blood flow to the ovaries and uterus

Most physicians and scientists accept the fact that massage increases blood flow. For centuries, people who receive massage have noticed that they leave therapy with a "reddish glow" at various areas of their bodies where blood flow has increased.

This increased blood flow is attributed to the theory that muscles relax during massage, allowing more space in arteries and veins. The additional space allows more blood to pump through the tunnels of these vessels.

Blood vessels exist throughout the body and provide nutrition to the brain, muscles, bones, organs, and their support structures. Blood is the fuel supply for most bodily structures; decreased blood supply equates to decreased function in most areas of the body. Increasing blood supply to any area will naturally increase its supply of fuel, thus increasing its ability to function effectively.

Because of their location and access to the outside environment, the vagina and cervix may be subjected to inflammation, infection, or trauma before and during childbearing years. The body's response to any of these tissue insults is to lay down cross-links, the building blocks of adhesions. When cross-links lay down in the vicinity of blood vessels, they can restrict the flow of blood to these delicate and vital organs, decreasing their ability to function. We believe that the increase of blood flow to the female reproductive organs is a primary reason that we have documented (and published) success in improving pregnancy rates for women who undergo in vitro fertilization after therapy.

Improve cervical mobility and ease of transfer

Adhesions deep within the cervix can pull the cervix out of its natural midline placement in the vagina. This adhesive pull can cause spasm and inflammation at the cervix. If the cervix is pulled backwards, forwards, or to one side, the pattern of adhesive cross-links within the cervix can create a recurring pull up into the uterus. This in turn can cause inflammation which increases incrementally with every step the woman takes. We have found this pattern can create an ongoing cycle of spasm-inflammation-adhesions. These initially tiny adhesions can tighten the cervix at the opening to the uterus, making sperm transfer (whether through intercourse, IUI or IVF) more difficult and sometimes causing pain with deep intercourse.

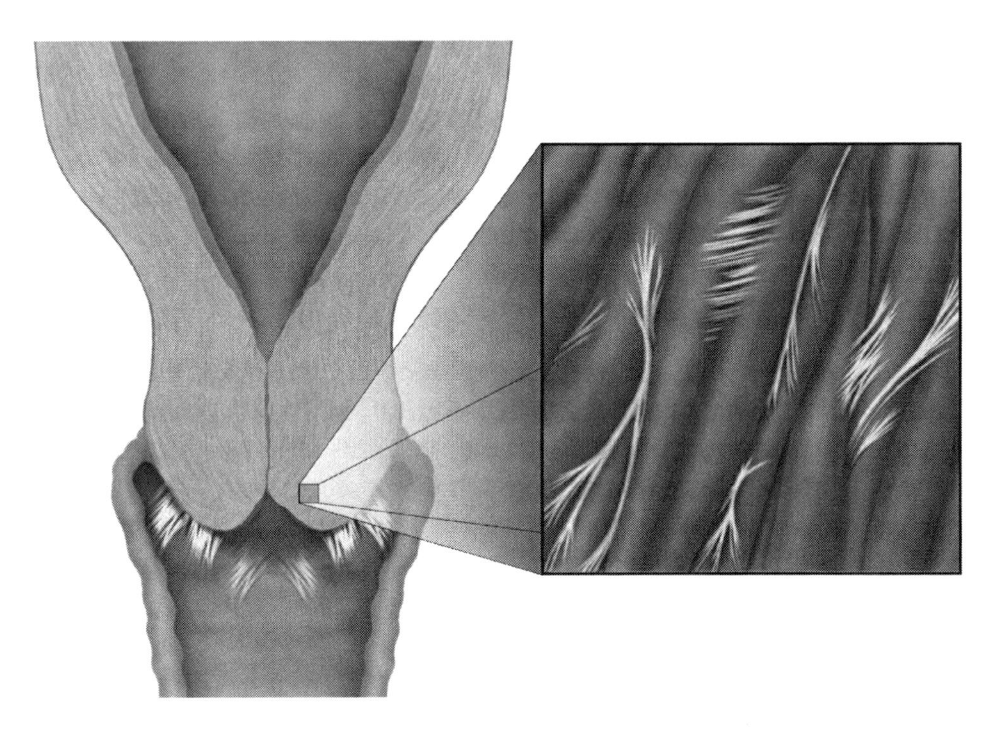

Adhesive cross-links can form outside the cervix, or deep within it, narrowing the opening for sperm, or causing pain with deep intercourse.

In fact, some women are first diagnosed with cervical stenosis (closing) or fibrosis (stiffness) when their physician evaluates them for a possible IUI or IVF transfer. After reviewing charts of dozens of patients, we feel that these tight or stiff conditions are caused by tiny adhesions that formed from earlier infections or medical procedures. The tiny adhesions appear to attach between muscle cells, deep within the cervix. When we treat this area, we find that positive changes are generally palpable to us and to the physician. IVF transfer becomes easier and implantation rates appear to increase significantly (per published studies) after therapy.

Improve receptivity of the uterine wall

The uterine wall is a complex structure consisting of smooth muscle fibers beneath delicate ciliated walls. Two of the primary functions of the uterine wall are to:

- create a surface suitable for implantation and
- gather the nutrients required to sustain a new embryo.

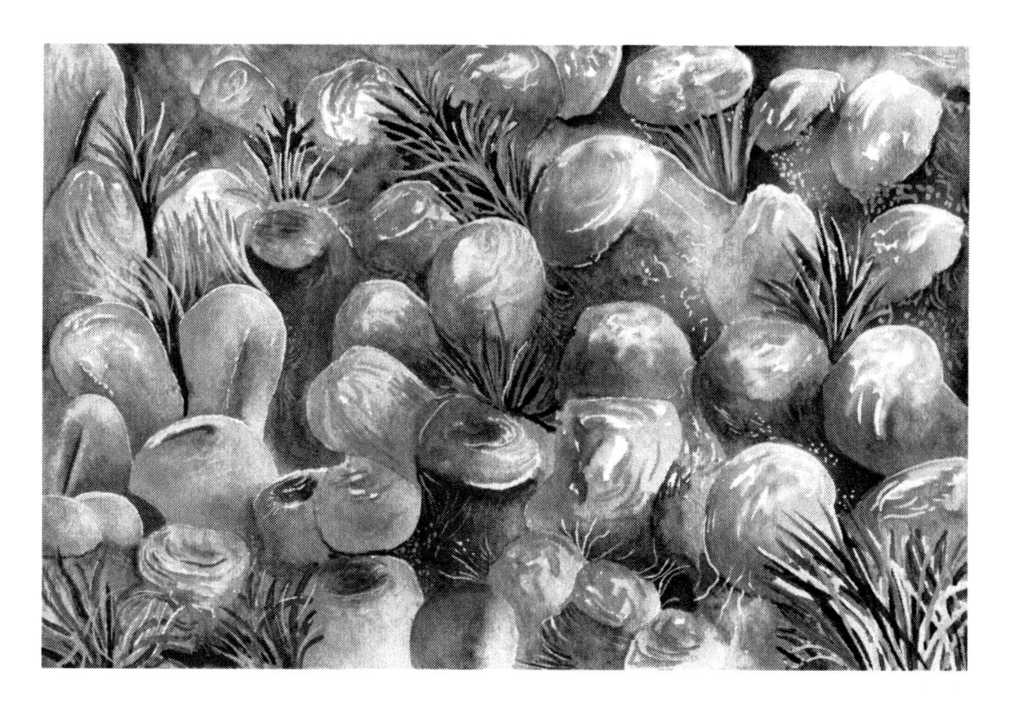

The uterine wall contains secretory cells (shown here, swelling after ovulation) nestled among delicate cilia

During the few days after ovulation, secretory cells swell as the uterus prepares to receive and nourish a fertilized egg. Thus, the surface structure of the uterine wall is of primary importance when the zygote (fertilized egg) enters the uterus, whether naturally or by IVF transfer.

The walls of the uterus are delicate, and they may be affected by several outside influences. Inflammation within the uterus can cause adhesions or increase temperature, killing sperm and creating a predisposition for miscarriage or failure to implant. In fact, intrauterine devices (IUDs) are used as a contraceptive device based on this principal; an IUD inserted into the uterine will create mild inflammation – enough to prevent a pregnancy.

As we have seen, the body's reaction to inflammation results in adhesive cross-links. These cross-links can lay down like a blanket over inflamed tissues to help prevent the spread of inflammation to other parts of the body. Even though the source of the inflammation has passed and the body has healed, the adhesive blanket that formed can remain on the wall of the uterus for a lifetime. This adhesive blanket can decrease the receptivity of the uterine wall to a fertilized egg.

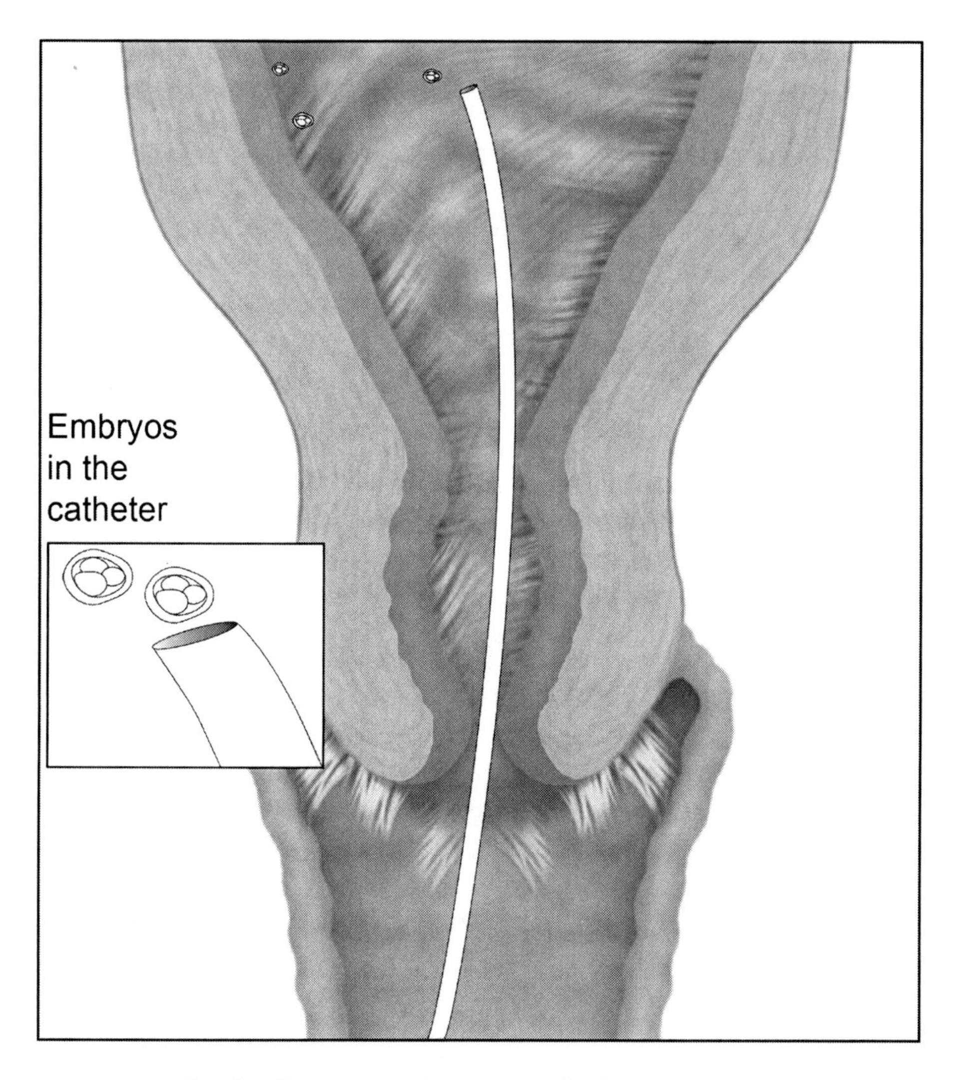

Small adhesions on the inner wall of the uterus can interfere with implantaion, whether natural or by IVF.

Adhesions affecting the broad, round and uterosacral ligaments can restrict the ability of the uterus to move freely within the pelvis. For example, if the ligaments are restricted on the right side, every step the woman takes with the right leg pulls on the uterus. This can create excess tension on the uterine wall, making implantation difficult.

Some of our primary goals as therapists for infertile women are to break down adhesive collagen into its individual elements, by separating collagenous cross-links from their neighbors. In doing so, we have found that implantation rates (clinical pregnancies) have markedly increased in the population of women who receive this therapy prior to in vitro fertilization.

Decrease adhesions & spasms in the reproductive tract

Adhesive processes occur in areas of the reproductive tract besides the uterus, including the ovaries, the fallopian tubes, and the delicate fimbriated fingers at the end of the tubes that are designed to grasp the egg from the ovary.

In muscular structures such as the uterus and fallopian tubes, this "gluing down" effect of collagen cross-links can cause spasm as tissues that are designed to be free and mobile become bound to each other. Restrained by tiny but powerful collagenous bonds, these organs are unable to undergo movements required to function normally. Thus restricted, the muscles can go into spasm as they strain against small but powerful, restrictive bonds as the woman goes through all of her normal daily activities, as well as during her menstrual periods or ovulation.

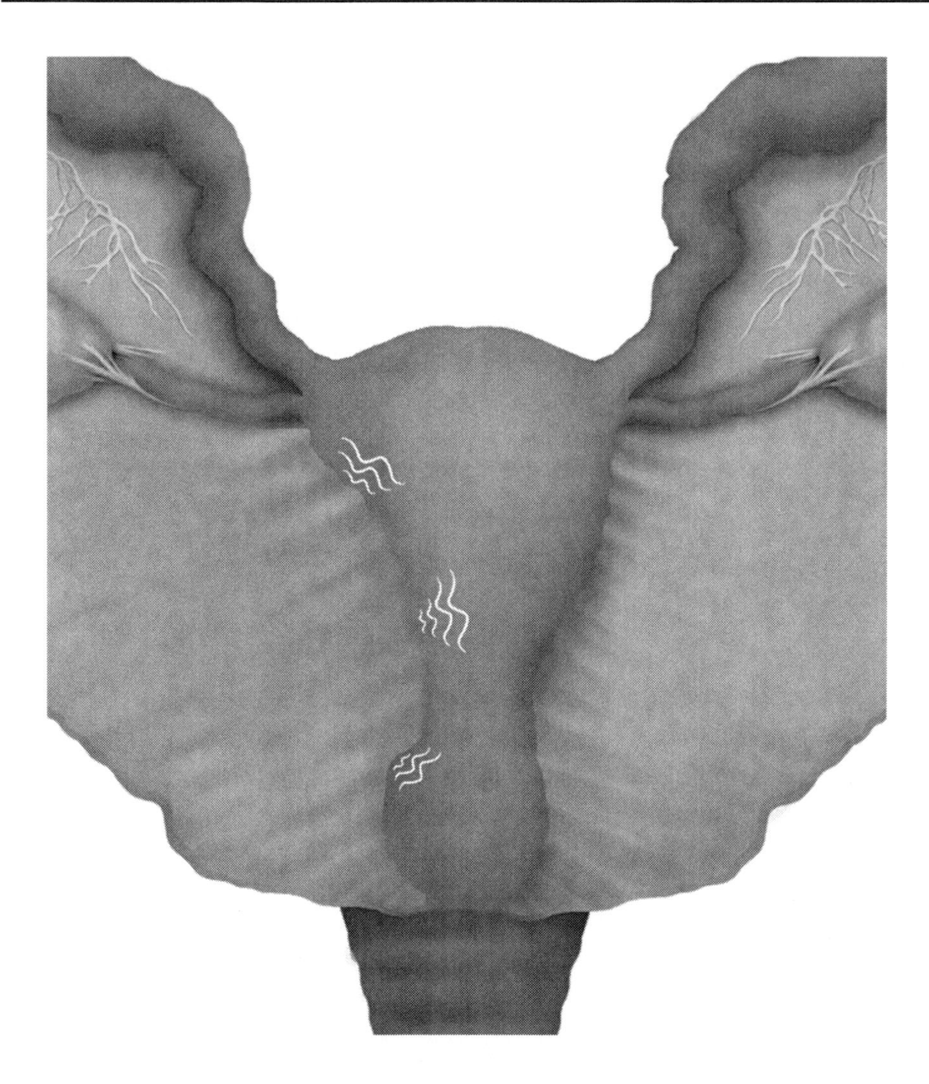

The uterus may go into spasm, decreasing its receptivity to a fertilized egg.

Improve hormonal function

As noted earlier in this book, we were surprised to witness natural pregnancies and improved hormonal function in women we treated who presented at our clinic with high FSH levels. We believe that some of this may be due to improved blood flow and mobility of the ovaries.

However, we were surprised to see dramatic improvements in FSH levels for women who arrived at the clinic with unusually high FSH — even menopausal levels, in several cases. Over time, we have come to believe that much of the problem of hormonal infertility can be reversed and function improved using the same mechanical process that appears to deform and detach cross-links elsewhere in the body. For more on this, please refer to Chapter Eight.

Age 43, Failed IVF, and Prior Ectopic Pregnancy

- Christine's Story

I yearned for children when I turned thirty-one, but Mr. Right was nowhere to be found and I wasn't really paying any attention to the tick-tock of the biological clock. It never occurred to me that I might have difficulties conceiving when I was finally ready to start my family. As an educated woman, I was woefully unaware of the term "advanced maternal age" and the exponentially difficult odds of conceiving as the years progressed. Mistakenly I thought women were able to conceive at the same success rate until menopause. Not until I entered my 40s did I learn that I might have problems due to my age!

I immediately decided to undergo IVF. After reviewing a chart with rates of successful pregnancies rapidly diminishing in my age range, I knew my age was an enormous challenge and that I needed to do everything I could to maximize my chances of success.

When my first IVF transfer ended in a chemical pregnancy, I rapidly began to look for alternative and complementary therapies. A couple years earlier, I had read a magazine article about the Wurn Technique®. I remember thinking how interesting it was, though I couldn't imagine ever needing anything like that.

Now faced with my own infertility, I researched my options online and again came across this special Wurn Technique®. I pored through the Clear Passage Therapies (CPT) website and called their headquarters for more information. CPT cited remarkable pregnancy statistics and offered many powerful patient stories: story after story of successful pregnancy after long periods of infertility. Learning that my chances of success could be increased relatively easily convinced me that I had to try this new kind of therapy. I wanted to know I had done everything I possibly could to help prepare my body (and mind) for a healthy, full-term pregnancy.

During my initial evaluation, I quickly discovered how knowledgeable my therapists were. Their level of attention to all of the parts of my body was extraordinary. They looked at how I stood, leaned, and sat, with my eyes open and closed. Even though I was an extremely healthy person (I always worked out, did yoga, and had run

As an educated woman, I was woefully unaware of the term "advanced maternal age" and the exponentially difficult odds of conceiving as the years progressed.

marathons in the past) they noted abnormalities in places I didn't know anything was wrong.

As they moved from examining my posture to examining my organs, they explained everything they discovered and felt. It was tremendously comforting; they had an intuitive sense of my body. I knew I had placed my body in the hands of highly skilled professionals.

When they began treating my fallopian tubes, they said that my left fallopian tube felt like it was folded sideways. It was a very profound moment, knowing a therapist could feel that deeply in my body and could manipulate and improve it. It became clear that this unique therapy was an entirely different level of treatment than I had ever experienced. As a previous marathon runner, I had seen plenty of physical therapists, but never with the level of attention and expertise that I was now receiving for my fertility.

By the end of my treatment, I just felt wonderful. I was walking better and more smoothly. I stood taller and overall felt better and happier. I felt a renewed sense of confidence. Before treatment, I had chronic pain in my back that would flare up after walking or shopping for an hour. I thought it was a normal part of aging. But after treatment, that pain vanished.

After I completed my therapy, I knew CPT was the best thing I could have done for myself, even if I didn't become pregnant. It helped put my body and mind in the right place; I was confident that it would increase my chances of pregnancy.

The week after treatment, I started medication for my second IVF cycle. It was indeed successful and I had a great pregnancy! I hadn't felt that good in a while. I was fortunate to maintain an increasing level of activity throughout my pregnancy. I followed the exercise instructions my therapists had given me and also did prenatal yoga and step aerobics. I kept my heart monitor on to make sure my heart rate didn't go above the recommended level and I was able to continue doing aerobics until the day before I delivered.

I know my therapy at CPT made a difference between my first and second IVF transfers. In fact, two physicians told me how great my uterus looked after therapy.

At the ripe age of 44, I delivered my beautiful, healthy baby. I know my therapy at CPT made a difference between my first and second IVF transfers. In fact, two physicians told me how great my uterus looked after therapy. I am sincerely grateful to have had the opportunity to experience this exceptional therapy.

Improve whole body function and communication

Reproductive endocrinologists and other infertility specialists have long recognized the existence and importance of the "pituitary-hypothalamus-ovarian axis." This term refers to the intricate communication loop of hormones during the reproductive cycle, leading to conception. While various theories have been postulated as to how the pituitary-hypothalamus (PH) complex (in the head) communicates with the ovaries (in the pelvis), the exact method of communication remains a mystery. Notwithstanding, the fact of communication between these distant structures is relatively undisputed. For example, the ovary signals the PH when it is ready to ovulate. The PH releases follicle stimulating hormone (FSH) to help the egg mature.

In our clinical experience, women who have high FSH or who frequently failed to become pregnant via IVF often present with physical restrictions between these two distant hormonal centers.

We find tightness in the structure of the body between the ovaries and the PH is a primary cause of failure to conceive, both naturally and via IVF.

In fact, most women who have failed one or more IVF transfers often present with one or more of the following structural abnormalities:

- Tightness in the neck
- Tightness at the base of the skull
- Headaches at the base of the skull, temples or top of the head
- Soreness at the upper trapezius or between the shoulder blades
- Tailbone pain, or pain with sexual intercourse
- Asymmetry of the lower aspect of the temporal bones (the

bumps of the bones under the ears) with one (usually the right) noticeably lower than the other

- Asymmetry of the cheek bones (under the eyes)
- Asymmetry of the two sides of mandible (jaw), or TMJ symptoms

Protected and surrounded as it is by the sphenoid bone (which runs through the cranium, from temple to temple) the pituitary gland is nevertheless in a very vulnerable position in the body. Any torsion, asymmetry, excess tension, or lack of mobility in the sphenoid (which surrounds the pituitary), will cause a consequent pull and tension on the delicate glands it contains, decreasing their function.

The 28 cranial bones (excluding the teeth) create the structure of the skull in a similar fashion to continental shelves that create the surface of the earth. Some cranial bones create the surface of the skull, such as the frontal and parietal bones at the forehead and the top of the head. Others descend deeply into the head, such as the sphenoid (between the temples) and the occiput (which starts at the base of our skull, but meets the sphenoid deep within the tissues of the skull). Because of their intricate attachments and close relationships with each other, any torsion, pull, or restriction of mobility in one of the cranial bones can cause an asymmetrical pull in other cranial bones. Like other areas of the body that are pulled from their normal orientation, we have to assume this happens in the brain as well, especially when we witness the positive results after treating in this area.

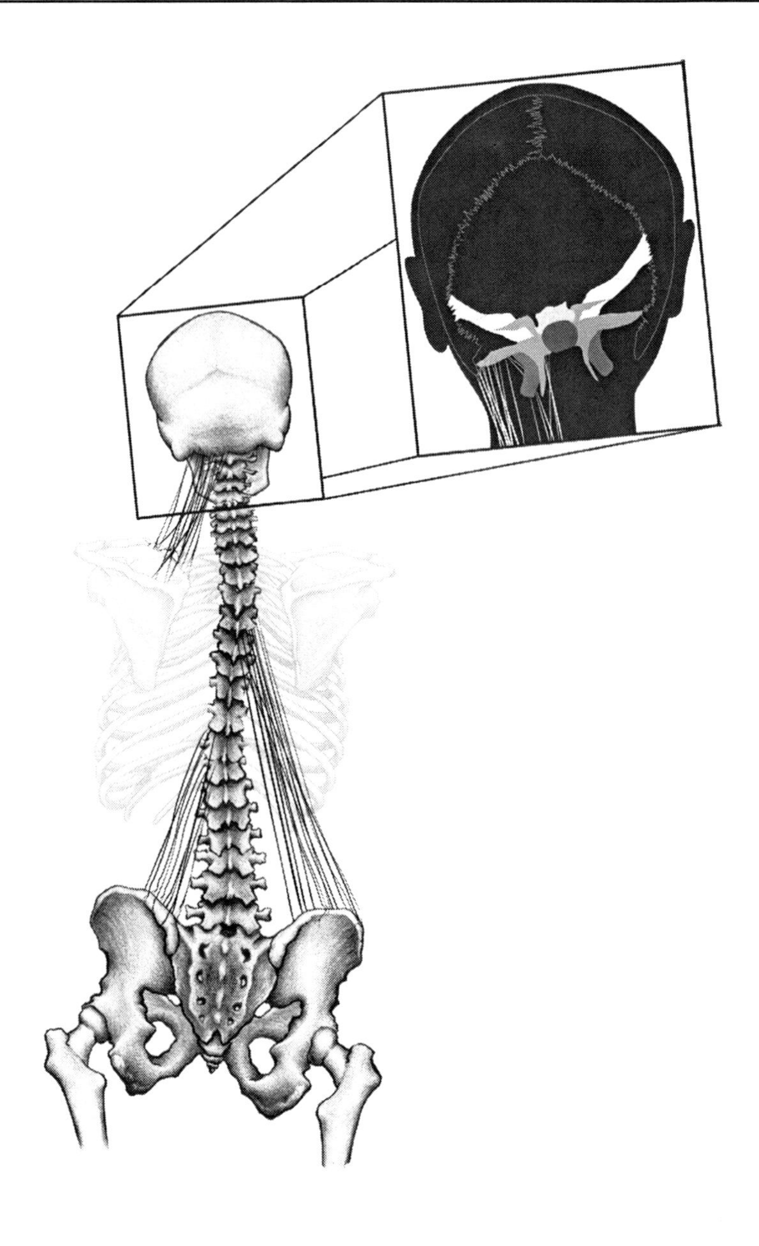

Large structures from the neck, shoulders or back can pull on delicate cranial bones, causing unusual tensions on tiny structures in the head.

As noted earlier, the sphenoid (which contains the PH complex) articulates with bones above, beside, below it and all the way through the center of the cranium to the occiput at the base of the skull. Thus, any unusual forces on any of those bones can pull the pituitary out of its normal midline alignment, compromising the sphenoid and thus the PH complex.

Moreover, the skull sits at the top of the neck, which rests at the top of the spine. The position of the spine is greatly dependent upon the position of the pelvic bones which form its foundation. If the pelvic bones are out of alignment, the spine starts its upward course at an angle, creating or contributing to a scoliosis. At the top of that chain is the skull and neck; at the center of that is the PH complex. Thus, external forces from other cranial bones and down to the spine into the pelvis can create torsion of the sphenoid, thus (we believe) adversely affecting the pituitary function in some people.

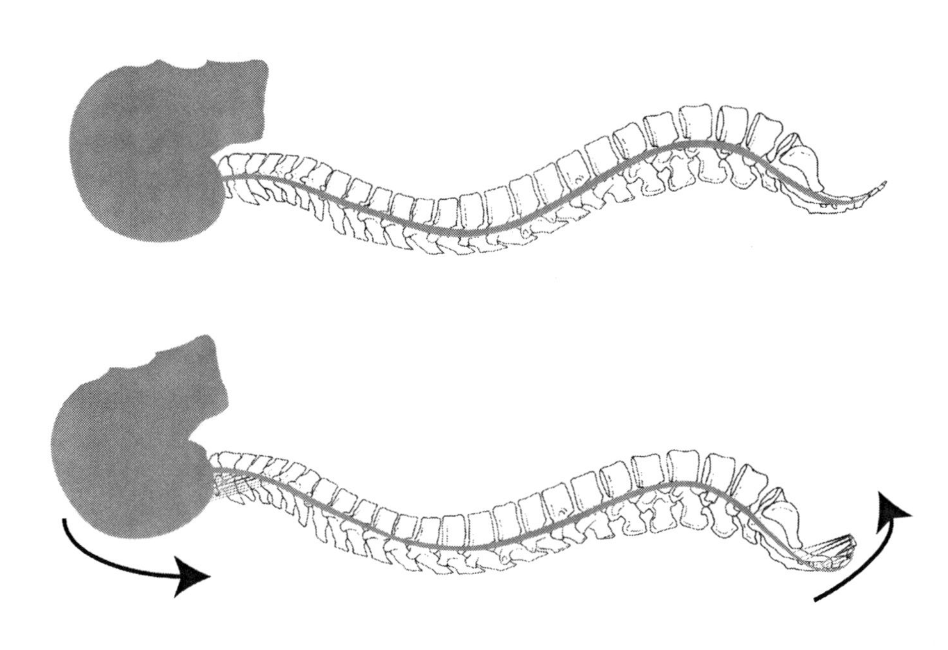

We note this because clinically, we often see these forces and biodynamics at work in women who present for therapy with high FSH. As noted earlier in this book, the vast majority of them exhibited significant improvement in FSH levels (or natural pregnancies) when we addressed this part of their biomechanics in therapy. (See Chapter Eight for more information and clinical trial results.)

Remarkable Patient Successes

For reproduction to occur, so many processes must happen simultaneously or in sequence that entire colleges of medicine are devoted solely to reproduction.

With so many processes occurring in harmony, it is no wonder that some things do not go as planned. The smallest disruption during any step of the process can cause failure of the entire process, and conception will not occur.

Similarly, many patients and their physicians find that a small change in the reproductive tract is all that is required in order for a previously failed procedure or process to succeed. The challenge is often finding the areas or processes that need to change, then doing what is needed to repair them without causing other problems or adverse side effects.

We have found that therapy improves function for women undergoing the remarkable process of IVF. Clinically, we have noted that introducing this manual therapy to treatment of the female reproductive organs appears to improve most of the processes involved in reproduction, whether natural or by IVF.

Blocked Fallopian Tubes and Scar Tissue after Chlamydia

- Wendy's Story

Wendy's struggle with infertility began in her early twenties. She contracted Chlamydia and went to her doctor immediately. The doctor told her that he could take care of it and she should be "fine."

Wendy didn't think anything of it again until she was thirty-five and wanted to become pregnant. She went to her doctor for tests and learned that her fallopian tubes were blocked. Her doctor informed her that Chlamydia was probably the culprit. Chlamydia is often known as a "silent" disease because it shows very few symptoms and carriers may not know when they contract it. In women, the bacteria travel through the cervix, uterus, and to the fallopian tubes, where it can cause inflammation and scar tissue to form, often causing the fallopian tubes to block.

Chlamydia is often known as a "silent" disease because it shows very few symptoms and carriers do not know when they contract it.

Wendy's doctor suggested she undergo surgery to open her blocked fallopian tubes, but after researching the success rates, Wendy decided she didn't want to undergo the procedure. Wendy told us, "I even considered IVF, but my health insurance didn't cover it."

She then researched different treatment options on the web. She found Clear Passage Therapies (CPT) and felt that it was a treatment option she was comfortable with.

Wendy made an appointment and flew down to our clinic for an intensive week of treatment. She told us, "Treatment was really great. I could feel all of the adhesions loosening. I felt much better afterwards."

Wendy and her husband tried to get pregnant naturally for a year after treatment and then decided to pursue in vitro fertilization. She told us, "My new insurance said they would cover it and we made the appointment right away."

The transfer was successful and Wendy became pregnant. She told us, "I felt very lucky that I got pregnant with my first try. While I was at the IVF clinic, there was another woman who was there and it was her sixth IVF. I really feel that my treatment at CPT helped me become pregnant with my first IVF."

Wendy later gave birth to a boy in perfect health.

Extensive Endometriosis

- Megan's Story

My husband and I had tried for a little over two years to get pregnant. When I finally got pregnant, I was thrilled, but was quickly depressed to learn it was ectopic. I had emergency surgery and one of my fallopian tubes was removed. The surgery confirmed my doctor's suspicion of endometriosis and he said it was pretty extensive.

My sister, a physical therapist, told me about Clear Passage Therapies (CPT), a clinic that could help reduce endometriosis and improve infertility. But I dismissed it — I am a prosecutor and am very skeptical.

After Clomid and artificial insemination both failed, my sister again mentioned CPT so I began reading up and watching the DVD. My sister was convinced that the bladder surgery I had when I was younger also made me a good candidate. I was very unsure what to do, since IVF was our last option and our insurance didn't cover it. I knew I only had one shot at IVF and we couldn't afford any other tries. I had never heard of in vitro working on the first try so I was discouraged. I had to decide whether to go straight to IVF or spend more money preparing for the cycle with CPT. All of my friends were pretty skeptical about their treatment, as was my husband.

Finally, I decided to try CPT because I didn't want to spend my whole life just wondering, "What if . . ." When my flight was the last one into Florida because of a hurricane, I decided that was a good omen.

I knew I only had one shot at IVF and we couldn't afford any other tries.

Once I began my treatment, my doubts were erased and I had a very good feeling. I could feel pulling sensations, so I thought something must be going on. I faithfully walked and drank water after each treatment, as instructed by the therapists.

I had treatment at CPT in July and then had my IVF transfer in August. I was thrilled to learn I was pregnant. My pregnancy went smoothly and I now have a beautiful, healthy baby girl. I look at her and cry because I feel so lucky to have her.

Using Intuition through Fertility Treatments

- Hana's Story

The first time I got pregnant, my husband and I had only tried for four months. As a physician, my husband knew that most couples needed about six months to a year to conceive, so we were happy to be pregnant. But then I miscarried at seven weeks. That's when I really started to think about infertility and read more about it.

As a physician, my husband knew that most couples needed six months to a year to conceive.

We didn't try again for another five months. When we did, we were dismayed to find that we could not achieve a pregnancy despite our attempts. It was strange because while we couldn't become pregnant again, I kept feeling like I was pregnant. I experienced all of the similar symptoms as before — my period would be a couple of days late, I experienced cramping, breast tenderness, sometimes I felt bloated, etc.

After five months of trying, we went to a fertility specialist and completed a full work-up. Everything came back looking just fine: my tubes, ovaries, hormones, and blood work all looked normal.

The specialists recommended we try an intrauterine insemination (IUI) in conjunction with Clomid, a fertility drug that improves ovulation. We tried three rounds, but again there was no pregnancy. However, each month I still felt like I was pregnant early on.

We then decided to do IVF. After they retrieved my eggs, my doctor said they all looked great and strong. The IVF team placed three embryos in my uterus, but all post-transfer tests came back negative for pregnancy.

At that point, I knew something else had to be happening. While researching different techniques and treatments, I came across Clear Passage Therapies (CPT). In the past, I had experienced interstitial cystitis (recurring pain and discomfort of the bladder). I thought that maybe whatever had caused this condition had also caused abnormalities in my reproductive tract that prevented a successful pregnancy.

I scheduled myself for treatment, but continued to search for other answers and possible causes for my infertility. After reading about genetic disorders, I asked my doctor to perform a karyotype test which could identify an abnormality in my chromosomes that would prevent me from becoming pregnant or cause me to experience frequent miscarriages. My doctor said it was expensive and not necessary, but I wanted to make sure there was nothing wrong.

After completing the blood work, we found I had a balanced chromosomal translocation. This somewhat rare condition decreased my chances of a healthy full-term pregnancy to 20%. I was told that 80% of the time, I wouldn't be able to conceive or I would have a miscarriage by eight weeks gestation.

My husband and I discussed our options and we decided to pursue preimplantation genetic diagnosis (PGD), a test that could determine if our embryos had a balanced number of chromosomes before they were implanted in my uterus. PGD is completed in conjunction with IVF. The ovaries are stimulated with hormones so they produce a large quantity of eggs, which are retrieved and mixed with sperm to form embryos. Afterwards, the PGD is performed to test for abnormalities and the healthy embryos are placed in the uterus. Although the procedure was extremely expensive, we decided to do it rather than to possibly suffer more miscarriages.

I was still scheduled to attend an intensive week of therapy at CPT before my IVF and PGD, and I decided to attend. I wanted to make sure my uterus and entire reproductive system were ready for my upcoming procedure. I had spent a lot of money and I wanted to increase my chances of success.

I attended therapy for a week in August and then began my IVF medication in September. The medication was intended to stimulate my ovaries, but my estrogen levels rose too rapidly (a condition know as hyperstimulation). In essence, I reacted too well to the medicine. My doctors were still able to retrieve 10 eggs, which were mixed with my husband's sperm. But because I had hyperstimulated, the embryos needed to be frozen and my transfer was postponed for one month.

We transferred that single embryo, and were thrilled to find that I was pregnant.

When my body was ready for the transfer, the embryos were thawed. One embryo did not survive the thaw. The PGD was completed on the remaining embryos and only one was balanced/normal, meaning it did not contain the unbalanced translocation. We transferred that single embryo, and were thrilled to find that I was pregnant.

My pregnancy proceeded without complications and I delivered my healthy baby boy via C-section at full-term!

Looking back, I cannot scientifically say whether I would have gotten pregnant without treatment at CPT. Although my main issue was a translocation, I did only have one embryo to be transferred, so my chances for a pregnancy were only about 30-50%. I wonder if the embryo (now my son!) would have adhered to the wall properly if I hadn't received therapy at CPT. Looking back, I believe the treatment I received at CPT set the stage for a successful pregnancy by preparing my uterus to accept the embryo.

It's important to listen to your intuition and your body, and investigate other options on your own.

I can only speak from my own experience, but I would say doctors don't always have all the answers. It's important to listen to your intuition and your body and investigate other options on your own. For me, I believe it was the combination of PGD and CPT that enabled me to become pregnant.

13 Years Infertile with Endometriosis

- Ava's Story

Where do I begin? I'm a 39-year-old mother of twins. I endured 13 years of disappointment without any medical explanation for my inability to conceive. The only obstacle I thought I really had to overcome was having only one fallopian tube. Years earlier, I had a tubal pregnancy and the doctors had to remove my tube during emergency surgery. Thus I understood that I would need more time to become pregnant than if I had both.

I felt I would be successful at some point within the first few years of trying to become pregnant, but that was not the case. I made a commitment to myself that I would not be consumed by conceiving. Being a person of strong faith, I knew there was a reason for everything and my first sign was the breakup of that marriage.

However, I was blessed to start my life over a few years later with my new (and adoring) husband Andrew. Prior to our vows, I made sure that Andrew knew my medical history and my years of infertility. He said, "I fell in love with you first and anything more in our time together would be a blessing." He has always put me above all else.

We tried the first couple of years to conceive on our own — still nothing. We decided to consult my gynecologist, who happened to be a fertility doctor, to get his opinion on where to go from there.

Unlike my first husband, Andrew was willing to undergo whatever tests were necessary to ensure he did not have a medical issue. All of his results came back fine. We were back to square one: exploring my reproductive health. Naturally, this was no surprise.

After about eight months and some unsuccessful tries by my gynecologist, he referred us to a specialist. Upon meeting the reproductive endocrinologist, we knew he wasn't going to waste any time answering our questions. His approach was no nonsense and very prompt. Our first meeting was in June, and by August I underwent surgery to confirm that I had stage three endometriosis, which is considered severe.

After he made this diagnosis, our specialist outlined our options and instructed us to make any decisions necessary by February. The urgency was due to the nature of my endometriosis and its rapid growth.

Over the next month we discussed our options, and how on earth we were going to come up with the funds needed for the procedures we were going to try.

Ironically, just as we were considering our options, a coworker of Andrew's shared an interesting column on infertility with him. Andrew researched it further before sharing the article with me; he did not want to get my hopes up with another treatment option.

What Andrew stumbled on was a new infertility therapy provided by manual physical therapists at Clear Passage Therapies (CPT). In our research on this therapy, it almost sounded too easy and too good to be true. The testimonials they shared on their website gave such hope to women like me.

It didn't take us long to decide it was something we needed. In my case, they were going to help me not only to become a mom, but also with some severe back pain that I learned later was associated with the endometriosis.

We made the arrangements and traveled to their clinic. The clinic ensured they had as much of my medical history as possible, prior to my arrival. Once at the clinic, they reviewed my information with me to create an individualized plan for me.

No drugs or surgery were a part of their technique. It was a combination of physical therapy and deep tissue massage and manipulation. That may have been why Andrew and I were a little skeptical at first. In today's age of modern medicine, we're generally programmed to expect anything effective to be intrusive and involve drugs.

I received therapy for five consecutive days for roughly four hours per day. I cannot say enough about the staff or the therapy. It was a very unique process and one I'll never forget. They felt that the adhesions from the endometriosis and surgeries were acting like glue in my pelvis, binding my reproductive organs and causing me pain.

The first thing that happened following my therapy is that the endometriosis pain I had lived with for over ten years completely disappeared.

The first thing that happened following my therapy is that the endometriosis pain I had lived with for over ten years completely disappeared. My body felt looser and somehow more free when I walked and moved.

They did so much for Andrew and me that I believe it was due to their therapy and God's blessing that my IVF procedure, done four months later, was a complete success. I was also able to become pregnant a second time and now have two children. CPT cares so much for their patients.

Secondary Infertility, Endometriosis and Failed IVF

- Erin's Story

My husband and I were married in 1995 and we started trying for a family right away. I thought it was going to be easy to become pregnant. I am a physical therapist and have studied physiology and the reproductive system in my course work, and I was confident we could get the timing right. Furthermore, I am one of six children and all of my sisters were able to get pregnant easily.

As a woman, I felt like it was part of my responsibility to be able to carry a baby, and I couldn't.

I went off my birth control and I thought I could tell when I was ovulating. After a year passed with no pregnancy, I went to see my doctor. I received the "try a bottle of wine" answer and finally consulted an Ob/Gyn for help.

He did some general testing, but everything came back normal. Shortly afterwards, I was pregnant, but dismayed to learn that it was a tubal pregnancy. I underwent emergency surgery.

Even though the surgeons were able to save my tube, I still wasn't able to become pregnant afterwards. It was a very lonely feeling — one that you cannot understand until you live with it. It was always painful when someone said, "I know how you feel," when they really didn't. My husband was very supportive of me and our situation, but I don't think he could fully understand the disappointment I felt as a woman whose body was not performing as it should. As a woman, I felt like it was part of my responsibility to be able to carry a baby, and I couldn't.

I finally saw an infertility specialist who checked my thyroid levels and found them to be abnormal. She was disappointed that my initial doctor had not checked my thyroid and immediately placed me on medication.

(As a physical therapist) I could connect with what Clear Passage said about the importance of having mobility in all tissues.

She also suspected I had endometriosis and scar tissue from my previous surgery. I agreed to undergo laparoscopic surgery and the doctor discovered I had stage IV endometriosis and scar tissue. She removed everything she could and I was able to get pregnant directly after surgery. Unfortunately, I miscarried again.

We then decided to do an IVF. I was fortunate enough to become pregnant and deliver my son.

When he turned eighteen months old, we decided to try again with IVF. My cycle was not successful, and my husband and I wanted to try a third time. But before we began, we wanted to make sure we had done everything in our power to ensure a successful transfer.

My husband is also a physical therapist, and we had both heard about Clear Passage Therapies (CPT). I could connect with what CPT said about scar tissue and the importance of having mobility in all tissues.

I decided to attend treatment and went for an intensive week of therapy directly before my third IVF transfer. I felt their treatment helped my body get back to a normal state.

I also underwent acupuncture treatments as a way to prepare my uterine lining and blood flow to the area.

My IVF transfer went well. My doctors decided to perform ICSI to ensure my eggs were fertilized and also did assisted hatching. When we learned we were pregnant with twins, we were so grateful our doctors had done everything they could to ensure our success and I had done everything I could to ensure my body was ready.

Results for Women with Prior Failed IVFs

After we published this study, we took a closer look at a sub-set of participants — women who had failed earlier IVF transfers. We wanted to see if therapy might help women who had not become pregnant by one or more earlier IVF transfers.

Criteria for acceptance into this pilot study were very tight. We accepted only those patients who had

- never had a clinical pregnancy in any IVF transfer they had ever attempted, and
- had undergone at least two prior IVF transfers.

Because of the narrow parameters of this study, only seven women fit the criteria for inclusion. When we compiled the data, the results seemed remarkable to several of us (though they did not seem relevant to our biostatistician). You may decide for yourself.

Before therapy, these women had failed a total of 17 IVF cycles, and none of them had ever had a pregnancy after any IVF. Thus, they came into the study with a 0% (0/17) success rate for both pregnancy and birth.

After therapy, these women (who had failed so many prior attempts) each underwent an IVF cycle. In that first cycle after therapy, five of the seven (5/7 = 71%) had a clinical pregnancy and four of them (4/7 = 57%) had live births. More specific results are shown in the two paragraphs below.

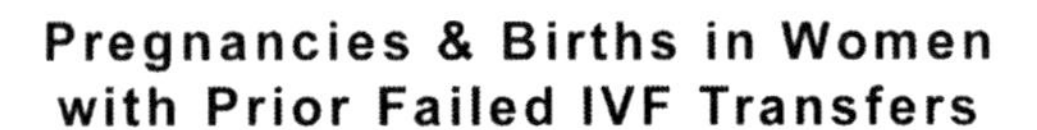

Pregnancies & Births in Women with Prior Failed IVF Transfers

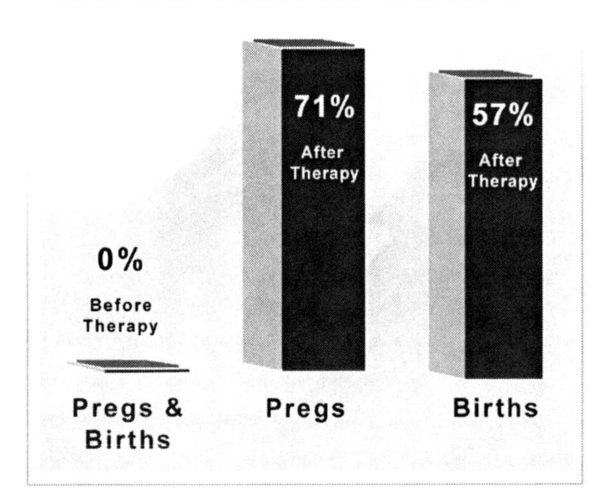

Based on these two studies, we feel confident of our ability to significantly increase pregnancy rates for most of the women we treat prior to IVF transfer.

Emergency Ectopic Surgery and Two Failed IVFs

- Amelia's Story

Three years into their marriage, Amelia and Jonathan were ready to start their family. "I was only 31," Amelia told us. "We never thought we might have difficulty conceiving. I had never had any gynecological problems at all."

But when months of trying turned into a year, Amelia looked for ways she could track and improve their chances for conception. She began charting her temperature and also casually mentioned her concerns to her doctor, who assured her no significant treatment was necessary at the time.

"We just kept trying and trying," Amelia explained. "We finally became pregnant three years later." She learned she was pregnant from a home pregnancy test.

I continued to have a lot of pain. I kept calling my doctor's office but they told me it was normal.

However, she began spotting within three days. She immediately called the doctor, who explained she was probably miscarrying. Three days later, Amelia had an ultrasound that confirmed she had miscarried.

"I continued to have a lot of pain," Amelia told us. "I kept calling my doctor's office but they told me it was normal." Two weeks passed and her pain became searing. "I didn't call the doctor again," Amelia explained. "I thought I would just be told the same thing."

That night, she woke up with the worst pain she had ever experienced and rushed to the hospital. The doctors discovered that Amelia's fallopian tube had burst. The pain she had experienced for the past two weeks was due to an ectopic pregnancy.

Amelia underwent emergency surgery and the doctors had no choice but to remove the tube. "It was a slow recovery," Amelia told us. "I had lost so much blood and was so weak. I also continued to experience pain."

When her pain did not subside after three months, Amelia changed doctors. Her new doctor suspected that her pain might be due to scar tissue and decided to perform an exploratory laparoscopic surgery.

During the procedure, the physician performed a dye test that showed her remaining fallopian tube was partially blocked. The doctor also found signs of endometriosis.

Amelia's fallopian tube had burst.

"They basically told me to stop trying to get pregnant," Amelia said. "They were concerned I might have another ectopic pregnancy because my only remaining tube was partially blocked, and I had endometriosis."

Amelia was referred to an infertility specialist, who immediately recommended IVF. "That was a scary day," Amelia recalled. "They talk about your eggs, your production, and all of that. By the end, it sounds like it will take a miracle to get pregnant."

Amelia and Jonathan decided to proceed with IVF. When it was unsuccessful, they decided to wait a cycle and try a second time. "I felt dejected when it didn't work the second time," Amelia told us. "We had long blown through the little bit of money our insurance gave us for infertility treatment. I was frustrated and scared. After all the disappointments, I didn't know if I wanted to continue with the infertility treatments."

They decided to take time off to make the right decision. "We weren't sure if we wanted to adopt or whether we should do another IVF cycle," Amelia said. "Personally, I never wanted to do IVF again. With all of the shots, weight gain, and emotional ups and downs, I just didn't want to consider IVF again."

While trying to make this difficult decision, one of Amelia's friends shared an article about Clear Passage Therapies (CPT) with her. After researching the treatment, Amelia and Jonathan decided it was something she should try.

Over the course of three months, Amelia underwent 20 hours of treatment. "From week to week, I couldn't feel a significant difference in my body because at that time I did not have any pain. But the therapy did give me a better sense of my body, and I knew the changes might not be something I would feel right away."

After treatment, Amelia and Jonathan decided to wait three months before they made any further decisions. At the end of that time, they considered their options again. Amelia told us, "My husband really wanted to do another round of IVF. Even though I did not think it would work, I reluctantly agreed to undergo the procedure."

When they consulted with the fertility specialists, they learned that the clinic had recently changed their fertility protocol and medications. "Even with the changes," Amelia said, "I still didn't think it would work."

It's hard to believe we went through so much to get where we are today. You have to listen to yourself, and consider all of the options.

But to their surprise, that transfer was successful and Amelia became pregnant with twins. "My pregnancy was a bit rough for a while, but I managed to carry my boys for 37 weeks." Joshua and Matthew were born healthy.

Now, Amelia's twin boys are three years old. "They are certainly high energy!" she told us. "It's hard to believe we went through so much to get where we are today. I really learned to keep an open mind and be assertive. I used to think that if the doctor says you have the flu, you have the flu. But, after my experience with infertility, I know you really have to listen to yourself and consider all of the options."

Unexpected Natural Pregnancies After IVF

Small changes in the reproductive process can increase IVF success rates. As the reproductive tissues are released from their glue-like bonds, the same small positive changes can also precede unexpected natural pregnancies. We have been pleased to see this happen in many cases.

Four Unsuccessful IVFs, then Natural Pregnancy

- Rachael's Story

My husband, Ethan, and I tried to have a baby for over five years with no success.

My physician told me my chances of a natural pregnancy were less than 10% due to severe pelvic adhesions that blocked my fallopian tubes. He also warned that even if I was able to become pregnant, there was a great risk for an ectopic pregnancy (a pregnancy that remains in the fallopian tube). For these reasons, my physician felt my only options were in-vitro fertilization (IVF) or adoption. He also stressed that I needed to make a decision quickly because of my age.

Adoption sounded wonderful, but the fact that I could not experience pregnancy was horribly depressing and I felt like I had failed our marriage. Fortunately, my husband was very supportive and told me that he did not marry me just to have children.

The fact that I could not experience pregnancy was horribly depressing and I felt like I had failed our marriage.

We waited a little over a year to do our first IVF. It required many visits to the doctor and all kinds of different medication. Many of the hormones I was given resulted in symptoms such as moodiness and weight gain. After three IVF transfers, I still had no success.

Afterwards, my massage therapist friend asked me if I had ever heard of Clear Passage Therapies (CPT). At that moment, I was not interested in learning about a new intervention for getting pregnant. I had been experiencing emotional highs and lows for many years and wanted to give my body a break.

A few days later, another friend of mine who was also suffering from infertility problems called me and said she was going to receive treatment at CPT. She asked me if I had ever considered going there.

I thought it was a strange coincidence that two good friends would suggest the same clinic in the same week. I interpreted it as a sign, and called to make an appointment.

I signed up for a consultation the next week and spoke to the physical therapists, who were very informative and compassionate about my drive to experience pregnancy and have a baby.

Since I was gearing up for my fourth IVF, the therapists put together a program that centered on preparing my body for the transfer. Because of my history, they also focused quite a bit of therapy on my tubes and ovaries.

After my CPT treatment, I completed my fourth IVF. Unfortunately, it was not successful.

We were disappointed, but we thought that God must have another plan for us. At this point, we opened the doors to adopting a child.

A few months later, I missed my period, but couldn't even bear to buy another pregnancy test. I finally bought the pregnancy test and to my utter disbelief, it was positive!

A few months later, I missed my period, but couldn't bear to buy another pregnancy test. I finally bought the test and to my utter disbelief, it was positive!

Ethan and I were so happy, but feared an ectopic pregnancy. We prayed that God would protect the baby, and placed our full trust in Him.

Nervous, we went to my infertility doctor a few days later to have an ultrasound, and to our amazing surprise, there was a healthy heartbeat.

Each step that we took in those five years, including our visits to CPT, got us closer to our ultimate goal of experiencing pregnancy and having a baby. I recommend CPT to women who are using medical interventions such as IVF or pursuing a natural course. They are performing many little miracles. Our little miracle is now five years old.

Endometriosis, Three Failed IVFs, Two Miscarriages, Then a Natural Full-Term Pregnancy

- Claudia's Story

When I was 27 I was ready to conceive. I was young and happy to be starting my family. I never thought that I would struggle with conceiving.

After two years and no pregnancy, I went to see my doctor. I had all of the typical fertility work-ups done, but they couldn't find anything. My doctor then suggested I undergo diagnostic laparoscopic surgery to see if she could find a cause.

During the surgery, she found endometriosis and multiple uterine fibroids. A few months later, I had a full myomectomy to remove everything she found that shouldn't be there.

After the surgery, I was able to conceive naturally, but then I miscarried. My husband and I continued trying to conceive naturally, but finally I returned to the doctor for some help.

I was prescribed Clomid and was able to conceive after the first dose. I anxiously proceeded through my first trimester and was happy when I finally made it past 12 weeks. But at 14 weeks, I miscarried.

Despite this great misfortune, my husband and I kept trying to conceive with Clomid and intrauterine inseminations.

Now in my thirties and still no success with inseminations, we decided to try IVF. The cycle medication went well and they were able to get two fertilized eggs. Although this was a low number for IVF, I was excited with the prospect of maybe having twins. However, the transfer didn't work.

I then took the time to really examine my life. I was the Vice-President of a large company in Canada and I knew I needed a break. I wanted to take a year off to resolve our fertility problems or finally let go of my desire to conceive.

We decided to move to the US, where I went to a fertility specialist and did two natural cycles of IVF — neither of which worked.

The costs of IVF were astronomical and I knew I couldn't continue trying forever. I finally found an IVF institute that would let me pay for three IVF treatments upfront. If none of them worked, I would get a large percentage of my money back.

I knew this was my last chance and I wanted to ensure my body was prepared. I had heard about Clear Passage Therapies (CPT) and I decided to undergo a week of intensive treatment there first.

I took that week to really reflect and meditate on healing my body. It was a very powerful experience... healing, physically and emotionally.

I took that week at CPT to really reflect and meditate on healing my body. It was a very powerful experience. I felt their treatment was healing, both physically and emotionally.

One month later, I went to the IVF institute. They gave me high doses of medication and were able to get one egg. I timed my transfer with acupuncture and through all of that, I was able to have my daughter.

It was hard to say what role CPT played in my body, but I knew it had calmed my body, as well as my mind and emotions.

To my surprise, six months after my daughter was born, I had an ectopic pregnancy. No one could believe it. We had all assumed I wasn't able to conceive naturally. Although the experience was a nightmare, I was happy to know my body could conceive without the assistance of medication.

The following year, my body took a beating as an underlying infection went undetected and I became septic. I had to have an ovary removed and nearly died. It was a very harrowing experience.

I explored all of the opportunities because I didn't want to have any regrets.

Two weeks later, I became pregnant naturally. No fertility drugs, no acupuncture, nothing. It's hard to say where my CPT treatment came into that, but I know it must have helped. I gave birth to my beautiful son after nine months.

Looking at my two children now, no one would realize everything that I went through. I did everything I could to conceive. I explored all of the opportunities because I didn't want to have any regrets. That was one of the reasons I went to CPT. Now I can say for certain that I have no regrets.

Improving IVF and Natural Pregnancy Rates

The process of reproduction is remarkably complex, involving the intricate interplay of various organs, glands, structural, and support elements as well as hormonal systems. IVF attempts to bypass many of the areas that could cause problems by inserting a fertilized egg directly into the uterus or fallopian tube.

We have been pleased to find that the addition of our unique deep tissue therapy improves IVF rates. In our published study, the Wurn Technique® improved fertility for women undergoing IVF. In many cases, therapy has resulted in subsequent natural pregnancies months or years after the initial IVF pregnancy or earlier IVF attempt.

Chapter Ten

Secondary Infertility

Secondary infertility can be one of the most confusing diagnoses for a woman trying to become pregnant. This term refers to a woman who has already conceived one or more children via natural pregnancy, but has since been unable to achieve another natural full-term pregnancy. In most cases, her diagnosis is coupled with the vexing adjective of "idiopathic" or "unexplained" infertility, also termed "no known cause."

Causes of Secondary Infertility

In assessing secondary infertility we have found it is important to review the childbirth and any other traumas, inflammations, or surgery since that event. Was there a C-section or an episiotomy? Has there been a direct or indirect trauma to the vagina, tailbone or cervix? Was there a subsequent vaginal or bladder infection? Any of these events may cause glue-like adhesions to form at areas of the female reproductive tract, vital for reproduction.

While the diagnosis of secondary infertility is often frustrating for the patient, we find that the causes generally fall into one (or both) of two categories:

- Adhesions related to biomechanical factors including post-surgical scars (often diagnosed as "unexplained") and
- Age or hormone related infertility.

With each healing event, tiny cross-links form to help heal the area that has been stressed. After healing, those adhesions remain as a permanent record in the scrapbook of healing that occurred.

Adhesion can exert close to 2,000 pounds of pressure per square inch. Thus, it does not take a tremendous amount of healing to severely compromise the delicate tissues of the female reproductive tract. Freeing those adhesions in a non-surgical manner, like peeling the runs out in a three-dimensional sweater, is a bit like going back in time for the tissues that have been bound by the straight-jackets of collagen that can form over time.

We have found that the following events may signal the onset of new adhesions that can bind down the delicate tissues and structures of the reproductive tract, causing secondary infertility:

- Surgery in the abdomen, pelvis (including cervix), hip, or low back
- Trauma (car accident, a fall, abuse, etc.)
- Infection (bladder, vaginal, yeast, etc)
- Inflammation (endometriosis, PID, etc.)
- Any new or increased pain in the area (hip, back, period, ovulation, intercourse, etc.)
- Sexual dysfunction or pain (decreased desire, arousal, lubrication, orgasm or satisfaction)

With a thorough history, evaluation, palpation, and range-of-motion assessment of the reproductive structures, we can generally find and address any mechanical contributors to decreased fertility. Then we develop a treatment plan specific to each woman, based on our findings, and on any sense she may have of what is standing in the way of achieving her continued success.

Episiotomy

An episiotomy is designed to assist vaginal delivery and prevent tearing of the vagina or perineum. In this procedure, the surgeon cuts the posterior aspect of the vaginal opening in order to enlarge it, to help the newborn exit the vagina during childbirth. The cut may be a vertical incision, running from the vagina directly toward the rectum. Some physicians prefer to create an angled incision, in part to avoid the perineal nerve. Thus, the incision will be more of a 5 o'clock or 7 o'clock rather than a 6 o'clock vertical incision. In either event, the surgery enlarges the vaginal opening to ease childbirth for the mother, and to allow for vaginal delivery. You can see both of these incision types in the drawings below

.

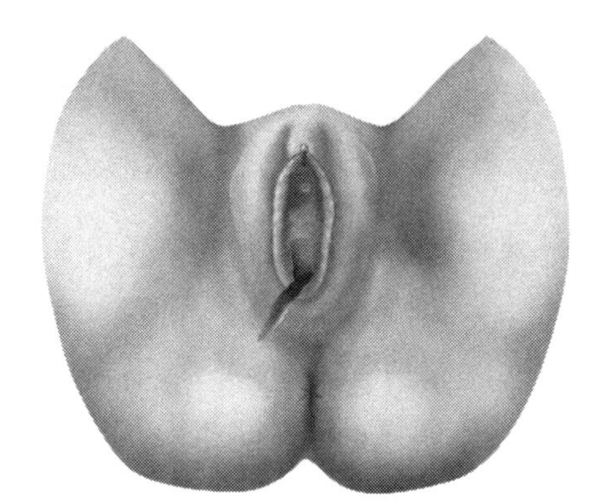

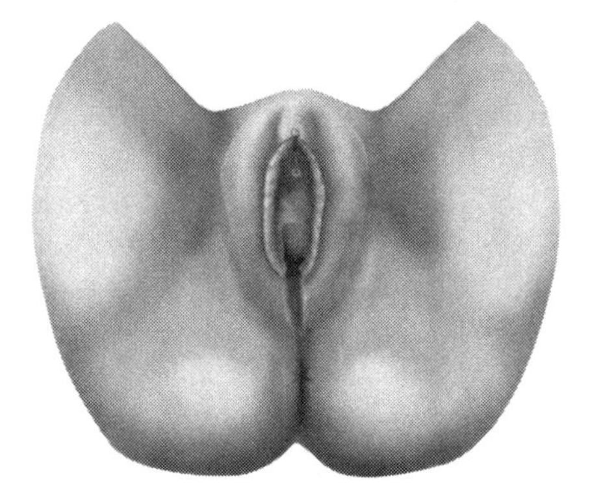

An angled incision (left) and a vertical incision (right) made for an episiotomy

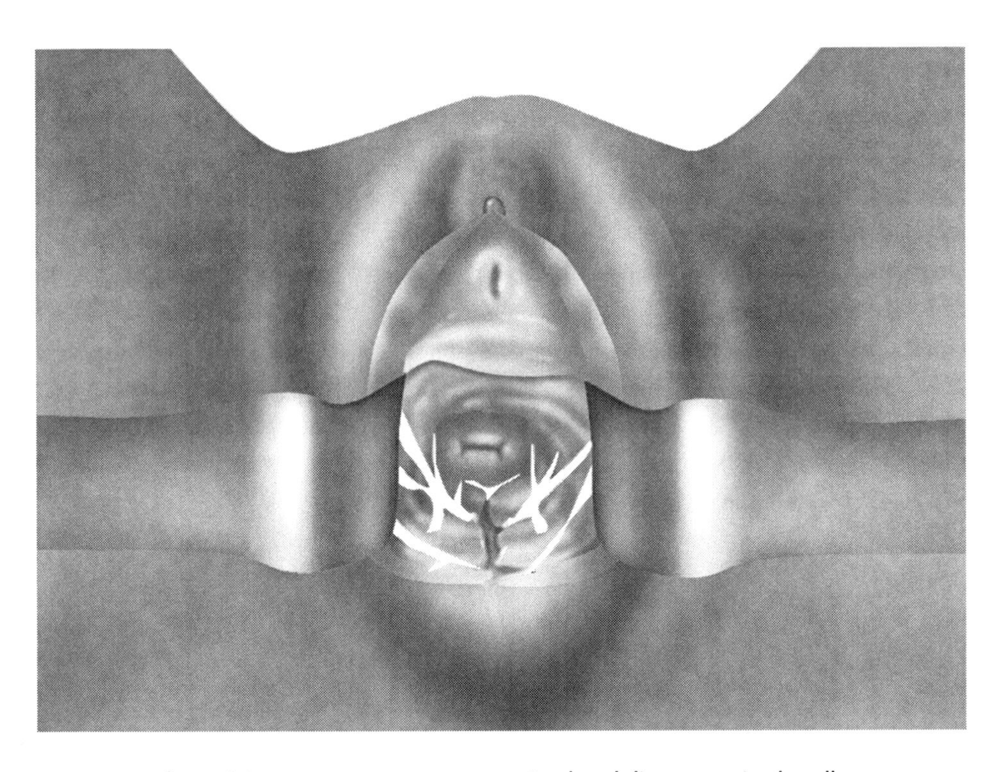

An episiotomy can create scars in the delicate vaginal walls.

All areas of the reproductive tract, including the vagina, need to have free mobility in order to function properly. If an area becomes cut, torn, or otherwise traumatized during the process of giving birth, adhesions subsequently form to help the area heal. In the perineum (the area cut by the episiotomy), the resulting scar can cause spasm or inflammation in the vagina, or up into the support ligaments of the coccyx (tailbone), sacrum, or the adductors on the inside of the thighs.

Inflammation can raise the internal temperature within the vaginal walls, causing a hostile environment for sperm. Furthermore, the gluing down of the vaginal wall and nearby structures (coccyx, sacrum, and adductors) can create unusual pulls throughout the pelvis, decreasing movement and causing pain or dysfunction, including infertility. We sometimes hear complaints of tailbone or intercourse pain at the vaginal entrance or with deep penetration after an episiotomy.

C-section

A C-section is a much more invasive surgery because it involves cutting much deeper into the body. To access the uterus, the surgeon must cut through the skin, superficial fascia, abdominal muscles, deep fascia, the peritoneum (a layer of fascia that lines and protects virtually all of the abdominal and pelvic organs), and finally, the thick walls of the uterus itself. The physician must create an incision in the anterior (front) wall of the uterus large enough to allow the newborn to emerge. Following C-section, the uterus is stitched closed; then the several structures that were cut to access the uterus need to be stitched closed, as well. The trauma of surgical cutting and repair to all of these tissues can create significant adhesion formation in or between any of these layers, as the body heals.

Low vertical incision

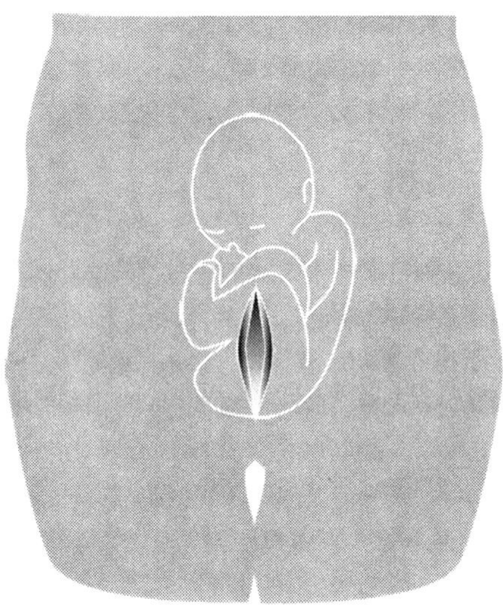

Low tranverse incision

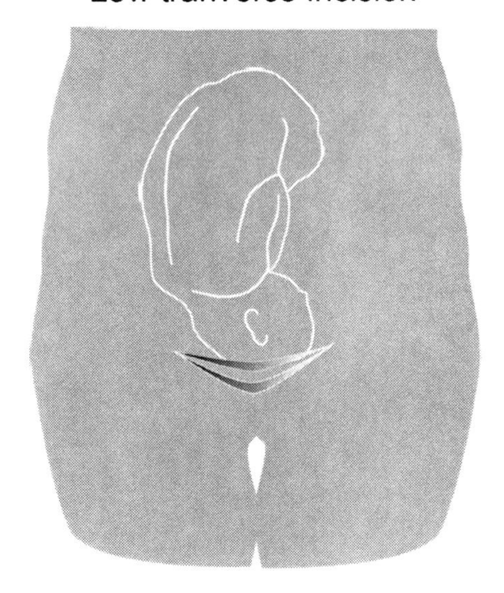

Classical incision

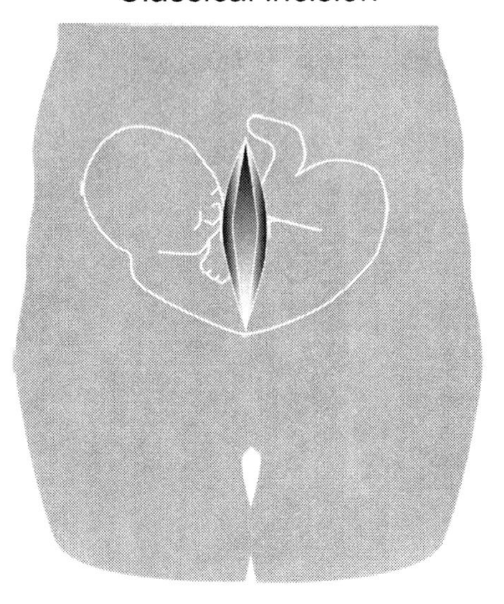

C-section surgery can assist childbirth, but may cause unwanted adhesions, as the body heals from the surgery.

As the body heals from a C-section, the adhesive process we have reviewed throughout this book occurs. Tiny but powerful collagenous cross-links rush into the area to help join and repair the cut tissues of the uterus and all of the other structures noted above. Adhesive scars form on the inside of the uterine wall and outside the uterus, as the healing process continues in the weeks following surgery. These adhesions act like glue, drawing nearby tissues and structures (such as the bladder, ovaries, or fallopian tubes) toward them by the very process of healing. The surgery and its adhesions may cause an unnatural state of immobility of the uterus. This immobility sets up the propensity for spasm, additional adhesion formation, and secondary infertility.

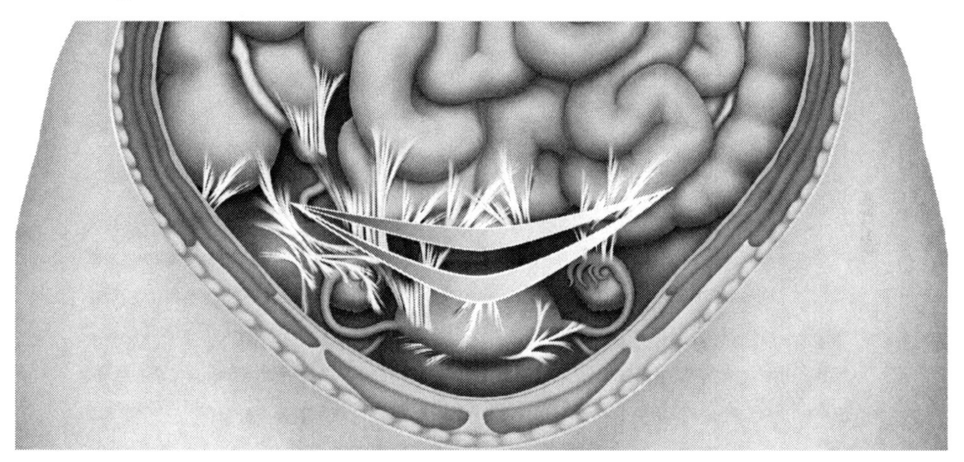

Adhesion formation after C-section

Just as an IUD (intra-uterine device) will prevent pregnancy by causing inflammation in the uterus that kills sperm, the scarring left by a C-section can cause a constant state of inflammation in the uterus with a similar effect. The consequent adhesive cross-links attach to the walls and prevent successful implantation of the embryo or cause a miscarriage. In our experience, we see secondary infertility relatively frequently in women who have undergone C-section or episiotomy surgeries.

C-section scars can also cause pain. Pain anywhere in the body is a signal that something is wrong. Perhaps nowhere is this as true as the pain that starts or persists at a C-section scar. Ongoing pain after a C-section indicates a significant amount of scarring – enough to cause a pull on the surface, or deep into the organ. The same scarring that is causing the pain is creating an abnormal pull on the walls of the uterus, generally where that structure healed from the surgery, as well as on nearby structures (such as the bladder).

One Fallopian Tube Removed, Remaining Tube Blocked after C-Section

- Ivy's Story

The first time I became pregnant I was 31 years old and it caught me by surprise. We had been trying for six months and I just had a period. I went in for my yearly Pap and told my doctor that my period had started up again early. She said I could be pregnant and it could be an ectopic — she was right. It was in my left tube and I received a Methotrexate shot to "dissolve" the ectopic. After that I had an HSG to check my tubes. It was uncomfortable, but the dye spilled.

My Ob/Gyn said to wait two months and try again, after which we did indeed have a successful pregnancy. I ended up having a C-section. My doctor said at the C-section that my left tube was pretty much disintegrated. I asked if that would be a problem in the future and he said no.

I breast fed our son for eight months and when my son turned one, we figured we would try again soon. In the meantime, I had only had one period since my son was born. I mentioned this to my new Ob/Gyn (as we had moved), so she started me on Clomid to return my periods and get the right progesterone level in preparation for a pregnancy. I took that about four times.

Interestingly, the month that I did not take Clomid, I got pregnant, but it was another ectopic in the little bit of my left tube that remained. I again had a Methotrexate shot. My doctor then removed the dysfunctional remnant of my left fallopian tube laparoscopically and we decided to do another HSG to check the status of my remaining fallopian tube. This time the HSG was extremely painful. My doctor called me with the results and told me it showed that my right tube was blocked. She said this was out of her scope of practice, which I interpreted to mean "go see an infertility specialist and get started with in vitro" — an option I really did not want.

My doctor removed the dysfunctional remnant of my left fallopian tube laparoscopically.

Feeling very disheartened, I used Google to look for a way to "open blocked fallopian tubes naturally" and came upon Clear Passage Therapies (CPT). Having a therapy background myself, I was convinced it would work and talked with my husband about it.

In the meantime, I tried some acupuncture locally as well as just trying and waiting, to no avail. I finally decided to go for it, applied with CPT, and was accepted.

My therapist was awesome, extremely knowledgeable and understanding. I felt great after getting all "loosened up inside." She even fixed an old running injury I had! When I returned home, I continued to practice the meditation and visualization techniques we worked on during the treatment as well. My last cycle was in July and the pregnancy was confirmed in August (not in the tube!).

The treatment really, really works — my husband and I are now expecting again!

The pregnancy went very well and our daughter was born in April 2007. I absolutely know it would not have happened without CPT! The treatment really, really works — my husband and I are now expecting again!

Hormonal Factors

We also look at age-related concerns. Is the patient 35 or older? Has she had her FSH levels tested? If a woman's secondary infertility is related to high FSH, we design a treatment specifically targeted to address this issue for each patient. We will not repeat treatment options for these conditions here, as they are already covered in Chapter Eight.

Successfully Expanding Your Family

Discovering the cause of secondary infertility follows the track of primary infertility, with a few additions. Because childbirth itself can be a traumatic event, we look for mechanical causes of adhesion formation. We then tailor an individualized treatment plan for each woman, enabling her specific issues to be addressed. We have found this approach enables many women to finally expand their families.

Adhesion Formation after C-Section

- Megan's Story

Megan and her husband waited until their son was three years old before they tried for another child. However, when a year went by and they were still not pregnant, they started to wonder if something was wrong. Before long, Megan started having severe abdominal pain during bowel movements on the first day of her menstrual cycle. Her gradual increase in pain with no medical explanation signaled the possibility of adhesion formation.

Her gradual increase in pain with no medical explanation signaled the possibility of adhesion formation.

Her doctor suspected her pain might be related to her C-section with her first child. He decided to perform a laparoscopy, now her second surgery. Once inside, he found scar tissue (layered adhesions) joining her abdomen to her uterus. The scar tissue helped explain both her infertility and her pain, because the adhesion attachments would be putting her uterus into a less mobile state, decreasing function and increasing the chance of uterine spasm.

Her physician also found an area close to Megan's bowels that he thought might be endometriosis, another condition that is closely associated with inflammation and adhesion formation. The doctor tried to remove as much of the adhesions and endometriosis as possible, but as medical literature has shown, the unfortunate probability was that the surgery itself would cause more adhesions to form.

Five months after her surgery, Megan still had not become pregnant. She began taking Clomid, a hormonal drug designed to increase fertility. When this proved unsuccessful, she sought an infertility specialist who increased her Clomid dose and performed two intra-uterine insemination (IUI) procedures.

When these efforts were also unsuccessful, the specialist decided to perform laparoscopic surgery again. During two hours of surgery, he found more adhesions, numerous cysts, and stage IV endometriosis – the most severe form of that condition.

Five months after her surgery, Megan still had not become pregnant.

Two months after her second laparoscopy (and the third surgery), Megan continued hormonal injections and IUIs. When none of those proved successful, the specialist concluded that Megan's fimbriae (the finger-like projections at the end of the fallopian tubes that grasp the ovary and help pull the egg into the tube) were not working. After all of her surgeries, it was likely they had become adhered.

Her physician then suggested she try in vitro fertilization (IVF). Megan and her husband had mixed emotions about IVF and decided to get a second opinion. Their new specialist wanted to start over, but after three surgeries Megan did not think her body could go through the entire process again.

She then began researching on the Internet for alternative methods to treat secondary infertility and she found our website. The testimonials of other women caught her attention and she was amazed at how similar some of their stories were to hers.

Megan underwent our five day fertility program; she received two hours of therapy each morning and two hours each afternoon over five days. Given her medical history, we focused on areas where we knew it was likely adhesions had formed. We focused much our work on her C-section scar, fallopian tubes, and fimbriae. We worked to return mobility to her uterus and her other pelvic organs.

When Megan started therapy, her abdominal area was noticeably tight and restricted. By the end of the week, it was very soft, pliable, and mobile. We were pleased with the results.

After treatment, Megan decided to let her body rest for two months before trying to become pregnant. When they started having intercourse in time with her ovulation the third month after therapy, Megan immediately became pregnant. Megan called us in shock and told us, "We tried ONE time and I'm pregnant!" Megan delivered a beautiful baby boy nine months later. One year later, Megan and her husband decided to try for one more child. They were so happy to find out they were pregnant two months after trying. Their third son was a welcomed addition to the family.

By addressing the adhesions that we felt had formed from her C-section, laparoscopies, and endometriosis, Megan's body was able to function much more as it did before being glued down by adhesions. In her case, she was fortunate enough to achieve the desired result.

Seven Years of Secondary Infertility

- Lyla's Story

I met my husband, Rodger, in the spring of 1997. I was a 25 year-old single mother of a 2½ year old boy, Paul, from a previous marriage.

We married in the summer of 2000. We talked of expanding our family and decided to start trying that following year. Many months and many pregnancy tests later, it started to wear on me. I wanted so desperately to have another child, but just couldn't figure out why it was not happening.

I wondered why I would put my body through a surgery causing more scar tissue, when ultimately that was the cause of all my troubles to begin with.

I was referred to a local Ob/Gyn, whom I hoped could help me find the cause and address it. He performed routine blood tests and an ultrasound, and Rodger's sperm levels were checked. I made weekly visits to the doctor's office after sex to see how my body reacted to Rodger's sperm. There was charting, waiting, and then waiting some more, yet still no answers to why I wasn't getting pregnant. Time was ticking and so was my patience. I thought, "How long do I wait with no answers as to why I'm not getting pregnant?"

After eight grueling months of getting nowhere, I decided once again to switch doctors — what did I have to lose?

I met with the new Ob/Gyn and right away she ordered a hysterosalpingogram (HSG). The following week I went in for the HSG. They were able to tell me right away my fallopian tubes were blocked. They explained to me that any kind of surgery, infection, etc. could have caused my "infertile condition."

I met with my Ob/Gyn and she thoroughly explained my options. One was surgery, where they would cut and repair the tubes so the blockages were removed. This would give me a small time frame to work with to get pregnant. I questioned this. Being a massage therapist and into health and nutrition, I wondered why I would put my body through a surgery causing more scar tissue, when ultimately that was the cause of all my troubles to begin with. (I had an appendectomy in 1992, accompanied by infection.)

I quickly got on the Internet and began to investigate my choices. Search engine upon search engine, "Clear Passage Therapies (CPT)" would pop up. I called and got detailed information on the program. It was all natural, no surgery, and would require me to spend a week in Florida. Sign me up! My Ob/Gyn was very supportive of my decision and wrote a prescription for the treatment.

In early 2003, Rodger, Paul, and I headed to Florida for my treatment. I knew that treatment would be intense, sometimes twice a day, but I felt that was exactly where I was supposed to be. Every staff member was so kind and loving. I had no discomfort, nothing but a wonderful experience.

After spending a week in Florida I was excited to come home and see the results of the treatment. My doctor scheduled another HSG. The test concluded the blockage had "moved" but was still in fact there. I was discouraged but hopeful. The therapists told me it could take a few months before I saw the full effects of therapy.

After more investigation on my part, I was led to a supplement that claimed to diminish scar tissue and improve women's reproductive health. I invested in a four month supply. If anything else I felt even more balanced, and knew even if I never had another child I was getting my body in the best health possible.

The left side was completely clear and the right side had some clearing with dye spillage. The doctors couldn't explain it, but I could!

It was December 2003 and I had scheduled my final HSG. Once again hopeful, but not expecting anything, I went in with a positive, loving attitude. This time, it was finally proven! The left side was completely clear and the right side had some clearing with dye spillage. The doctors couldn't explain it, but I could! I ran home with my news. We had company in for the holidays: Rodger's brother, his wife, and two kids. Rodger was busy playing video games with his brother. I barged in to proclaim the news, having him not even look up. I was disappointed, but let it go.

The months went on and we continued to "try." Nothing. My obsession with becoming pregnant lessened as Rodger dove more into work and I let go and decided to get my individuality back. I was really at a point of "just being." After two years of wanting another child so badly, I was just thankful to have one. During this time I discovered my love for horses, horseback riding, country line dancing, yoga, working out and traveling. I really was at peace. I began to question why I should obsess over something I had no control over. I loved my life with or without baby number two. I expressed this to Rodger, who was not happy with my "new found freedom." The wedge between us grew over the next year and a half.

I took another test and it was also positive! How could it be? Trying for years and nothing, and then just one day ...

Neither of us were happy and we divorced in 2005. That same year I met a wonderful man, Myrl. We grew close very quickly. We shared a lot of the same interests and philosophies on life. I told him about my infertility. Not having any children of his own, it could have been a huge deal, but he was willing to accept not having kids to be with me.

It was late January 2008 when both my sister and I suspected that I was pregnant. Her period and mine were days apart. She started hers, mine never came. A week later I took the test, and it was POSITIVE! Two days later, I took another and it was also positive! How could it be? Trying for years and nothing, and then just one day ...

After the initial shock wore off, we welcomed our own miracle and blessing. On October 6, 2008, our baby boy, Ryly was born at home with the assistance of a midwife. Weighing 9 pounds and 21 3/4" long our healthy baby is everything we could ever want and more!"

Two Miscarriages then Two Children

- Dana's Story

As a newlywed couple, we made the decision on our one-year anniversary to try and have a baby. With me at home and my husband working, we thought surely there would be three of us in no time. I went off the pill immediately. I had only been on it a year and I had one normal cycle and then didn't have another. I was so happy, yet scared, thinking I'm already pregnant! So, I finally told my husband and my mother and went to her Ob/Gyn.

Boy, were we wrong. Not only was I not pregnant, I wasn't having a menstrual cycle — and the doctor couldn't find anything wrong. I decided to find a new doctor.

"Welcome to the world of infertility" may as well have been written on the front door of my doctor's office. After numerous tests, I was given hormonal medications and scheduled for diagnostic laparoscopic surgery. The surgery went well and my doctor found no reason why I couldn't become pregnant. He referred me to a specialist. "Well, here we go to the Big Boys," I thought.

My specialists determined I wasn't ovulating. I was given numerous medications to help me to menstruate and ovulate. Our nurse taught my husband how to give me daily shots of hormones and we coupled these medications with intrauterine inseminations.

We had many unsuccessful IUIs, but in March of 1997 our miracle happened. We were getting ready to eat with some friends and I decided since I had never had a cycle after our last insemination I would take a pregnancy test. It was positive. I went to the doctor the next week to find I was eight weeks along.

Our little son, Ethan, was born at 36 weeks by emergency C-section. I had holes in my placenta and was leaking amniotic fluid. My doctor said we were touched by God that day — if I hadn't kept my regular appointment the baby would not have made it through the night inside of me. One week later the hospital released Ethan and we came home.

Our (first) son was born at 36 weeks by emergency C-section.

After Ethan's birth, I had a normal cycle. When Ethan turned two we decided to try for baby number two. In just a few months I found out I was pregnant without any medications. We conceived on our own. However, the day before my first doctor appointment, I started having severe abdominal pain and started spotting. I called the doctor and kept my next day appointment, but I had a miscarriage. I was eight weeks along. The doctor tried to remain positive and told me, "At least we know you can get pregnant and now you can focus on that."

Being the stubborn and determined person that I am, I didn't want to wait. We went back to the Big Boys.

Wow, had infertility advanced since I was last there. I was placed back on hormonal injections. We went on to have another miscarriage at two weeks. They monitored me closely and I had laparoscopic surgery to remove a cyst off my right ovary. I then had a tubal pregnancy at thirteen weeks. My tube was okay and not blocked afterwards, but my husband decided he didn't want to go through anymore. Physically and emotionally we both couldn't handle any more. We were blessed with our son Ethan.

From the age of four on, Ethan prayed every night that God would give him a sister. After my second miscarriage, he made up an imaginary friend he called "little girl" and even tried to buy her some purple flip flops. I told him if she couldn't try them on, then we couldn't buy them for her. He finally put them back on the shelf and said, "Okay mama." I cried all the way home.

(The test) was positive. I went in and sat in the closet for an hour and cried. My boss and my friend joined me in the closet and we prayed God would let this one be okay.

A friend of mine from work saw a clip about Clear Passage Therapies (CPT) on the news one day and brought me the phone number. I called my husband and asked him if he cared if I went for a consultation. He said he didn't care, but he wasn't going to give me any more shots. If God wanted us to have another baby, He was just going to have to make it happen.

After my consultation, I decided to schedule the treatment. I completed my treatment within six months. A few months later, I was sitting in my office feeling absolutely miserable and realized it had been two months since I had a cycle. I went to the store at lunch, came back, and took the test — it was positive. I went and sat in the closet for an hour and cried. My boss and my friend joined me in the closet and we prayed God would let this one be okay.

I have been married 16 years. Thirteen of those years we spent trying to grow a family.

The next day I went to the doctor and he did an ultrasound. His nurse, who I had known since high school, was in the room and cried when we saw that little heartbeat.

Ruthie was born at 36 weeks. Ethan, at age eight, finally got his little sister and bought her some purple flip flops.

I am 35 years old now and I have been married 16 years. Thirteen of those years we spent trying to grow a family. We are convinced totally that miracles can happen and that Clear Passage was the open door to help it along — especially now because I just gave birth to a second baby girl!

Miscarriage After C-Section

- Madeline's Story

In my first pregnancy, I became pregnant relatively easily. I gave birth to my wonderful baby girl via C-section in 2003.

When my husband and I were ready to have another child, we once again became pregnant easily. To our surprise, we were naturally pregnant with triplets. My pregnancy was rough though, and two died through miscarriage. At 24 weeks, I went into early labor and my third baby died shortly after birth.

I was determined to get pregnant as soon as possible and I began trying just two months later. When we were unable to conceive after three to four months, I saw my Ob/Gyn. She then referred me to a fertility clinic.

In 2006, we did various infertility treatments that didn't work. At the end of November of 2006, we did IVF and that didn't work either.

I decided I needed to step away from western medicine. I saw an acupuncturist and did some research on the Internet for natural treatments. I found the Clear Passage Therapies (CPT) website and felt I would be a good candidate for their treatment because of my previous C-sections.

I began treatment in February of 2007. I noticed some immediate improvements during therapy. I no longer experienced pain near my C-section scar. I also no longer experienced tailbone pain that occurred after my second pregnancy. With these results, I was optimistic the treatment would help with my fertility.

A few months after treatment I started intrauterine inseminations with medication. I did two rounds without a pregnancy. I was in such a hard place emotionally that I began taking antidepressants. I knew all of the treatments I was receiving were good, but I needed to be in the right place emotionally and mentally.

I no longer experienced pain near my C-section scar (or the) tailbone pain that occurred after my second pregnancy.

When I went in for my third round, they found I had already ovulated and thus wouldn't be able to do the insemination. I was disappointed, but then surprised when my husband and I were able to get pregnant naturally that cycle.

My pregnancy was perfect. I was a little bit anxious because of what had happened before, but I went to a high-risk pregnancy clinic that monitored my progress. After I made it past 24 weeks, I felt better. I made it all the way to 37.5 weeks.

Losing my babies was tough, but the infertility was even harder in some ways. . . .

From the beginning, we had planned to have a C-section. But I went into labor a week early and gave birth naturally — without drugs! That was quite a shocker. I was too far along for an epidural, and after five hours, I gave birth to my beautiful daughter who was 6.5 pounds and 19 inches.

Afterwards, I was actually glad I didn't have to do the C-section because I didn't want to have more scar tissue.

Now, with my beautiful daughter, I am making up for all of the pain and frustration I went through. Losing my babies was tough, but the infertility was even harder in some ways. When you lose a baby, you go through the grieving process and you work towards finding peace with it. But with infertility, you never know when it is going to end.

Having this baby provided closure for me. I was finally able to close the door on two years of hell. I feel like I have more perspective on life now and I really appreciate what I have.

Chapter Eleven

Unexplained Infertility

In the United States, infertility is defined as the inability to conceive after 12 months of unprotected sexual intercourse. Internationally, the time frame is generally longer: 24 months. Of the 6.1 million infertile women in the United States[55], it is estimated that 40% have medical or hormonal infertility, 40% have mechanical infertility, and 20% have idiopathic (unexplained) infertility.[21]

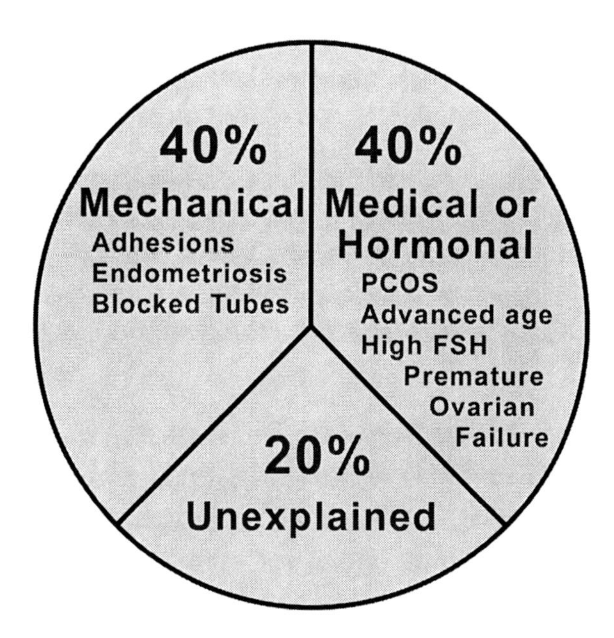

INCIDENCE OF FEMALE INFERTILITY IN THE UNITED STATES

Source Stephen EH: Projections of impaired fecundity among women in the United States 1995 to 2020 Fertility & Sterility. 1985,86, no 2205

The Confusing Diagnosis of Unexplained Infertility

Sometimes, despite all the best efforts of modern medicine and the array of diagnostic tests and procedures to find a cause, physicians arrive at a diagnosis of idiopathic (unexplained) infertility.

The mystery of unexplained infertility is truly no mystery. There is always a cause of infertility; discovering the cause and finding the treatment (or treatment combination) that works best is often a challenge.

A Hidden Cause of Unexplained Infertility

Physicians are equipped with a vast array of tests for hormonal and medical infertility. When none of these show a cause and there is no tubal blockage, we find that it is likely these women have unexplained infertility due to tiny cross-links or adhesions.

Adhesions are constructed of the same collagen that surrounds and separates literally every structure in our body, from the largest muscle and organ to the most delicate cilia on the walls within the fallopian tube. Like these cilia, adhesions and cross-links may be microscopic in size. Adhesions can be extremely difficult to diagnose when

- they are within the body of the organ, binding that structure's cells where they can't be seen, impairing function, or
- they reside undetected on the surface of organs where they bind or cover organ surfaces like a blanket, decreasing function and sometimes causing pain.

Wherever they form, cross-links act like glue within the structure, binding down tissues that should be mobile in order to function the way they did in our youth.

We have found that adhesions often go undetected or overlooked by reproductive endocrinologists and other fertility specialists. Adhesions do not show up on x-rays. The smallest of them are not even visible by a physician under surgery, nor are the ones that reside within organs or muscles.

Adhesions can impair infertility by forming in any of several important locations. We will examine each of these in the following pages.

Adhesions that form in the following areas can impair fertility:

- On internal and external uterine wall ligaments
- At distal ends of the fallopian tubes
- On the surface of the ovaries
- At proximal ends of the fallopian tubes
- On or outside of the fallopian tubes
- On and within structures of the cervix
- On the pituitary gland, or nearby structures

On internal and external uterine walls and ligaments creating inflammation and spasm. Adhesions can form on the inner walls, especially in women who have had an IUD, abortion, D&C, or uterine surgery. In these cases, irritation within the uterus can increase the possibility of uterine spasm or inflammation, creating implantation problems or leading to recurrent miscarriage.

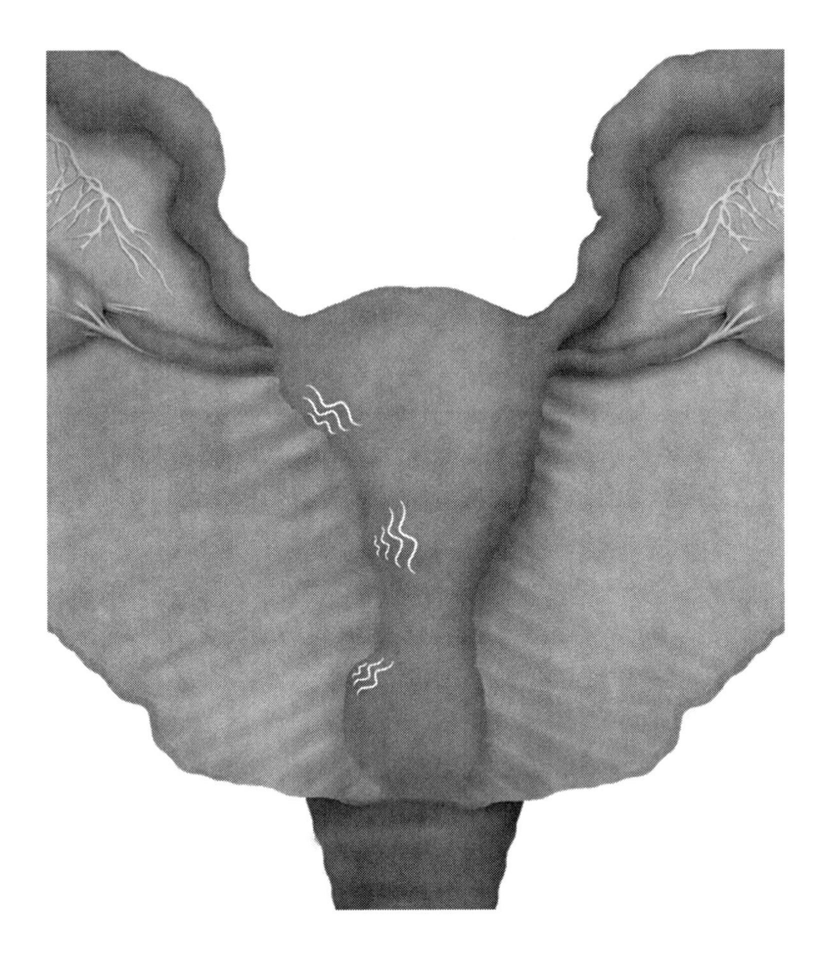

Adhesions that form on the inside or outside of the uterus can cause spasm and decrease the opportunity for lasting implantation.

We have found that adhesions which directly or indirectly attach reproductive organs to nearby support ligaments of the uterus or muscles (such as the psoas of the low back, or the adductors on the inside of the leg) can create strong recurrent pulls on the uterus. Thus, the uterus is literally pulled with every step a woman takes, creating a state of spasm, inflammation, or tension in an organ that should be relaxed in order to support a pregnancy.

At the distal end of the fallopian tube (by the ovary). Adhesions at this location can restrict the tentacle-like grasping of the egg by the delicate fimbriae, hence increasing the risk of the egg being wasted in the abdominal cavity.

On the surface of the ovaries. When adhesions cover the surface of an ovary, they can prevent exposure of the ovum, making transfer to the fallopian tube difficult or impossible. We find this condition to be especially prevalent in women with PCOS and those who have had ovarian surgery, such as a cyst removal.

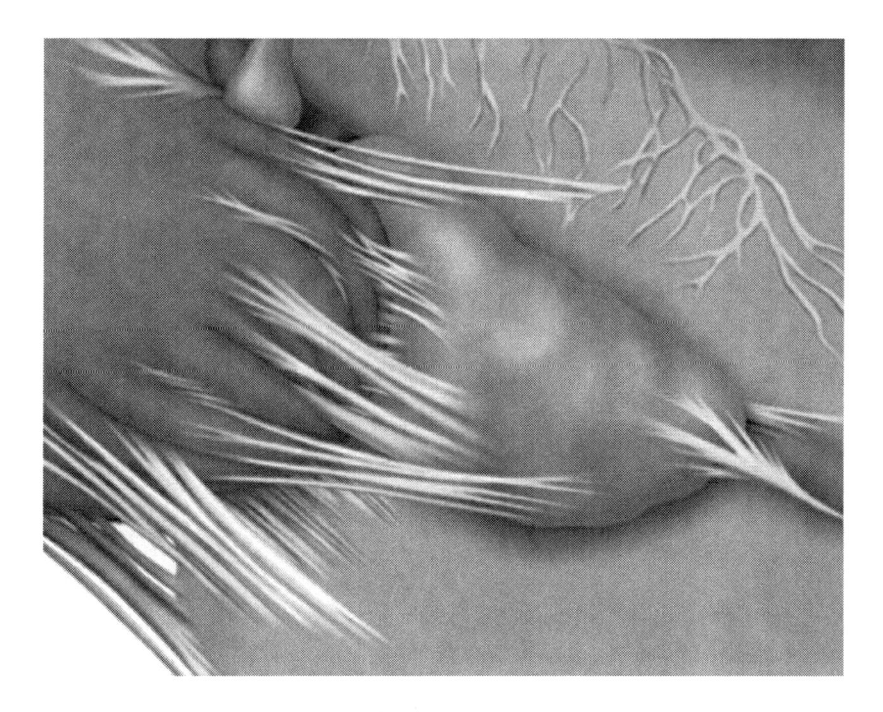

The ovary and distal fallopian tubes are delicate tissues that do not respond well to glue-like adhesions.

At the proximal aspect of the fallopian tube (near the uterus). When adhesions form near the uterus, they can prevent sperm and egg from meeting. Adhesions at this location are especially prevalent in women who have had fibroid surgery, pelvic inflammatory disease (PID), or any sexually-transmitted disease.

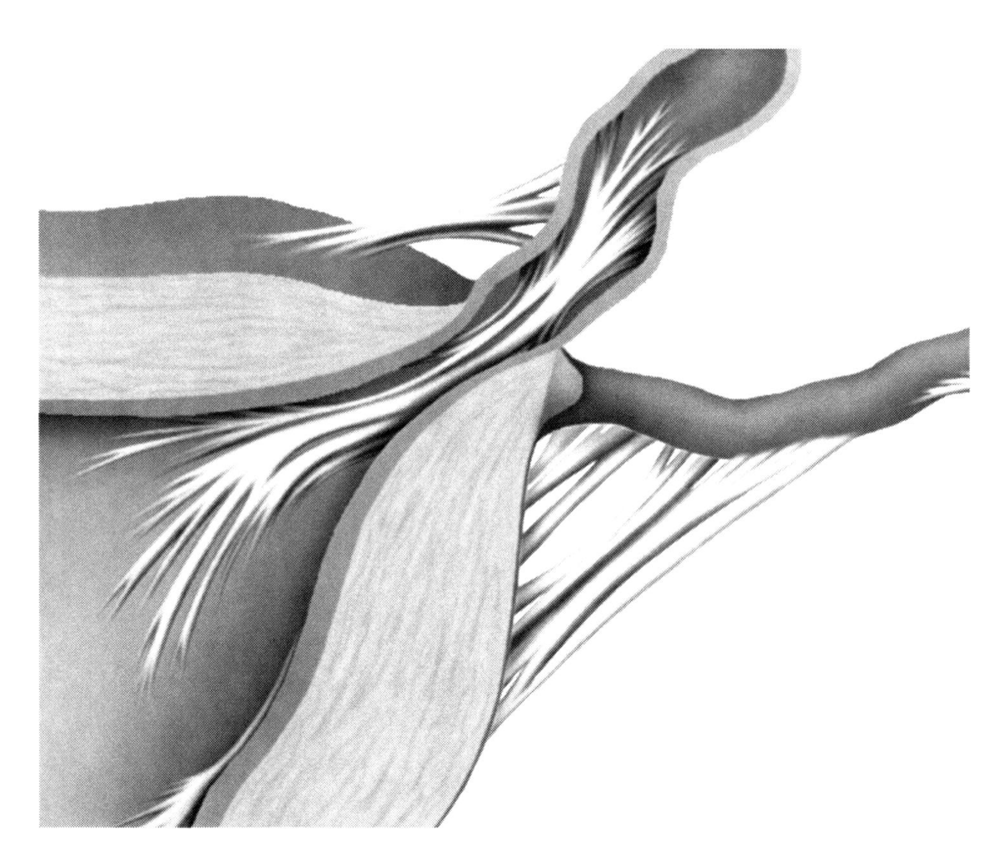

Proximal tubal adhesions often form after an inflammation, infection, or sexually transmitted disease (STD).

On the inside or outside of the fallopian tube. Adhesions at this location can cause spasm in the tube or decrease the ability of egg and sperm to easily travel the length of the fallopian tube unhindered. Tubal adhesions also decrease the opportunity for conception and increase the chance of an ectopic pregnancy.[9-11]

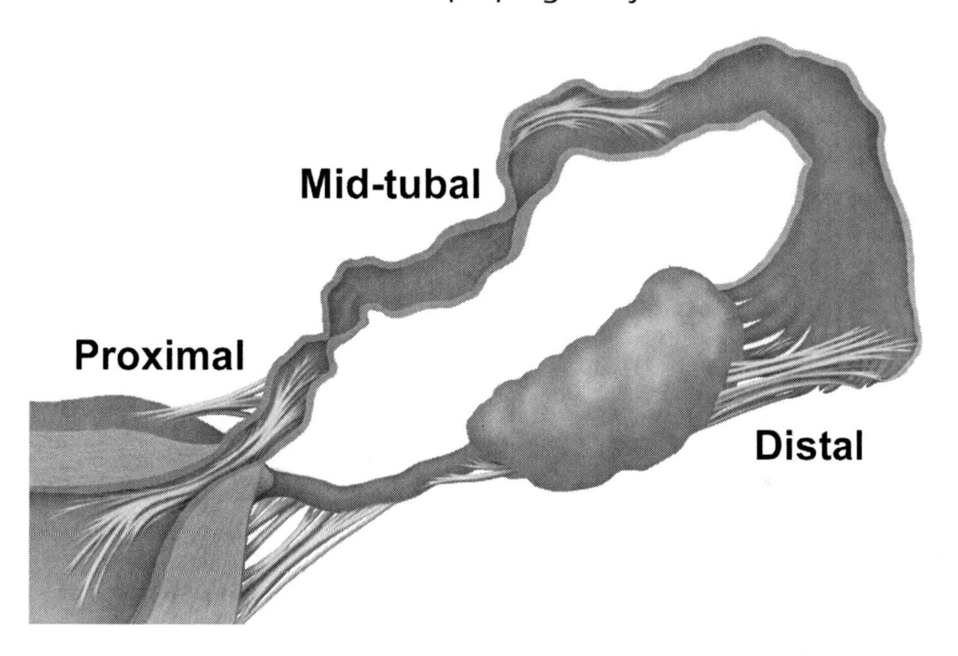

The entire fallopian tube is vulnerable to adhesions and spasm. Above are three main locations of adhesions.

On and within the tissues of the cervix. Adhesions on or within the cervix can create stenosis (closing) or fibrosis (stiffening) of the cervix, affecting its mobility and normally relaxed midline position, contributing to uterine spasms or complicating sperm transfer to the uterus. We find this condition frequently in women who have pain with deep penetration during intercourse.

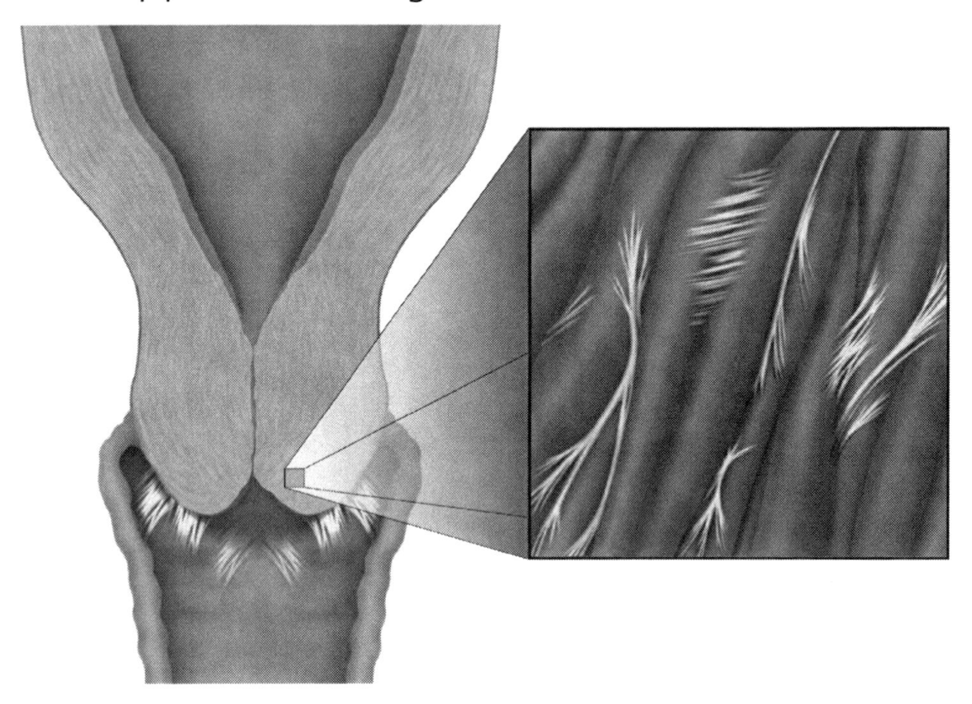

Adhesive cross-links can form outside the cervix, or deep within it, narrowing the opening for sperm

On the pituitary gland, or nearby structures. Adhesions can pull on osseous structures (bones) of the cranium, putting unusual pressures on the pituitary-hypothalamus complex that is encased within the sphenoid bone. When this happens, adhesive cross-links within the cranium or the support structures of the upper cervical spine appear to create unusual tensions on those structures, causing disruption in the normal communication loop between pituitary, hypothalamus, and ovary.

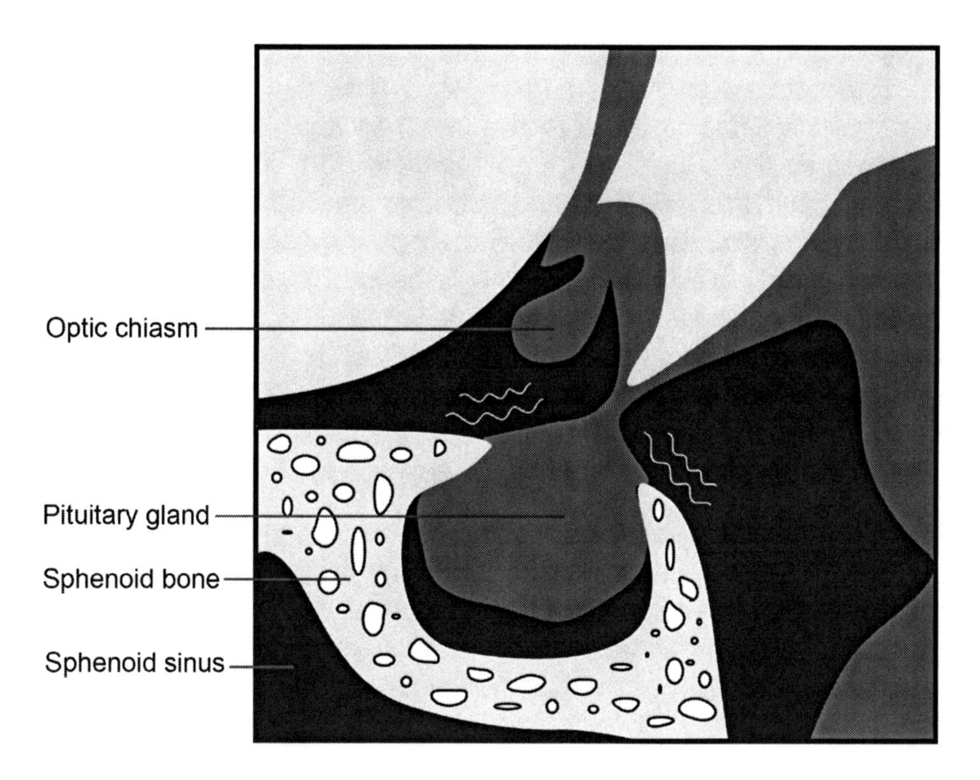

A poorly aligned sphenoid may pull on the pituitary gland, restricting its mobility and decreasing its function

Treating the Cause of Unexplained Infertility

Many of the women that had natural full-term pregnancies in our first published infertility study were diagnosed with unexplained infertility. They came to us frustrated, confused, and exhausted from years of searching for answers and for a solution to their infertility. For a large number, the manual physical therapy we were using to treat adhesions appeared to be just what they needed to find success.

In evaluating a woman with unexplained infertility, we look first to her history for adhesion formation. What hints can we gather there? Was there an early trauma to the pelvis or hip? Was her leg overstretched to the side doing a split during athletics when she was younger? Did she undergo any event or trauma to the pelvis that might cause adhesions to form at the pubic bone and perhaps into the uterus or vagina? Was she a gymnast, or horseback rider? Did she fall on her bottom or receive a trauma to the coccyx, where tissues attach to some of the reproductive structures? Did she receive a trauma to her head or neck, such as a whiplash injury that may have affected the alignment of her cranial bones, thus torsioning her sphenoid bone and pituitary (see Chapter Eight)?

Asymmetries of the pelvic bones and tightness of the ligaments associated with reproduction are not generally assessed and are certainly not treated by most reproductive specialists. Yet we have seen the importance of symmetry, balance, mobility, and motility to all of the structures in the pelvis and their function, including fertility.

Simply put, if structures are being pulled out of their normal positions in the body, spasm and inflammation will often result. While spasm, inflammation, and adhesions do not generally show up on most diagnostic tests, we have found them to be a major cause of unexplained infertility. Addressing these structures with a site-specific manipulative therapy has proven to be very effective for many of the women who came to us with unexplained infertility.

Five Years Infertile and 13 Unsuccessful IUIs
- Terri's Story

In 2001, my husband and I decided we wanted to have a child. But after a year, we were still unable to conceive. I was 35 and did not want to waste any time, so we spoke with my doctor right away. We completed a series of tests and all of the results came back normal.

My husband and I continued trying to conceive, but we still had no success. Our diagnosis of "unexplained" infertility was extremely frustrating because at least when you know a cause, you can find an answer, or you have something to battle against. I, on the other hand, didn't even know where to begin.

I looked into natural treatments for infertility and tried everything I could find. I saw an acupuncturist, tried different fertility diets, and tried massage to help relax my body. I strived to remain calm, but the more I thought about my inability to conceive, the more I stressed.

Our diagnosis of "unexplained" infertility was extremely frustrating because at least when you know a cause, you can find an answer, or you have something to battle against.

After some time passed, my husband and I decided to see more infertility specialists and started intrauterine inseminations. The insemination process was difficult because it depersonalized the act of making a baby — the wonderful part of making love with your husband. It soon became an effort, a job, a chore, and that was very sad. We did thirteen inseminations, but none of them worked.

I continued reading fertility books and read a great one entitled, *Taking Charge of your Fertility*. The book helped me learn more about my body and my treatments. I decided to find a new doctor. He examined our history and felt that IVF would be our best choice. However, that wasn't an option for us because our insurance did not cover it.

About that time, I read about Clear Passage Therapies (CPT) online. When I read about their treatment, it just clicked with me. I felt that it made sense and it could work for me. I waited until their clinic opened in New York and attended in 2005.

My treatment went extremely well and my therapist helped me to think positively about becoming pregnant. I think a huge part of the success of any treatment or becoming pregnant is believing that it will work.

My treatment ended in early September and my period started September 10th. I was concerned that this meant the therapy didn't work. I knew I was getting older and my "time was running out." My husband and I decided to return to the doctor and discuss IVF. We decided to go through with the cycle and

The insemination process was difficult because it depersonalized the act of making a baby — the wonderful part of making love with your husband.

my doctor said he would start me on medications after my next period.

The entire month, I kept thinking, "Please just start your period so we can get going with IVF." I kept waiting and when my period was late, I decided to take a pregnancy test; that's when I learned that I was pregnant. I didn't have to do IVF. CPT worked!

Our beautiful baby was born in 2006. After her birth, my husband and I didn't think about contraceptives. We decided that if something happened, then something happened.

In 2008, at age 40, I became pregnant naturally again. We recently learned we will be having another girl.

I am grateful for the work I received at CPT and that I am able to share my story with other women. When other women shared their stories with me, it helped me explore different options. I know CPT is not a "cure all treatment," but it worked for me, and other women need to know it is an option.

Terri's story is not unusual. It seems relevant to us that after so many years of infertility and failed treatments, she became pregnant naturally after therapy and carried that child to a full-term delivery, and then had another full-term natural pregnancy at 40. We suspect that the therapy broke down tiny cross-links that were binding structures, thus allowing her to become pregnant and achieve her goal of motherhood — twice!

Suspected Adhesions

- LaRue's Story

As a physical therapist who worked with premature babies and pregnant women, I commonly heard, "You are so good with children, when are you going to have a baby?" It was always a difficult question for me but how could they know I was surrounded by exactly what I couldn't have?

At 25, my husband and I decided to start our family. He was an Ob/Gyn, so we were well aware of the time it takes most couples to become pregnant. But when we still weren't pregnant after a year, we knew something was wrong.

We both went through tests and the doctors told me everything was fine with me. They discovered that my husband had some antibodies in his sperm. We knew the chances were low, but we decided that we would just keep trying naturally.

Each month, my hopes heightened, and then when my period came, it was like another failure. We had both succeeded at everything else in life and I always thought, "Why can't I succeed at this?" To make matters worse, I was surrounded by pregnant women at work who could not understand my struggle.

This was an extremely trying period for us. In fact, my husband even cried during a delivery once. While the family thought it was out of happiness for them, he confessed to me that it was because the mom reminded him of me and the child that we were not able to have. It got to the point where I actually dreaded going to baby showers. I finally accepted I would never be a mother.

It was not until years later, after my husband tragically passed away, that I thought of having children. I remarried and my present husband traveled a lot, and although we tried when we could, I knew our chances of conceiving weren't high. We tried for a year or so, and I became concerned that nothing had happened.

Because I was in my thirties, I wanted to make sure my hormones were at the right level. I went to see my doctor for a series of tests, which all came back normal.

My doctor recommended we try an IUI to increase our chances for conception, but when it was unsuccessful, my husband didn't want to continue with infertility treatments. He already had children and did not understand my desire to have my own.

Because I am in the medical field, I knew that adhesions beget adhesions.

For a couple of years we pursued no treatments, but I finally decided I was not okay with this option. I wanted children of my own and I decided to see a specialist.

The specialist suspected I had adhesions from three surgeries I underwent as a teenager. She suggested I have another surgery to remove the adhesions.

Because I am in the medical field, I knew that adhesions beget adhesions. As a physical therapist, I had already heard about Clear Passage Therapies (CPT) and asked my doctor if she felt their treatment might be beneficial. I even provided her with a brochure detailing the treatment that was available. She told me, with some skepticism in her voice, "I suppose it is worth a try if you feel strongly about it."

I decided to attend treatment for an intensive week of therapy. The first day of treatment, I knew right away this wasn't typical physical therapy. The therapists evaluated my entire body and they soon found a spot that, when stretched, elicited exactly the kind of pain I experienced during my menstrual cycle. If I had not been a physical therapist, I would not have understood that this was a good sign. Even though this aspect of treatment was somewhat painful, I knew if they could find the area that caused my pain, they would then be able to resolve that pain.

After my first day of treatment, I must have gone to the bathroom at least ten times. It was like their treatment helped clear my bowels and bladder.

By the time treatment was over, the majority of my aches and pains were gone. In fact, I never had menstrual cramps again after that one week of therapy.

I decided to give myself six months to become pregnant, and sure enough, that sixth month I became pregnant.

It is nice to see a natural treatment help women achieve their dreams.

After our beautiful baby girl was born, I knew I didn't want her to be an only child. My husband thought that one child was enough. But one day, he saw her sitting and playing by herself and thought she looked so lonely.

We decided to have another child and were able to become pregnant again the next month! I couldn't believe that after all of my years of struggling with infertility, it was that easy. I gave birth to our son nine months later.

A year after his birth, I was able to become pregnant again. Although I lost that pregnancy as a miscarriage, I know that a single miscarriage is not uncommon for a woman to experience.

I still think it is incredible that I was able to have three successive pregnancies because of CPT. It is nice to see a natural treatment help women achieve their dreams.

Seven Years of Infertility and Chronic UTIs

- Jennifer's Story

My husband and I attempted unsuccessfully to get pregnant from the very beginning. Upon attending Clear Passage Therapies (CPT), I had been married for six years.

I come from a large family with five siblings, including a twin sister. I love being from a large family, so I have always wanted many children. My husband has three siblings and feels the same way.

I felt intuitively that the intercourse discomfort and pain must be connected to my infertility.

We married just a week shy of my 30th birthday, so we started working on a family right away. Early in our marriage, I suffered from discomfort and sometimes pain during intercourse. Months, and soon years, went by and I was not getting pregnant despite the fact that I had never used any form of birth control. I felt intuitively that the intercourse discomfort and pain must be connected to my infertility.

I decided it was time to visit my gynecologist to gain some understanding of the problem. My doctor said that after two years of unprotected sex and no pregnancy, I was officially "infertile." Wow, I never thought that it would happen to me! But sure enough, that diagnosis became part of my life.

I then began the next step, trying a fertility drug called Clomid. I tried three months of Clomid with no success. My doctor then suggested that I undergo some diagnostic tests to see if there was a physical problem.

I went through the typical battery of tests. In fact, my HSG was done on the morning of September 11, 2001. It was a bad morning in many ways to say the least! The doctors told me that I was not getting spill of the dye into one side and they suspected one of my fallopian tubes was blocked. However, because of where the blockage occurred, they could not be certain that it was totally blocked. They encouraged me not to worry because, "Sometimes this procedure opens things up, and women often get pregnant afterward."

I left with a bittersweet feeling. I had a blockage on one side, but it could be "opened up." Although I was hopeful initially, months went by, and I still was not pregnant. I then went back to my gynecologist, who sent me to the local infertility specialist.

During consultation, he suggested that I had two primary options; I could either do in vitro fertilization (IVF) or artificial insemination. He said with the statistics, IVF was the most likely method to produce results. As a practicing Catholic, I knew this was not a good choice for me.

I decided to speak with several Catholic priests about this. They all suggested that even though we do not always understand God's plan, or the church's "rules" on sanctity of life, we must still obey as Catholics. We cannot "pick and choose" which rules to obey and which not just because they do not fit into our lives. I knew this was a spiritual lesson for me as well, and my responsibility was clear.

As a practicing Catholic... this was a spiritual lesson for me as well, and my responsibility was clear.

I thought about adoption, and would be open to it, but my husband was not fully on board. He felt that God would give us a baby one day, and that we should wait longer. Easier said than done!

I decided to buy the sticks that would tell me when I was ovulating and keep trying naturally. I used those sticks nearly daily for four years! I also tried the "basal temperature/natural family planning" method, but I didn't have success with it either.

In the meantime, I was having chronic urinary tract infections (UTIs). I went through a battery of tests regarding this, and even received antibiotic treatment for six months. All testing was inconclusive or negative, yet the UTIs continued.

Through all of this, I couldn't help feeling that these issues were all somehow connected to my infertility. After all, they were in the same general part of the body. How could I have occasional discomfort during intercourse, chronic UTIs, and infertility all generally unexplained? I also knew I had chronic back pain from two accidents I was in. I asked my doctors if these were related, and most said no. But I still was not convinced.

My emotions during this process were difficult to bear, Any time a friend would tell me she was pregnant, I received an invitation to a baby shower, or a baby was born, I would feel happiness for the friend, but incredible sadness that it was not me.

My twin sister married several years after me. I warned her to try to get pregnant right away if she wanted a family. After all, I was having such a difficult time and we were twins. Wouldn't you know, she conceived on her honeymoon! She miscarried a month later, and re-conceived again within two months. Two pregnancies within three months!

Finally, in 2004, my sister-in-law was working as a medical director in a medium-sized hospital. She was receiving medical journals online, and found an article regarding the efficacy of treatment by Clear Passage Therapies (CPT). She forwarded the article to me, and I felt that this may just be the answer that I was looking for. Many of their patients also had chronic UTIs and infertility, as well as pain during intercourse. This sounded familiar!

I thought this may be an answer to my prayers, and I contacted them immediately. They gave me a medical history form to complete in order to determine if I was an appropriate candidate for treatment. The closest treatment center at the time was in a city about 2.5 hours north of my home.

When I was accepted into the treatment program, I set up my first 10 hours during a holiday break. My family doctor specialized in physical medicine, and he readily gave me a script for "physical therapy" due to chronic pain, which ultimately helped to alleviate some of the cost of the program.

I began my treatment the week after Christmas in 2005. I am in the rehabilitation field myself, and have worked alongside physical therapists, so I had an inkling of an idea of what was to occur, but did not know fully, so I was slightly nervous.

The process consisted of both typical physical therapy maneuvers, but also "internal" maneuvers. This was uncomfortable at first, but it proved to be one of the most beneficial parts of the process. It was kind of like going to the Ob/Gyn for a check-up. The therapist was thoughtful and described what she was doing, why, and what she was finding in her assessment, and during treatment. She also explained why I may be feeling pain during intercourse on occasion.

Many of their patients also had chronic UTIs and infertility, as well as pain during intercourse. This sounded familiar!

I left feeling filled with hope. Because of my work schedule, I had to complete my remaining 10 hours six months later. In the meantime, the clinic that I went to closed! I was devastated. However, CPT contacted me, and helped pay for my transportation to their Florida clinic since I had already paid for the treatment. I was relieved, and looking forward to completing the process.

Six months later in June of 2005, I went to Florida, and completed the final 10 hours. I had multiple therapists, all of whom were professional and caring. The halls of the center were filled with baby pictures, and a new mother was there showing the therapists her child. I started to cry. I felt hope and anxiety at the same time. Would this really work for me or was I just a hopeless case? Why would this work after six years of no success? Just because there are some success stories doesn't mean it will happen to me. I was 36 years old now.

As I completed my treatment, they gave me some suggestions and materials for preventing pain during intercourse. When I returned home, I was eager to see my husband. We had a wonderful night, pain-free and pleasurable! I had a new intimate life with my husband! This was an unexpected bonus!

By September of 2005 (three months later), I took a home pregnancy test at my sister's house because I suspected I could be pregnant. It was positive! I never cried so hard in my entire life! I felt so relieved and so filled with joy and excitement. I couldn't wait to tell everyone. I wanted the world to know — I didn't care about "waiting until the first trimester is over just in case." I just couldn't hold it in. I gave my husband a "Parents" magazine with a positive test inside to tell him our news. He was elated as well. We were finally going to be parents.

We had a wonderful night, pain-free and pleasurable! I had a new intimate life with my husband! This was an unexpected bonus!

However, we were not out of the woods yet. During the pregnancy, I contracted "fifth's disease" while working at a school with young children. I had never heard of it before, but apparently it is one of the diseases on the "don't get this when you're pregnant" list. So I had to have weekly ultrasounds. It was another blessing in disguise because I had a chronicled picture history of my daughter's development in-utero.

In June of 2006, we had a beautiful, healthy baby girl 8 pounds 6 ounces. She was the most beautiful thing I have ever seen. I was 37 years old at her birth, and I finally had the child I had always wanted my entire life. I can't even look at her without crying tears of joy. I am so grateful to God and to the caring, skillful therapists at CPT. They not only helped me conceive my daughter, but also conceive again naturally — I'm 11 weeks pregnant! They truly changed my life!

Unexplained Infertility, Despite Multiple IUIs and 3 IVFs

- Nicole's Story

Being diagnosed with infertility is like being asked to walk a tight rope. It's all a balancing act – having faith you will conceive but not holding on to your dreams too tight. All around you, well-intentioned friends and family offer advice and it's hard to not be consumed by infertility charts, tests, and procedures. Ultimately, my efforts resulted in my beautiful daughter – but I had to learn to trust my own instincts and do what I felt was best for my body.

I was a year into my efforts to conceive when I realized there might be a problem. I consulted one of the top infertility specialists in the country. After all of the testing, he couldn't find anything wrong; I was given that lovely diagnosis of "unexplained infertility."

He decided to put me on Clomid for a couple of cycles to see what would happen. However, the medication made me an insomniac. I normally am a great sleeper – and I need that sleep. After two months, I couldn't function with the side effects of sleep deprivation so my doctor suggested I move straight to IVF.

I had to learn to trust my own instincts and do what I felt was best for my body.

Instead, I really felt I needed to treat the cause of my infertility, so I decided to consult another specialist. My new specialist felt laparoscopic surgery would enable him to find the cause of my infertility. During surgery, he found that the tiny fimbriae at the ends of my fallopian tubes were adhered. He told me, "Your fallopian tubes are still clear on the inside, but your fimbriae and tubes are stiff and not moving. I tried to remove as many adhesions as possible, but I did not want to damage your fimbriae."

I tried to become pregnant naturally afterwards, but suffered a miscarriage. My doctor and I decided to continue with different forms of hormones. I was able to become pregnant once again, but then I miscarried again. We even tried several IUIs to help the sperm reach my uterus, but I was only able to become pregnant once and then miscarried again.

Finally, two years into my struggle to conceive, I proceeded with IVF. At 38, I did my first cycle and was able to become pregnant, but again miscarried. I did two more IVF cycles at 39 and 40, but I didn't get pregnant at all.

By this time, the infertility specialist told me that the "grade of my eggs" was low because of my age and encouraged me to pursue donor eggs. I didn't agree with his assessment because I always responded well to the drugs and produced high quality embryos – my inner voice was telling me that there must have been a problem with implantation.

It was then that a friend mentioned Clear Passage Therapies (CPT). I looked it up online and was intrigued. I was already familiar with massage and physical therapy because I have scoliosis. I had tremendous success with these treatments and I hoped manual physical therapy could help my infertility.

Before I attended treatment, another friend of mine suggested a doctor who specialized in finding causes of infertility. As I wanted to cover every possibility I went to see him. The doctor found I was positive for mycoplasma, which he could easily treat with antibiotics. It is a bacteria/virus that is hard to find and in some can cause infertility. He also found that my natural killer cell count was a little high and may spike at the time of pregnancy. Natural killer cells are the "special forces" of the immune system and they see an embryo as a parasite and try to kill it. High levels of natural killer cells are usually found in people who have fought cancer – and that was definitely me. When I was 20, I was

My inner voice was telling me that there must have been a problem with implantation.

diagnosed with cervical cancer and had to have a portion of my cervix removed. My doctor explained that when I became pregnant he could test me for the natural killer cell levels and give me medications to prevent my immune system from killing the embryo.

My doctor felt (CPT) treatment made sense.

I spoke with my doctor about CPT and he felt their treatment made sense. I scheduled the therapy and explained my extensive history to the CPT therapists. When they examined my cervix, they found it was very tight and hard, leaving only a small opening. This was an important finding as it was yet another key to a cause of my infertility. My evaluating therapist said that they would add a special focus for treatment in this area during my sessions.

Since there was a CPT clinic where I lived, I scheduled my remaining sessions over the next few months. Each session, they worked to reduce the scar tissue around my cervix and fimbriae. At the same time, my therapists greatly reduced my upper back, neck, and shoulder pain.

I became pregnant naturally after 16 hours of therapy and before I was finished with the antibiotics course for the mycoplasma. I immediately went to my doctor who gave me the medication I needed to suppress my immune system. He also noted that the tightness in my cervix was greatly reduced. My preg-

When they examined my cervix, they found it was very tight and hard.

nancy was phenomenal and I delivered naturally – eight days after she was due! She has been amazingly healthy.

My success was a combination of my doctor's efforts and CPT. I am so grateful that I was able to become pregnant naturally. I think CPT created the possibility for my body and reproductive organs to work properly, and then my doctor resolved the conditions with my immune system that were impeding a full-term pregnancy.

My struggle with infertility showed me that my body functions as a whole entity … You cannot just treat your infertility; you have to treat your entire body.

My struggle with infertility showed me that my body functions as a whole entity. Everything is connected. You cannot just treat your infertility; you have to treat your entire body. Exercising, living cleanly, and eating healthy food will help, but sometimes we need additional help clearing out the psychological and physical damage of the past. I think my CPT treatments helped me do that. They rejuvenated my body and prepared it for the greatest natural miracle.

Myomectomy and One Blocked Fallopian Tube

- Nyamekye's Story

I thought I had planned the "perfect" life. I got married at 18 years old, and went to college on a full scholarship. I got my first teaching job right out of college. When things settled down for my husband and I financially, we decided to try foster care by a referral of a friend. My husband and I loved working with children and we thought we would welcome a few in our home. We enjoyed the fostering so much that we decided it was time to start our own family. We thought the fostering had given us great experience with the full-time nature of parenting.

I stopped taking birth control pills and started taking prenatal vitamins. I was ready! We tried for a couple of months, and got pregnant! I surprised my husband with the news by buying a bib that said, "I love my daddy!" When my husband saw it, he was just as happy as me.

The next day, I started bleeding. I read on the Internet that some women bleed in pregnancy so I decided to take it easy at work, but it did not stop. I immediately called the doctor and told her. She tested my blood and said it did not look like a viable pregnancy. She confirmed it during a vaginal ultrasound when she could not find anything in my womb. I was devastated. The doctor encouraged us to keep trying.

We tried for many months after that loss. Intercourse started to become monotonous, scheduled, and meaningless. After more than six months of trying with no success, we went back to the doctor. She told me that she could begin running some tests.

All of the blood tests came back normal, but the HSG showed my uterus was covered with fibroids and I had a blocked fallopian tube. She immediately referred me to a specialist. The specialist recommended surgery to unblock the fallopian tube and to remove the fibroids from my uterus in order to become pregnant. My world simply shattered. For many months, our moods were very down and I thought my chances for pregnancy were nil! My husband could not help but blame me and vent to his relatives overseas.

In December of 2004, I consented to have a myomectomy, even though my husband was out of the country on a pre-scheduled trip. My sister-in-law came to stay with me and comfort me. This was my first major surgery!

The surgery was successful in removing the fibroids, but she was unable to open my tube. I was told to recover for six to eight weeks and then come to her office to discuss the next steps. My husband returned and we decided to return to the specialist. She told us that we could try some less expensive alternatives, like insemination. Now that the embryo could stick to my uterine wall, we just needed to bypass the tubes. Okay, we decided to give this a try!

This test showed significant problem with the sperm and that we would need a miracle for it to produce a pregnancy.

We got started with all of the testing of my ovulation, the drugs to stimulate ovulation, and the testing of the quality of my husband's sperm. The test showed a significant problem with the sperm and that we would need a miracle for it to produce a pregnancy. Again, our spirits took yet another dive. My husband really struggled with this news! He had been putting pressure and venting on me until this day. He broke down emotionally.

The specialist suggested we consider a sperm donor. I remember looking on the website for a donor. My husband was crushed and refused to participate. He said there was no way he would ever let us consider that option. We talked about adoption, but we just could not wrap our brain around the fact that we were an infertile couple.

We went through two cycles of insemination with my husband's sperm, even though the doctor said it was highly unlikely to work with his sperm. I took Clomid and other drugs to boost my ovulation. Neither cycle worked! At that point, my infertility benefits were depleted. We were convinced the inseminations were not working, and we needed more options. The specialist said that our only remaining option was in vitro fertilization (IVF). She told us to visit with the financial counselor who may be able to help us find a way to pay for it.

I was not convinced and I did not want a home equity loan on our house. I got on the Internet and wanted to do more research. I had researched previously and saw a website about blocked fallopian tubes. I did a search again, and typed in "blocked fallopian tubes." Again, the same website, Clear Passage Therapies (CPT), came up first that had appeared when I was researching the surgery.

This time I decided to really analyze and look at the website again. I read all of the information on the website, ordered the brochure and video, and talked with my husband. I wanted to really see if there was a possibility in this technique or if it was too good to be true. On my next visit with the specialist, I asked her about the treatment. She said she had one patient who went to the clinic, but she was unaware of the outcome and she did not know about it personally.

We watched the video and read the results over and over. We were inspired by the story of Larry and Belinda discovering this miracle procedure that was helping women get pregnant. We were touched by the individual stories of success when there seemed to be no hope, so we started listing the pros and cons.

The cost was drastically cheaper than IVF, and it could also help to make IVF more successful if we had to go that route. The only cons were the time away from work for both of us (I was not going to go alone), and the travel expenses. We made the decision to go for it. The week before school started in August, my husband and I traveled in faith to Florida. We stayed with my husband's cousin, a medical doctor. We asked her to look over the CPT materials and see what she thought. She said to give it a try and just pray for a blessing.

Each morning, we drove to the clinic. My husband came to all of the sessions with me and came in the room to give me support. The CPT staff was very welcoming and encouraging. Each night we would walk and pray for a miracle. The stretching in the sessions made me tired and sore, but I didn't mind!

We came home hoping to get pregnant really soon. Nothing happened in September. In the beginning of October, my breasts started to grow. I knew I was pregnant. I took a test. We were pregnant! I knew not to get excited yet, because of what happened the first time. This time proved to be different! We were really pregnant on our own!

I had a very smooth and easy pregnancy. I delivered a son on July 13, 2005, weighing 8 lbs., 2 oz., and 21 inches long. We were parents!

This time proved to be different; We were pregnant on our own! When he turned four months old, we were pregnant again . . . on our own with no assistance. Our parents and supporters were shocked at the rapid turnaround.

We enjoyed our baby boy and when he turned four months old, we were pregnant again! We got pregnant on our own with no assistance. CPT had definitely cleared my tubes! I delivered a baby girl, August 31, 2006, 6 lbs. 0 oz., and 20 inches long. Our parents and supporters were shocked at the rapid turnaround.

My husband's cousin, the doctor in Florida, is now referring her own infertility patients to CPT after seeing our results. We are forever appreciative to CPT for their part in making our family!

From IUD to Infertile

An intrauterine device (IUD) is a "T-shaped" or spiral birth control device. It is inserted into the uterus using a minimally-invasive technique. The IUD is designed to kill or immobilize sperm, to thicken the consistency of cervical mucus, and/or to create inflammation on the walls of the uterus, thus increasing the temperature and creating an inhospitable surface for implantation.

Sometimes, the IUD does its job as an irritant all too well. Belinda and her physicians noted that her cervical cancer started at the exact point in her uterus where her IUD had slipped out of place and became imbedded in her uterine wall.

IUDs create inflammation, which in turn creates adhesions. These adhesions can create a blanket-like effect on the wall of the uterus, often interfering with implantation of a fertilized egg, in our experience.

The copper used in some IUDs is toxic to sperm. While IUDs are considered safe by many physicians, our retrospective experience with these devices makes us concerned by the placement of a toxic irritant within some of the most delicate tissues of the female body. In our clinical experience, we have begun to observe a correlation between IUDs and subsequent infertility, even after the device has been removed.

Infertile after IUD

- Mia's Story

"My infertility is unexplained," Mia told us. "My doctors have never been able to find a cause."

Like thousands of women, Mia was frustrated with her diagnosis and wanted to find answers. Her infertility struggle had begun years earlier, and as she explained, her experience was different from many infertile women, "I am in a same-sex relationship, so for us, natural conception means home inseminations and intrauterine inseminations (IUI)."

At 29, Mia tried for a year to become pregnant with a friend. Then they tried with the help of IUIs, but after three unsuccessful attempts she decided to take a break.

A few years later, Mia and her partner decided to resume their efforts, but this time they pursued in vitro fertilization (IVF). "I was devastated when it didn't work," she told us. But after a while, she realized that she needed to move on and began researching other options. That search eventually led her to Clear Passage Therapies (CPT). Hoping to improve her body's ability to conceive and carry a child to term, Mia scheduled a one-week course of therapy.

When Mia arrived, we reviewed her history to look for possible areas of adhesion formation, which we have found to be a frequent cause of unexplained infertility. Among other things, we noted that she had used an intrauterine device (IUD) years earlier — a contraceptive device that is inserted through the cervix into the uterus, where it prevents pregnancy by creating inflammation. We suspected that Mia had adhesion formation in her cervix and uterus that was interfering with implantation. Our therapists worked to dissipate those adhered tissues, and restore normal mobility and receptivity to the area.

As we worked with Mia in this process, we explained each step. Mia said she appreciated our informative approach and later told us this helped her learn to "experience and understand her body on a whole new level."

Three months after treatment, she tried another IUI with Clomid. When it didn't work, she tried again two months later, with frozen donor sperm. While many physicians and researchers have found that frozen sperm yields lower success rates than fresh sperm, in Mia's case, it worked! Mia told us, "I believe the work I received at CPT was very beneficial."

We suspected that Mia had adhesion formation in her cervix and uterus that was interfering with implantation.

Thirty-three weeks later she gave birth to a son. "Luc was born premature," Mia told us, "but he was fine. He's almost two years old now, and doing great!"

Causes of Recurrent Miscarriage

Miscarriages are known to occur normally and are not necessarily a cause for alarm, or for assuming that there may be a problem. However, when miscarriages occur repeatedly, doctors suspect there must be an underlying cause. There are a number of reasons for recurrent miscarriage. Many of these, such as genetic chromosomal defects, autoimmune disorders, and male factors are beyond the scope of this book and our practice.

Physicians do note that age, hormonal factors, adhesions, and uterine factors are implicated among the causes of recurrent miscarriage. We address age in Chapter Eight and several other factors in the various chapters of this book.

It is estimated that 50% of all miscarriages are unexplained. We believe that many of these unexplained cases are due to adhesions and collagenous cross-links. Uterine problems can occur when tiny (even microscopic) cross-links form on the inside surface of the uterus. There, they can create a less hospitable surface for implantation and lead to miscarriage. When cross-links form on the outer walls of the uterus or its support ligaments, they can create spasm, preventing implantation or causing miscarriage.

The effectiveness of treating recurrent miscarriage is difficult to research scientifically, due to the retrospective nature of miscarriage and the near-impossibility of creating a control group. Because of the difficulty of conducting research in this area, we do not have (and are not likely to get) clear scientific data on the ability of manual therapy to reverse the condition of recurrent miscarriage. However, several stories in this book address women who underwent multiple miscarriages before success, including two stories that follow.

Age 42, Five Prior IVFs, and Three Miscarriages

-Ashley's Story

My husband, Aaron, and I met and married in our mid-30s. We knew that we wanted children, so after roughly six months of marriage, we began trying to conceive. Little did we know the long, difficult journey on which we were embarking. In the beginning, we were very excited about trying, and each new month brought with it the renewed anticipation of achieving a pregnancy. We couldn't wait to become parents!

After several months of trying without success, we began getting a little worried. I made an appointment with my Ob/Gyn in order to have things checked out. She ran a series of tests on me and on Aaron. My test results indicated no hormonal problems and no blockage in my tubes. Some problems were found in Aaron's semen analysis, but none of the problems would ultimately prevent conception, only make it more difficult to achieve. Because of my age, she referred me to a reproductive endocrinologist. Now, we were officially on the roller coaster ride of our lives.

The RE ran some additional tests. I passed the Clomid Challenge Test (a test in which Clomid is used to measure if the woman has decreased ovarian reserve), so we were ready to pursue IVF. We began completing the required checklist of items in preparation for IVF, including training on giving shots. As we worked toward the completion of the checklist of requirements, we couldn't wait for the day to arrive to begin the procedure. Once again, we were full of hope, and I found it refreshing that the doctor and nurses were now in charge. I could stop charting my temperature and monitoring each day of my cycle. I didn't realize until much later how much stress my body was being put under, simply due to this constant reminder of our fertility struggles at the start of each day.

The day finally arrived to begin our IVF cycle. The next few weeks were comprised of giving myself shots, taking pills, having blood drawn, and ultrasounds. The day of retrieval finally arrived and it was a success. Several eggs were retrieved, and the next day we were informed that ten had successfully fertilized. Things were looking good, and on day three, the doctor transferred four embryos of good quality.

Aaron and I felt good about how things had gone. We were experiencing feelings of hope and excitement, but I couldn't help also feeling fear and anxiety in anticipation of taking the pregnancy test.

On the scheduled date, I showed up at the doctor's office to have blood drawn for my pregnancy test. Afterwards, I drove to work and started the waiting game again. Every time the phone rang, I fearfully answered and thought to myself, "Is it the doctor's office calling with the results?" When it finally was a nurse, I heard the words, "You're pregnant." We did it! I was finally pregnant! I called Aaron with the news.

I had to reach the point of hopelessness before I could hear the guidance for which I had been praying.

I can't even begin to describe the way that we felt, but unfortunately, the joy wouldn't last. At about seven weeks

I miscarried, and the emotional roller coaster continued. We went from the highest of highs to the lowest of lows, and I began asking God, "Why?"

We met with the doctor to discuss our options, and we decided to try IVF again. Once again, the retrieval was a success. Two blastocysts of high quality were transferred to my uterus and six remaining blastocysts were of high enough quality to freeze. The cycle was going very well, and Aaron and I were very excited. Once again, a pregnancy occurred with one embryo, and we were back on an emotional high.

We were thoroughly enjoying watching our baby grow in the ultrasounds until about week ten. It was at this ultrasound that our nightmare began again. The doctor could no longer find a heartbeat. I had miscarried for a second time. He scheduled me for a follow-up ultrasound a few days later to confirm the miscarriage before going forward with another D & C.

Aaron and I turned to one another as we searched within each of us to deal with the grief of losing another baby. We later found out that the baby was a boy, and he miscarried due to a chromosomal abnormality. While it didn't lessen the pain, it was good to have an answer, and fortunately, the problem was not highly anticipated to recur.

After some time, we met with our doctor and discussed our options yet again. We decided to do a frozen embryo transfer. The decision was made to transfer three embryos, and fortunately, the first three thawed well, leaving us with three still frozen. Again, I beat the odds for someone my age, and I became pregnant with one baby. Now, each ultrasound brought with it fear and anxiety, as we waited each time to hear and see the heartbeat. Only after finding the heartbeat each time could we relax and enjoy seeing our baby grow. Near the end of the first trimester, my RE released me to my OB's care.

Finally back under my OB's care, we breathed a huge sigh of relief when I made it to the second trimester. The pregnancy continued progressing well, and we found out that we were having a boy at the 20 week ultrasound. Aaron and I were feeling really good about everything as we headed into the holiday season. We traveled a few hours to my parents' house for the weekend to celebrate Christmas. It was there that our nightmare began yet again.

After we arrived, I couldn't shake the feeling that something was wrong, and I had noticed a decline in the baby's movement. The morning we were leaving, I told Aaron that I thought we should call the doctor. The nurse tried to reassure us that everything was probably fine, but if we would like, we could go straight to the hospital when we got back into town to have the baby checked. When we arrived, the doctor could not find a heartbeat. I had never before felt such a deep pain and sense of loss in my life. I can still see the image of tears running down Aaron's face. The pain never completely goes away. Even now, four and a half years later, recalling these memories has brought tears to my eyes.

> ***Even now, four and half years later, recalling these memories has brought tears to my eyes.***

The next day, my doctor began inducing labor, and our son was stillborn on December 23, 2003. He was beautiful, our little angel, and we were given the opportunity to hold him and to say goodbye. The doctor and nurses allowed us to keep him with us for the night. I am eternally grateful for this time with him.

Aaron and I had a very quiet Christmas, and we found ourselves questioning our faith once again. I can remember feeling completely empty inside, and as we prepared for our son's funeral, I found myself longing to be with him. I knew that I couldn't begin the healing process until the funeral was behind us. Grieving is a process of steps, and the next few months were spent reading books about coping with the loss of a child and about trying to understand God's purpose. In time, I began getting my faith back on solid ground and praying to God for guidance.

After some months had passed and with no explanation found for the death of our son, we went back to our RE to discuss our next step, while I also continued praying for guidance. We decided to go through another fresh IVF cycle, and so the routine (shots, lab work, ultrasounds, etc.) began again. By now, I had grown to hate the process, but I was also feeling very desperate. My 40th birthday was approaching, and the doctors, unfortunately, do us no favors mentally, emotionally and physically with the way they paint very negative pictures for women in this age group. The stimulation went well and they retrieved 13 eggs. It was at this point that the cycle turned bad. Only one egg had fertilized overnight, so the embryologist performed ICSI on six more eggs. The doctors could find no explanation as to why this was happening because the eggs and sperm had looked fine. Ultimately, only three actually fertilized, and on day three, two were still of a good quality when the transfer was done. This time, my pregnancy test was negative. Aaron and I were crushed and truly no longer knew where to turn. We were afraid to simply try again, and all of the treatments were beginning to take their toll on my body. I was actually beginning to experience menopause symptoms.

I didn't realize until much later how much stress my body was being put under.

It was at this point that I began being open and receptive to more natural methods of enhancing fertility. In past research, I had come across the benefits of acupuncture and types of foods in relation to fertility, but at the time, I was not yet receptive to such unconventional measures. I had to reach the point of hopelessness before I could hear the guidance for which I had been praying. I began researching these topics more, and read a book by a doctor specializing in acupuncture, diet and herbs (Traditional Chinese Medicine) to enhance fertility. It was fascinating, and I found renewed hope.

Aaron and I began seeing a fertility specialist, originally from China, who was a Doctor of Traditional Chinese Medicine. We saw her and her husband for nearly a year, driving eight hours round trip for each appointment. Using the knowledge I had gained from the TCM book that I had read, we also became very focused on the type of foods we included in our diet. While we noticed favorable changes in our health, including the disappearance of my menopause symptoms, we unfortunately did not achieve a natural pregnancy, and so once again, we geared up for another fresh IVF cycle.

We went into this (our fifth IVF cycle) with very high hopes because of the TCM and our very healthy diet. Much to the surprise of the RE, because of my age of 40, I stimulated very well and a good number of eggs were retrieved. I attribute this to the natural measures we had taken. Unfortunately, no pregnancy occurred. Our TCM doctor was just as surprised as we were. Aaron and I somehow held onto our faith, and I continued praying for guidance.

I had decided to jump right back into the acupuncture and herbs, but God had another plan for us. Conflicts on weekends kept occurring, preventing us from traveling to see the TCM doctor. By the time a month had passed, I had gotten the courage to pursue another natural way that I had uncovered in past research.

Through the Internet, I had discovered a couple who, after much research, had finally succeeded in conceiving naturally twice by changing their diet and adding certain vitamins, supplements, exercise and meditation to their daily regimen. The objective was to address the health of the whole person (mind, body and spirit). It seems the mind can have a very powerful effect on the body and how it performs, and anyone struggling with fertility issues and the all-consuming desire to have a baby, has most likely had a lot of negative influences (test results, medical statistics, poor prognoses, etc.). So our new journey began. We had already improved our diets and were exercising regularly. I came up with a vitamin and supplement regimen for us to follow, and I began working on my mind with meditation, visualization and positive affirmations.

Several months went by, and while we knew we were healthier and felt better, no pregnancy had yet occurred. I was now 41 years old. I continued praying for guidance, and some new information always seemed to come my way when I needed it most. I read a book by another woman who had been diagnosed with high FSH and who conceived naturally after addressing the health of her whole being. As a result, I made a few minor modifications to my regimen. I also began practicing yoga and Qi Gong geared toward enhancing fertility, and getting monthly hour-long massages in an effort to reduce stress and improve blood flow to my reproductive organs. Prior to ovulation, I would massage my lower abdomen to improve blood flow to my ovaries with the goal of improving the quality of my eggs.

It seemed to address a problem that could be affecting me: scarring from D&Cs after my miscarriages and stillbirth and from an appendectomy in my youth.

Months came and went. If a biological baby were to be in our future, I needed a booster shot of hope, and I got it. Not long after praying for more guidance, I came across a link on the Internet to the Clear Passage Therapies (CPT) website. I found the information fascinating, and I wanted to learn more so I requested additional information. I was so excited when the information came in the mail. I read the information, and it seemed to address a problem that could be affecting me, scarring from the multiple D&Cs that I had after my miscarriages and stillbirth and from an appendectomy in my youth. I was excited about the possibilities, but at the same time, I was hesitant to spend even more money chasing our dream. I put it aside for a while, but the therapy was always in the back of my mind.

My 42nd birthday was fast approaching, and I still wasn't pregnant. I brought the topic of the therapy up again with

Aaron, and we decided to go for it. We thought if nothing else, I would be doing something good for my body, and we would get a vacation out of it. I scheduled the therapy and off to Florida we went in the Spring of 2006.

The treatment was wonderful, and the therapists were friendly, professional, and knowledgeable. They put me at ease right away, provided a lot of interesting information, and made the sessions very relaxing. They found a lot of tightness in my reproductive area, and I learned that organs must be free to move in order to function at their best. They worked on me from my head to my toes.

By the time I left, sex no longer hurt in one position, my appendectomy scar felt completely different, and my tailbone was more properly aligned. No matter what happened after we returned home, I knew that I was feeling better both mentally and physically, and we had spent a wonderful vacation together.

Heading into fall of that year, I put my BBT thermometer away after Aaron told me to stop taking my temperature and leave it in the hands of God. It was so out of character for him to speak so frankly and pointedly to me that I couldn't get it out of my mind. I truly felt as if God were speaking through Aaron and telling me to trust in Him. It wasn't until I stopped taking my temperature that I discovered just how much stress that morning routine was putting on my body. It was truly liberating to retire my thermometer.

I was now 42 years old, and I felt like we needed to come up with a plan once again. Finally, I discussed my feelings with God, then with Aaron. I told him that if I were not pregnant by the end of the year, I thought we should try our remaining frozen embryos. If that didn't work, I thought we should pursue adoption. I was done with fresh IVF cycles, and I was ready to move on in our lives. He agreed. The remaining weight was now gone from my shoulders.

That was the month I became pregnant naturally, roughly seven months after my therapy at CPT. At 42, I gave birth to a beautiful baby girl.

I truly believe that the therapy provided by CPT was the help that my body needed to be receptive to a pregnancy.

My advice to others facing fertility issues would be to keep an open mind and don't think of it in terms of "infertility." That alone has a very negative connotation to it. Medical science and what doctors have been able to achieve is wonderful, and many couples have had their dreams of having children fulfilled with the high tech procedures. ART did help us to achieve three pregnancies. Just remember that doctors are not God, and if you are open to other ideas, you might just still achieve your dream. There are no guarantees, but there can be hope outside the realm of medically assisted techniques such as IVF.

I became pregnant naturally, roughly seven months after my therapy at CPT. At 42, I gave birth to a beautiful baby girl.

39, Multiple Miscarriages, and 12 Years Infertile

- Makayla's Story

As a young married couple, the thought of not bearing children never entered our minds. As a matter of fact, on our third date we named our children and over the course of our union, we prayed for them by name on a regular basis. Whenever we spoke of our family's future, we always referred to our children by the names we gave them, some 20 years ago.

The thought of not bearing children never entered our minds.

After our first two years of marriage, we miscarried our first child early in the first trimester. Laparoscopic surgery was performed on me, but the doctor insisted that there wasn't any reason for alarm. He told us that miscarriages happen without concrete medical reasons in most cases and one to three miscarriages were not unusual before delivering your first child.

After a brief mourning period, life continued. With the growing pains of marriage and career changes, life progressed. After seeing a holistic doctor for basic health reasons, the iridologist (after looking into my eyes for less than five minutes), told me that I had had a miscarriage and that my left tube was blocked. Both my husband and I went on a detox regimen and took specific herbs to increase our chances to conceive.

By our 12th year of marriage, we were faced with the reality of not having children.

Over the next ten years, I had several early miscarriages, yet our faith sustained our belief that our children would be born.

By our 12th year of marriage, we were faced with the reality of not having any children. Amongst our peers and family, we were the only couple in our age group that had not produced any children. Needless to say, there was constant questioning and in some instances taunting that challenged my husband's manhood. After a near restaurant brawl with one of our closest friends (whose wife was six months pregnant at 42), the incident provoked us to seek medical advice.

Through our HMO, we took the necessary fertility classes and tests. To the relief of my husband, there was no conclusive evidence of why we couldn't conceive (in other words, his sperm count was GOOD!) All hormone levels were normal! I did remember to tell our fertility doctor about the holistic examination done several years prior, but he was not a believer in those methods. Yet after several months of more testing, it was "medically" determined that I had a blockage in my left fallopian tube. Doctors performed a second laparoscopic surgery, and once again we were cleared for conception.

A year after the surgery, my husband and I were still determined to conceive. We tried various tips: eating oysters, rotating days, ovulation tests, and even the upside down method (don't laugh — it seemed logical). Nothing, nothing, nothing. Over this process, I was really in tune with my body and could feel certain pains emanating from the left ovary. By this time I was 39, and I attributed most of my pains to the aging process.

Around this time, the external pressure started to tamper with our parental psyche. We were bombarded with the same old question, "When are you going to have children?" There was constant prayer at our church; every time there was a healing line for couples wanting children, people would drag us to the front of the line. Finally it became so overwhelming to me that I made the decree that by the age of 40 I would deliver my first child, it would be a girl (who we had already named years ago), and I even got specific with other physical attributes. No one ever asked me again; they just prayed!

One day I was watching the local news and I saw an exposé on Clear Passage Therapies (CPT). I called a girlfriend, who was struggling with conception as well, and told her about the news story. She immediately called and requested more information.

Once I received my information package (which was quite impressive), I was convinced that the treatment offered at CPT would benefit my plight. Over the next several months, I gathered all the required information necessary for the treatment. After obtaining my surgical notes from the previous year, I noticed that the doctor had discovered a "nabothian cyst" two inches in diameter. Not only had he just left it there, he failed to even mention it to me. I sought medical attention from my gynecologist, who said the cyst should have no bearing on my ability to conceive.

My body was back in alignment, and the constant pain in my left ovary was gone.

By this time, my CPT treatment was days away. Upon my arrival in Gainesville, the staff at CPT was great. I had missed my original flight and arrived a few hours late. They restructured my schedule and began treatment. I was so overwhelmed with their personal attention, their knowledge, and just their overall kindness. The facility was pristine and the atmosphere was peaceful. By day three, I was calling all of my close friends to recommend the treatment for body realignment, peace of mind, and just an overall treat for self-improvement.

My sole purpose for the treatment was to increase my chances of getting pregnant, but by the time I left, the colors in the spectrum were more vibrant, my body was back in alignment, and the constant pain in my left ovary was gone. I felt more in tune with myself than ever . . . it was liberating.

Within months of my treatment, I conceived and by my 40th birthday I was entering my second trimester! Today, at 43, by the grace of God, I have a beautiful and extremely busy three-year-old little girl!

Within months of my treatment, I conceived (naturally) and by my 40th birthday I was entering my second trimester!

Without question, I attribute the miracle of having a child to my Heavenly Father, but I am certain that He blessed the minds and hands of those at CPT to provide a balanced, more feasible approach to conception for those of us with the desire to bear children.

A New View of Unexplained Infertility

Unexplained (or idiopathic) infertility means "no known cause;" it does not mean "no cause." There is always a cause for pain or dysfunction, though the cause(s) may not be evident.

When infertility remains unexplained despite the best efforts of fertility specialists, it may be prudent to step back and take a broader look at the body as a whole. As we saw early in this book, a hip injury can cause adhesions to form at the ovaries or fallopian tubes, just a half-inch away. A fall onto the tailbone or tightness at the base of the skull may disrupt reproductive function in ways that gynecologists may not consider — or may not have the tools to treat.

Over the years, we have found that by working together with their gynecologist and a knowledgeable physical therapist or other healthcare professional with a "whole body" view, and by bringing their own intuition into the equation, many women have found answers to their search that were simple and obvious. It was necessary to stand back and take a longer view — one that included histories of trauma, infection, inflammation and surgery over their entire lifetime.

Seven Years of Infertility

- Barbara's Story

My husband and I married in 1985. I was 29 and my husband was 33. We knew from the beginning that we wanted to have a family and decided to not use any birth control.

Becoming pregnant wasn't our main focus at the time and we weren't concerned when two years passed by without any pregnancy.

After the third year, we began wondering, "Why aren't we pregnant?" We considered going to a doctor, but we had just moved to Florida and didn't know any.

By our fourth year, we found a doctor and went through basic testing. We were counseled on the normal things: Don't wear boxer shorts, don't be in a hot Jacuzzi, etc. He really made us feel that we had nothing to be alarmed about.

We kept trying, and also decided to focus on healing my body. In 1986, 10 months into our marriage, I had a severe car accident. For years I had sought help from physical therapy, orthopedic doctors, and chiropractors in Colorado. Now, in Florida, I had continued this process. I was still experiencing pain and severe headaches on a daily basis when my chiropractor recommended I see Belinda Wurn, head of a new physical therapy clinic that had recently opened. At first, I was skeptical, but I was told that she had a new physical therapy technique and, as a massage therapist, I knew her manual treatment could only help.

I started attending treatment with Belinda and my body improved greatly. Over time, my one lingering complaint was severe headaches. Belinda explained that the dura runs from the base of the skull all the way to the tailbone. She felt that my car accident caused my dura to be pulled, leading to constriction and headaches at the base of the skull. She wanted to loosen the scar tissue around my sacrum and tailbone to see if it would help reduce my headaches.

After her explanation, I agreed and she performed the techniques to reduce scar tissue. Because I was a massage therapist, she also showed me how to perform some of the techniques myself.

Within eight to ten hours of therapy, my headaches disappeared. But the most astounding side effect was one I never expected — I was pregnant! After seven years of infertility, I was finally pregnant! When I told Belinda, she cautiously asked me, "Did you want to be?" When I explained my story she breathed a sigh of relief and told me, "Oh, I'm glad. I was afraid you might be upset. I've been using this technique and women who were infertile are getting pregnant! Some people are very shocked!"

Within eight to ten hours of therapy, my (chronic) headaches disappeared. But the most astounding side effect was one I never expected — I was pregnant!

Intrigued by yet another pregnancy, Belinda asked me a series of questions about my history. Because the technique reduced scar tissue within the reproductive tract, she was looking for probable causes of adhesion formation in my past. I told her that my doctors once thought I had pelvic inflammatory disease (PID), but they never did anything to treat it. They also told me that I had some endometriosis, which also wasn't treated. I had also been sexually abused as a child.

Three months later, we conceived again. At age 40, my second son was born.

Belinda explained that these events could have caused adhesions to form that prevented me from getting pregnant. When I told her that the painful intercourse I experienced before treatment had also gone away, she felt that the adhesions were the likely culprit of that pain as well.

My beautiful son was born in 1993, when I was 36. After his birth, my husband and I wanted to have more children. We tried many times, but we never had success. Finally, I suggested to my husband that we try the scar tissue reduction techniques that Belinda had shown me, and we got pregnant immediately afterwards! We miscarried that little one, but using the technique, three months later, we conceived again. At age 40, my second son was born.

I have since been able to get pregnant two more times. We are not sure what caused those pregnancies to end in miscarriage, but I still think it is incredible I was able to become pregnant five times. Furthermore, it was only after I used the techniques Belinda showed me that I was able to become pregnant.

As I look at my two sons now, I remember what Belinda told me during therapy: "Embrace the car accident. It happened to you, but look at all it is affording you." Because of the car accident, I was able to receive the funds for counseling and physical therapy. Through counseling, I discovered I was sexually abused as a child, which my parents later confirmed. I was also able to become pregnant through Belinda's physical therapy. God orchestrated something bad into something completely wonderful.

When I look at Belinda's own history, I can also see God's divine nature. She went through the tragic experience of cancer and was unable to have children afterwards. Yet, because of her cancer, she discovered a treatment that is directly responsible for my two children and dozens of others.

Releasing Emotional Pain

- Molly's Story

Let me first say I always wanted children and I always wanted to have a family. I never thought I wouldn't. My struggle to have children began with personal issues from my childhood. I had to change my thinking before my body and emotions would allow me to get pregnant and have a baby.

When I married at age 22, I was ready to start a family. However, my husband and I wanted to be in the right emotional and financial state. It was until New Years Eve of 2000, when I was 35, that we finally decided to start our family. My husband had a new job, I had a master's degree, and our new home was finally completed.

My husband and I flushed my birth control pills together down the toilet. We then went to an open field and lit fireworks together to celebrate our decision to have a baby. We moved into our new home and couldn't believe how wonderful everything with my husband was.

However, my body now wanted to stop my heart from joy...we could not get pregnant. Every month, we kept seeing my period. I was completely devastated.

Every month we kept seeing my period. I was completely devastated.

Christmas Eve of 2001 marked one year since we tried to get pregnant. We didn't have the money to see a fertility specialist, but my parents offered to pay for it.

In January of 2002, I turned 37 and all tests came back saying there was no reason I couldn't get pregnant: my tubes were clear, my FSH was 6, I did not have fibroids, my periods were normal, etc.

The doctor advised we begin Clomid ...nothing. We also tried IUIs and injectables, but no baby. Our doctor said it was time we try IVF, but the lab was closed for the next six months.

In the meantime, my mother came across an article on Clear Passage Therapies (CPT). She told me, "You know while you're waiting for your IVF this will keep you feeling proactive and help your uterus be nice and cozy for the new baby." I am crying as I write this for my mother and her support and love and finding this article.

My husband and I went to CPT from August 27-29th for 10 hours of treatment. We were so impressed with everyone there. My husband was even in the room during some of the treatments where they tried to show him how he could do the massages at home.

For the first time I loved my body, and released the emotional pain from my heart

I then went by myself for an additional 10 hours from September 3-6th. I had a lot of time to reflect, and one of my therapists explained how we hold past emotional trauma within ourselves and how we need to release it somehow. It got me thinking that maybe I was holding on to my past and even though everything seemed to be okay now, deep down I was still hurting.

That night, I went back to my hotel room. I started thinking about the messages from my past and how they could be holding me back. I vowed to start loving my body and see what other things I could do to get ready for IVF in January. I felt rejuvenated – all the way to my uterus and cervix. For the first time I loved my body and released the emotional pain from my heart that I did not realize was there.

When I got home, I decided to start acupuncture and eliminated bad carbohydrates from my diet. In November, I returned to the IVF clinic for a consultation and the doctor was amazed by how clear and smooth my uterus looked. I told him about CPT and he scoffed at the idea - but I knew CPT helped! CPT allowed me to start taking notice of my body and emotions as a whole. I learned that I needed to take care of my body and emotions in order to achieve a pregnancy.

In January I returned to the IVF clinic for my transfer. I was shocked when they told me my FSH was 16! My IVF cycle was canceled and the doctor told me my only option was donor eggs. The doctor said I had a 1% of ever conceiving with my own eggs. I fell to pieces. I left the clinic so angry and mad – I could not believe I had another obstacle. It was the worst day of my life.

My IVF cycle was canceled and the doctor told me my only option was donor eggs.

I was soon able to rationalize the experience with myself though. Even though he was a doctor, I knew he was not GOD and did not know everything. I knew my body was healthy.

I remembered that CPT told me to let go of internal anger. I got on the internet and started searching and came across a book by Julia Indichova called *Inconceivable*. I ordered it with a two day RUSH!

I remember so clearly the day it came in the mail. There were two packages – one with egg donor information from the fertility clinic and one with *Inconceivable*. I opened the egg donor info and was angry that all these girls had their eggs and were so young and healthy. When I was their age, I wasted my time and now I was too late.

I called my mom and she told me not to worry about it. She suggested we go on a cruise together to take our mind off everything. Her idea made me feel better so I dried my tears and got out the book. I read it straight through.

Afterward, I took a long hot bath and thought about my past. From my soul I cried just like the CPT therapist talked about. I could feel such love wash over me. I realized that I was meant to have a baby. *Inconceivable* talked about these same things and how women can ALLOW themselves to have a baby. I visualized that I could either walk down the road infertile with no baby or that I could walk toward my husband and the baby he had in his arms. I also visualized my mother, father, husband, and everyone whom I loved all around me smiling and wishing me to have a healthy

I visualized I could either walk down the road infertile with no baby, or I could walk toward my husband and the baby he had in his arms.

pregnancy. Even my sister who died at birth was there. It felt so good to see these images in my mind.

My husband and I made love that night, we did not try to get pregnant we just loved each other.

Later that week, my mother and I left for our cruise. I turned 38 while on ship. The day I got off, I took a pregnancy test and it was POSITIVE!!!!!!! My husband, my parents, and I were all there together in shock! We all cried and laughed and celebrated!!!! Then my husband and I drove back to our home a few states away with a little baby in my tummy.

Just 17 days earlier my doctor had told me that I had a less than 1% chance of ever getting pregnant with my own eggs. He never would have guessed that just nine months later, I held my beautiful little boy in my arms – born out of pure hope and love.

Nine Years Infertile Myomectomy and Failed IVF

- Addison's Story

For nine years, I tried to get pregnant — five years with a previous marriage and four years with my current husband. During the first five years, I did not pursue any invasive treatment. However, with my current husband, we were willing to try anything to have children.

I had several surgeries to remove fibroids and tumors on my ovaries and in my uterus. Afterwards, we tried Clomid and other hormone treatments, but nothing worked.

We made the decision to try IVF, however, my body did not accept the medications and it ended up costing double what we had anticipated. We chose not to try IVF again, and believed that God's plan for us must be to adopt, so we registered with a local agency.

Several months passed while we waited to hear from the agency. One day, as I was listening to the radio, I heard an ad that Clear Passage Therapies (CPT) would be featured on the news that evening. That night, I was fascinated with what I saw.

I told my husband about CPT, and he figured it was just a scam. After all that we had been through, he was not willing to lose any more money.

A few weeks later, my husband saw CPT featured on the news and became interested. We asked for more information and received a packet.

We tried Clomid and other hormone treatments, but nothing worked.

A month later, we saw another interview with CPT on the news. We started to feel that there must be a reason we kept hearing about it, and decided to pursue treatment immediately. After all of the heartbreak we had been through, we decided to go in with a mindset of decreasing my intercourse pain, rather than getting pregnant.

Our experience at CPT was wonderful. I received 20 hours of treatment over a 10 week period. The two hour drive up and back gave my husband and I quality time together. We usually took an entire day off for the trip — eating in the area and walking after treatments. We felt like the whole staff became family during our journey.

Upon completion of our treatment, we determined that it was well worth the money and time since my pain had been tremendously reduced. In addition, my therapist found and relieved problems that none of my previous specialists could.

Shortly after we completed our treatments, we received a call from the adoption agency. They told us that a couple had chosen us to be parents for their unborn child. We were ecstatic and hurried to meet the birth parents. Our meeting went well and the agency, the birth parents, my husband and I thought it was a perfect placement.

We decorated the nursery in lilac with butterflies. Everyone was so excited and happy for us that we had three baby showers! We were completely prepared and all we had to do was wait for the call.

We finally received the call in October. We rushed to the hospital, and were then taken into the nursery to meet our new baby girl. She was precious, and the nurse allowed me to stay with her in a special room for adopting parents.

A representative from the (adoption) agency told us "I have some bad news." My heart sank — I knew immediately what that meant.

The nurse told us she would be released the next day, so we hurried home to gather everything we would need to bring our daughter home. When we returned to the hospital, a representative from the agency came in and told us, "I have some bad news." My heart sank — I knew immediately what that meant. She proceeded to say, "The birth mom is having second thoughts."

I could not move, and the nurses came in to remove the baby from us. I fell to the floor in tears. My husband was devastated and so angry, but was trying to stay strong for me. For weeks, I refused to speak to anyone.

I was not about to give up, however. I proceeded to search the Internet for information on International Adoption. In a matter of days, I had completed most of the paperwork and set appointments with doctors for all of the medical requirements.

The day before our doctor's appointment, I was feeling really strange. I felt nauseated while driving back home. I couldn't recall the last time I had my period because I had been so busy working on the adoption process. I stopped at the store on my way home and picked up a pregnancy test, thinking that one more letdown wouldn't hurt.

I hurried to get home and take the test before my husband came home. I did the test, and it immediately changed to positive. I thought I had a faulty test because I had never seen one change to positive.

When my husband came home, I told him what happened, but told him not to get excited because I had bought a cheap test. I went out that night and bought two more tests. I did one that night and another in the morning — still, they were all positive.

I said, "Well, we have a doctor's appointment today anyway, I'll have them do a pregnancy test before they administer the medical tests for the adoption."

We explained the situation to our doctor and she went ahead and did the pregnancy test. She came in a few minutes later and confirmed that I was in fact pregnant. We were so shocked, we didn't tell anyone for several months due to all of the heartache that we and both of our families had already endured.

I thought I had a faulty test because I had never seen one change to positive.

However, everything turned out just great. I had a very easy pregnancy and Abraham was delivered six weeks early in June 2004. He was very healthy at birth despite the early arrival, and is doing very well today. We are so grateful to everyone at CPT for making our dreams come true!

Two Prior IUIs and a Failed IVF

- Paulina's Story

I never expected to have any problems getting pregnant. My mother had four children, and each of my two sisters have one son. So as I faced my mid-thirties, I kept wondering what was wrong with me, what was wrong with my body, why was this happening to me? I am healthy. I take care of myself. I try to eat right and exercise. Why is getting pregnant so hard?

"Trying" to have a baby, definitely took the fun out of having sex with my husband. After two years of "trying" on our own, we decided to get some professional help. We started with tests and then more tests without much explanation other than the fact that I had one blocked fallopian tube (the other was still functional).

I am a believer in natural body remedies, so I started acupuncture and Chinese herbal medicine and continued with this treatment for the next year.

My Ob/Gyn recommended Clomid to help with my ovulation. Unfortunately, I was on this drug for about six months with many unpleasant side effects, but no luck.

My Ob/Gyn then referred me to a fertility specialist, one of the top doctors in NYC (and one of the most expensive). After more tests for my husband and me, we discovered we were both healthy, no real issues — only a closed fallopian tube.

Of course, the fertility specialist immediately recommended the most aggressive treatment — IVF. He still had no real answers why we could not get pregnant. I never really felt comfortable with that doctor, as he would always address my husband, not me, when we consulted with him. I really felt like this was way too much and way too fast, without any explanation.

The fertility specialist immediately recommended the most aggressive treatment – IVF. He still had no real answers why we could not get pregnant.

Before agreeing to IVF, I wanted other options. We tried intrauterine insemination (IUI) twice, but it failed both times. After a few months of frustration and feeling the pressure of getting older, I agreed to IVF treatment, which became the most difficult process I had encountered. I had a lot of ups and downs on the meds and never felt quite confident it was going to work. I always felt this was not the way I was supposed to have a baby. Yet, I stuck it out and went through it all.

We spent our savings on IVF and fertility treatments, and it was devastating for both my husband and I when it did not work. After this treatment failed, we certainly didn't receive any sympathy from our doctor. His advice was we needed to do IVF again and we shouldn't wait too long.

At that point, I just decided I needed a break from treatments. I started researching and reading many books about infertility and diet and ways I could make changes in my life to help my body prepare for a baby. During this time I discovered Clear Passage Therapy's (CPT) website and read the personal stories from their clients. I thought it was amazing, but was too good to be true. However, there was something about how the women told their stories, the sincerity and honesty. The stories really created an emotional response in me. Unless you have experienced how devastating it feels not to be able to get pregnant, then you just don't understand how desperate you are and how you are willing to try anything.

I wrote to CPT and was fortunate to discover they were opening an office in NYC. So I decided to get their information, apply, and set up appointments when they opened. I was

Emotionally and physically I was exhausted.

very pleased to have such a wonderful therapist. I knew there was no guarantee with this treatment, but I was willing to try it and especially glad that I would not have to take any more meds.

Treatment with CPT was painful at times but my therapist always took the time to explain the treatment and what we were going to do. She was always aware and sensitive to my pain tolerance. The treatment definitely took a lot out of me. Emotionally and physically I was exhausted after each treatment and I started writing about my feelings. This helped me deal with my feelings of failure because I could not get pregnant.

After treatment ended, I felt better, with less pain in my uterus overall. I also noticed my cycles were stronger and healthier.

After the treatment, I wanted to talk to another fertility specialist to get a second opinion. My specialist was really insightful and explained why my previous IVF treatment failed. I told her about CPT and my acupuncture treatments. She was very open to alternative treatments and basically supported anything that I believed would help me. She really wanted to help me find the cause of my infertility.

She suggested, given my medical history and closed fallopian tube, I may have endometriosis. She did not recommend any drugs or any treatments until she knew more. I agreed to exploratory laparoscopic surgery to clear up scar tissue or any problems in my uterus. I was scheduled for surgery in December and performed the routine blood tests required before surgery.

A week before I was scheduled to undergo the surgery, I received a call from my doctor, informing me that I was not a candidate for surgery because my blood tests confirmed I was pregnant! I was in complete shock and could not believe it. I asked them if they were sure because it was not possible — I had a regular menstruation cycle last month. "Yes, we are positive because of your blood work," they told me. "It confirms you are pregnant." I needed to get in there for a sonogram immediately, she said.

I received a call from my doctor informing me that I was not a candidate for surgery – because I was pregnant!

Well . . .
the rest is just a happy ending. After years of infertility, I gave birth to my daughter, Teresa, who is my greatest gift and blessing in life. She is our miracle and has given us such complete joy and happiness that we have never known before.

I am very grateful to my therapist and CPT for all of their work that not only helped me, but continues to help many women with their fertility issues. No treatment can guarantee success, but at least women have an option without drugs or surgery. This manual physical therapy does much more than just massage therapy . . . it gives us hope, and in my case, a beautiful daughter despite years of infertility.

Section Three

Sexual Dysfunction and Pain

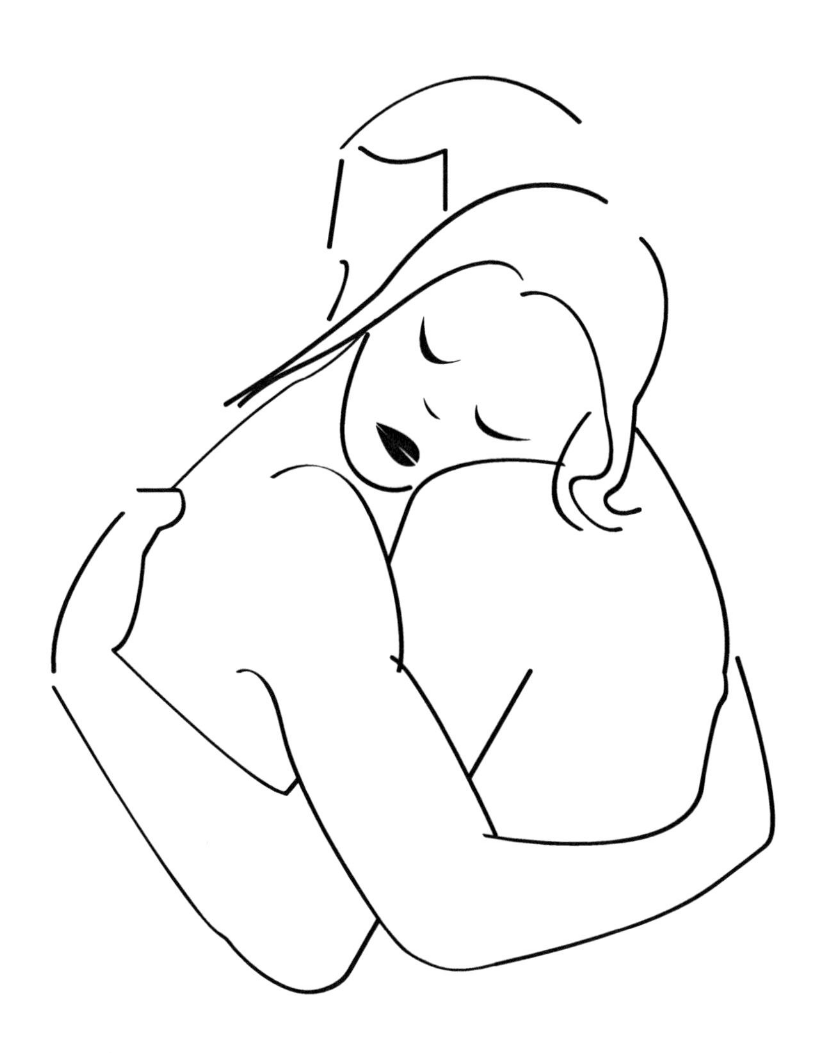

Chapter Twelve

Painful Intercourse

Millions of women suffer needlessly from intercourse pain. Today, we understand that there is no longer any need for most of these women to forego intimacy or undergo pain, especially at the times they should be experiencing pleasure.

- Belinda Wurn, PT

Is Intercourse Pain Normal?

Although few women speak of it, intercourse pain (dyspareunia) and sexual dysfunction impact the lives of millions of women. The journal *Urology* reported that 50% of all US women experience some form of sexual dysfunction during their lives.[22] Over 70% of women surveyed in a large study in the *Journal of Family Practice*[23] reported painful intercourse, and 60% of US women reported intercourse pain at some point during their lives, according to the *American Family Physician*.[24] Yet despite the high prevalence, women frequently do not discuss their sexual concerns with their physicians, according to the journal.

Sexual concerns and dysfunction include intercourse pain, anorgasmia (the inability to have an orgasm or to reach a full orgasm), and decreased desire (libido), arousal, lubrication, and satisfaction. For many women, intense orgasms are a myth, a thing of the past, or something that will never be.

Many women feel that "sex hurts" or that it has never been the pleasurable sensation they thought it would be, from their very first experience. Others note an increase in pain, sometimes accompanied by a decline in desire and vaginal sensation as years go by. In this chapter we will examine intercourse pain (dyspareunia) and treatments available.

Adhesions and Intercourse Pain

During the course of life, the vagina and female reproductive tract may be subjected to traumas or surgery. In addition, the opportunity for infection or inflammation can occur because the vagina is open to exposure from the outside environment via tampons, sexual partners, sexual abuse, and self-exploration. The dark, moist environment of the vagina is also a perfect environment to nurture bacterial growth — and bacterial infections.

When infection or inflammation occurs on the walls of the vagina, cervix, or nearby structures, the body's first response is to lay down collagenous cross-links, the building blocks of adhesions.

When adhesions form within the vagina, the delicate and sensitive tissues of the vaginal walls or opening can become restricted by tiny collagenous bonds with a strength of nearly 2,000 pounds per square inch. Bound down by small adhesive straight-jackets, these highly innervated tissues become much less mobile and pliable. During intercourse, they can be stretched beyond their ability to move. Fixed in place by tiny, glue-like bonds, they can pull on nerves and cause a significant amount of pain as intercourse begins.

For others, the adhesive process occurs much deeper in the vagina, at the cervix, and the pain occurs with deep penetration. This is experienced by some women as a broader, deeper pain. Other patients report that "it feels like my partner is hitting something." Some women have a combination of initial and deep penetration pain, sometimes accompanied (quite understandably) by pelvic and uterine cramping. We treat these conditions clinically every day as we have for twenty years. We have published solid data on effective treatment of this biomechanical cause of intercourse pain.

Our therapy is quite different from the psychological counseling that has been Western medicine's usual response for the last several decades. The "it's all in your head diagnosis" can be damaging to some women who then feel they must be crazy to be feeling pain. While we value psychological counseling, we find it necessary to physically address the mechanical causes of most intercourse pain

Pain at the Vaginal Opening

Direct trauma

The most common cause we see of introitus (vaginal entrance) pain is a direct trauma earlier in life. Sometimes, this can be traced to a single traumatic event, such as a fall onto the pubic bones or coccyx (tailbone) [e.g. from playing on a jungle gym or slipping on ice and falling onto the buttocks] or sexual abuse. Trauma may occur later in life, such as a nearby surgery or a cut at the entry to the vagina such as an episiotomy, when the back of the vaginal opening is cut to aid vaginal delivery.

In other cases, we find that an injury which caused overstretching of the adductor muscle (on the inside of the leg attaching to the public bone) causes adhesions that pull directly into the vaginal entrance and perineum.

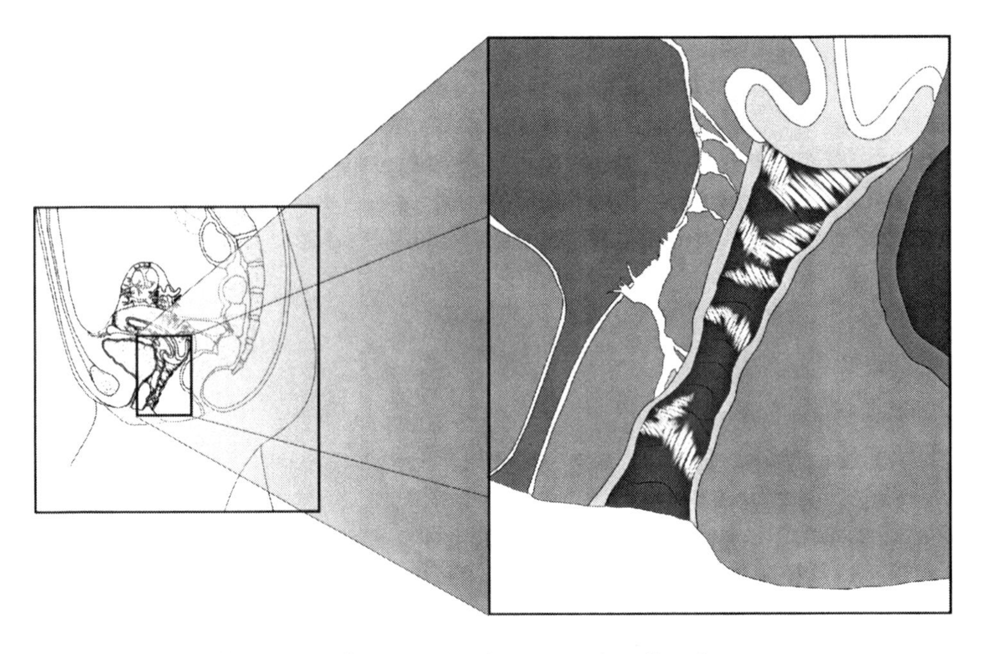

We find tiny adhesions on the vaginal wall to be common.
These can bind pain-sensitive tissues, causing intercourse pain.

In many cases, we find that pain at the vaginal entrance is a result of multiple traumas or events over life. Repeat traumas from gymnastics, bicycling, or horseback riding account for many instances of introitus pain we treat regularly.

Unfortunately, physical and sexual abuse are fairly common. Although the abuse or trauma may have ended years or even decades earlier, the effects remain in the tissues for a lifetime due to the cross-links, adhesions, and scars that formed to help the tissues heal so many years ago. We discuss this in further depth in Chapter Fourteen.

Infection/Inflammation

The entrance to the vagina is subject to bacterial infection, and we often see one or more vaginal or bladder infections in the histories of women who present with entrance pain or decreased sexual response. We surmise that as the body began healing from the infection and inflammation, tiny cross-links formed in the area, binding some of the vaginal tissues. Unable to move freely and attached to nerves, these tissues can elicit significant pain at the entrance of the vagina when a woman attempts sexual intercourse.

Psychological trauma

Less common, but just as debilitating, we sometimes treat women whose vaginal muscles have been "guarding" against traumatic sex or pain for most of their lives. Whether the patient is protecting herself against a tormentor who is no longer a threat, or is holding onto beliefs taught in childhood that sex is dirty, bad, or a sin, or for a host of other reasons, the muscles of the vagina can shut tightly, in a state of near-constant spasm. This condition is referred to as "vulvodynia" or as "vaginismus."

Early in our marriage, I suffered from discomfort and sometimes pain during intercourse... When I returned home (after therapy) I was eager to see my husband. We had a wonderful night, pain-free and pleasurable. I had a new intimate life with my husband!

- Jennifer, mother of one and currently expecting after struggling with infertility, intercourse pain and chronic urinary tract infections.

Over time, inflammation develops from the persistent spasm. The consequence generally includes adhesions that create, perpetuate, and even intensify the pain. This spasm can be so severe that it can prevent vaginal penetration by anything — a tampon, finger, gynecological exam, penis, or even the smallest dilator.

Pain at Deep Penetration

The Tailbone

Falls onto the buttock are common throughout life, and the coccyx (tailbone) is a common recipient of that trauma. The tailbone can be pushed forward or to either side by any fall in the area. If the fall is mild, the tissues generally recover and the tailbone becomes mobile again. When it is mobile, it can move out of the way during a bowel movement, and during sexual intercourse. But if the tissues and ligaments around the tailbone have been sufficiently injured, they can pull the tailbone forward and it can heal in that abnormally fixed position with mechanical restrictions to its mobility. The tailbone can then become a physical block to intercourse and/or bowel movements.

> ***By the time I left (CPT), sex no longer hurt, my appendectomy scar felt completely different, and my tailbone was more properly aligned.***
>
> *– Ashley, mother of one after struggling with infertility*

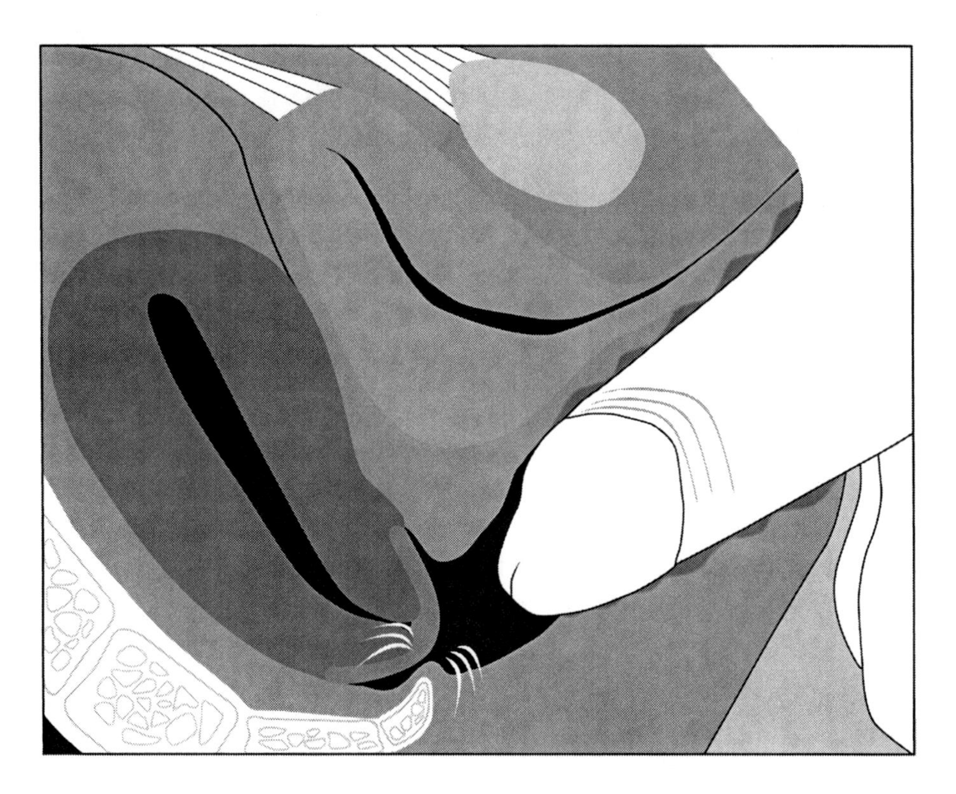

A fall or surgery can move the coccyx forward, causing a physical block to deep penetration.

When this happens, we hear such complaints as pain with deep penetration or bowel movements, chronic constipation, diarrhea (less frequently), difficulty sitting for long periods, and/or persistent headaches. These headaches often occur at the top or base of the skull or at the temples where the dura and spinal cord (which begins at the tailbone) attach to the skull. This phenomenon is explained more fully in Chapter Sixteen.

The Cervix

In its natural state, the cervix is situated midline in the vagina, at the entrance of the uterus. There, it comes in contact with everything that passes by: tampons, sexual partners, infections, and inflammations. In its position in the center of the vagina, the cervix is also in the center of the melee when problems arise.

The cervix is held in its (preferably midline) position by ligaments that attach to it at the front, back, and sides. Because of its unique position, it is vulnerable to adhesive cross-link formation at the various ligaments designed to hold it in place whenever the vagina undergoes a healing event — be it from trauma, infection, inflammation, or surgery.

When healing occurs at or near the cervix or neighboring structures, powerful adhesive cross-links form as the first step in the healing process. This causes the cervix to be pulled from its mobile, midline position, as it attaches via adhesive bonds to structures that lie in the direction of the healing mechanisms.

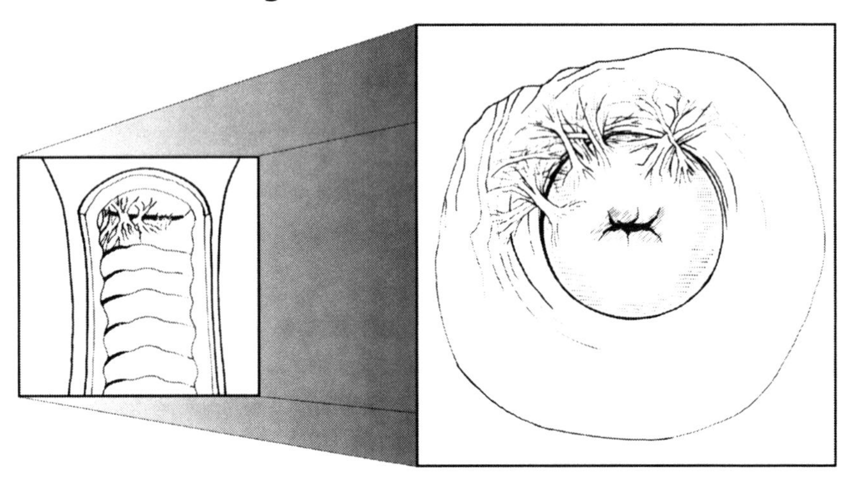

The cervix can become adhered to the vaginal wall, causing pain with deep penetration.

The cervix may be pulled towards the sacrum or tailbone by adhesions on the uterosacral ligament. In this position, it can tighten, close, or elicit pain with deep penetration. When the cervix is not in a fixed position, it can easily slide out of the way during intercourse. But when it is fixed in position by adhesions, it can be hit by the penis during intercourse. Unable to move and fixed in position against a thrusting partner, deep pain can occur for the woman.

The cervix may be pulled (and often is) to one side of the vagina, where it can attach via adhesive cross-links to the vaginal wall. When parts of the vaginal wall are glued to the cervix or tightened by glue-like adhesive cross-links, they do not stretch. Unable to attain their normal pliable and mobile state, the nerves within the vaginal wall may elicit pain when they are impacted by deep penetration.

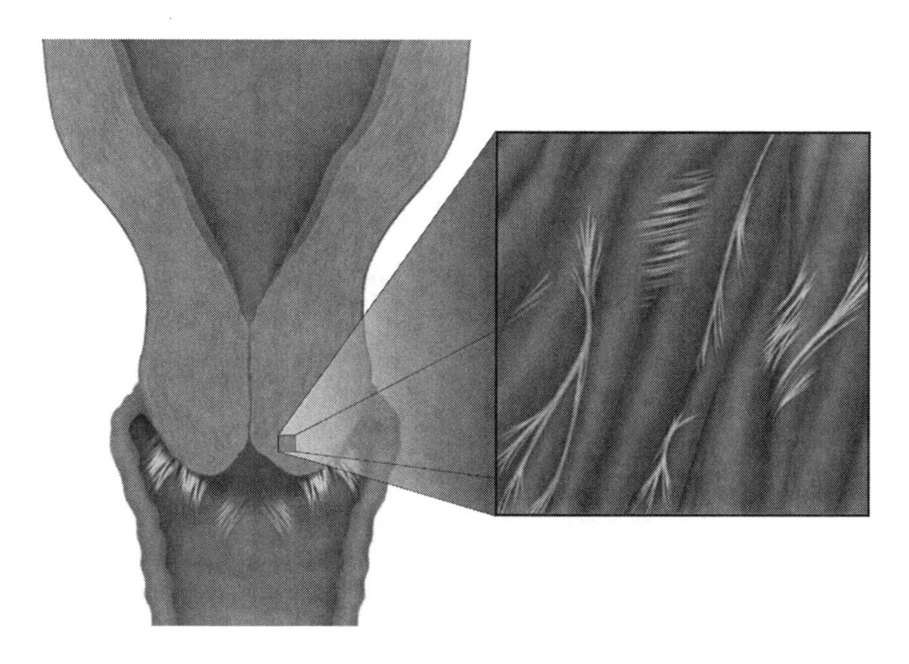

Tiny but strong cross-links can stiffen the cervix, or pull it out of a relaxed, midline position.

The cervix may also be pulled forward. We commonly see this in women who have suffered bladder or vaginal infections, abuse, or trauma to the anterior vaginal wall. This position of the cervix is often accompanied by additional sexual dysfunction, such as decreased desire, lubrication, or orgasm, due to its proximity to the G-spot and (through the vaginal wall) the clitoris. Some women also experience pain with urination due to adhesions between the anterior vaginal wall and the urethra.

Other conditions we notice quite frequently include cervical stiffening (fibrosis) and narrowing or closing (stenosis). In these situations, the adhesive cross-links may form deep within the cervix, between the cells of this highly muscular structure, as shown on the preceeding page. Upon palpation, the cervix may feel stiff, hardened or immobile. In some cases, the cervix may curl to the back, the front, or sides.

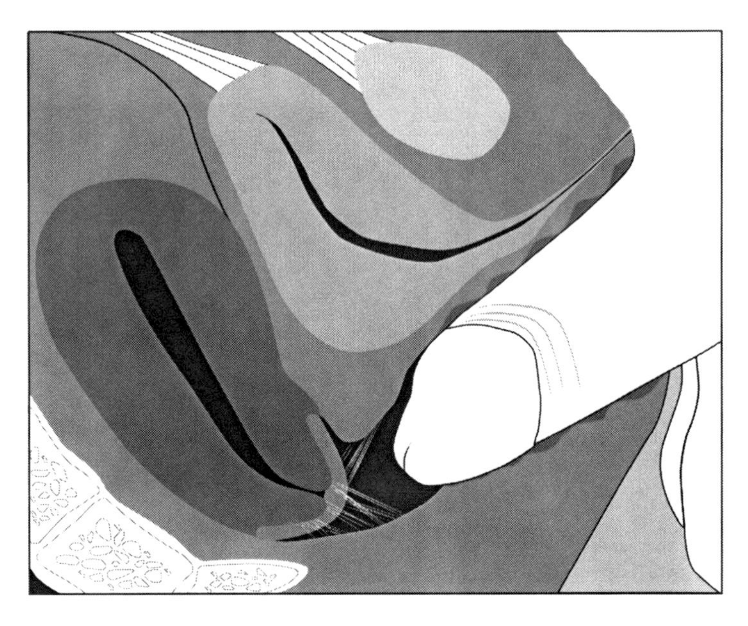

When a partner hits a stiffened cervix, deep pain is often the result.

The internal cross-links and scars within the structure of the cervix hold it in position. No longer pliable or mobile as it was during youth, the cervix becomes a fixed structure at the entrance to the uterus.

This can make it difficult for sperm to enter (naturally, or by catheter during IUI or IVF). In this position, it also becomes vulnerable to pain with deep penetration.

> ***When I returned home (after CPT), my husband and I were elated to find that there was no longer any pain with sex.***
>
> ***My husband joked that he would send me back for more treatment in a heartbeat.***
>
> *– Madison, mother of one who struggled with endometriosis, pain, and infertility*

Adhesions attaching within the muscle of the cervix or attaching the cervix to the nearby structures, including the vaginal walls, can also create an unnatural pull on the largely muscular uterus above. This can create spasm and inflammation when the woman has intercourse, walks, or has a period. Uterine spasm and inflammation are direct causes of infertility, and frequent causes of miscarriage in our experience.

> ***When I told my therapist that the painful intercourse I experienced before treatment (at CPT) had gone away, she felt that adhesions were the likely culprit of that pain.***
>
> *– Barbara, mother of two after struggling with infertility and intercourse pain*

As the reader may know, intrauterine devices (IUD) were designed to prevent pregnancy by creating inflammation within the uterus. The same biomechanical process occurs when the cervix or uterus becomes inflamed naturally. Adhesions form within the uterus and can bind it to other structures, causing a pull with every step a woman takes. This pull can create or perpetuate a cycle of adhesion-inflammation-adhesion as the woman proceeds through life.

The Vaginal Walls

As noted earlier, the vagina is subject to influences from the outside environment. Infection, inflammation, and trauma can cause adhesions to form, binding down areas within the highly innervated tissues of the vaginal wall.

In their natural state, the delicate tissues of the vaginal walls are pliable and mobile. But, when they become glued down by adhesions and collagenous cross-links, they lose their mobility and elasticity.

We often find tiny but powerful cross-links on vaginal walls of women with dyspareunia (intercourse pain).

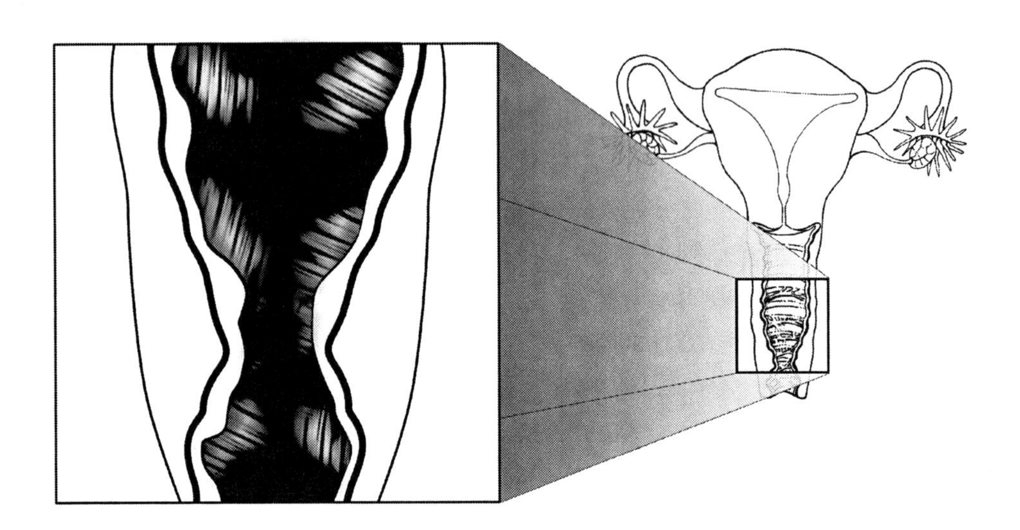

Still infused with thousands of tiny nerve endings, the now adhered vaginal walls can be pulled or stretched during sexual intercourse, causing moderate to severe pain.

Prior medical procedures

Surgeries performed anywhere in the pelvis can cause adhesions as we heal from the trauma of surgery. After viewing countless medical histories of our patients, we have found that medical procedures such as IUD placement and removal, D&C, surgery to the cervix, and dilation of the urethra to diagnose or treat urinary problems may also cause adhesions to form.

Intrauterine devices (IUD) are placed inside the uterus to prevent pregnancy. Their mechanism of action is to create inflammation within the uterus. Often, they do their job all too well. Inflammation creates adhesions and adhesions decrease mobility, often pulling into the cervix. The consequent adhesions can cause pain with deep penetration, or infertility. A dilation of the cervix or procedure at or near the vaginal opening can cause inflammation in some women, creating microscopic adhesions to form affecting tissues near the clitoris, urethra, and vaginal opening. This can cause pain with intercourse or urination, and can decrease sensation, libido, and the ability to orgasm.

Endometriosis

Sexual intercourse pain is a common complaint among women with endometriosis. Endometrial tissue creates inflammation wherever it is found. Inflammation causes tiny adhesive cross-links to form, binding the endometrial tissue to the underlying structures. Endometriosis within the vagina causes the same adhesive reaction as any other inflammation. As the body heals from inflammation, adhesions form. Whether found on the vaginal wall, the cervix, the coccyx, the entrance to the vagina (introitus), or at surgical scars, these adhesions pull on nerves during intercourse, causing pain. A thorough discussion of endometrial pain is presented in Chapter Seventeen.

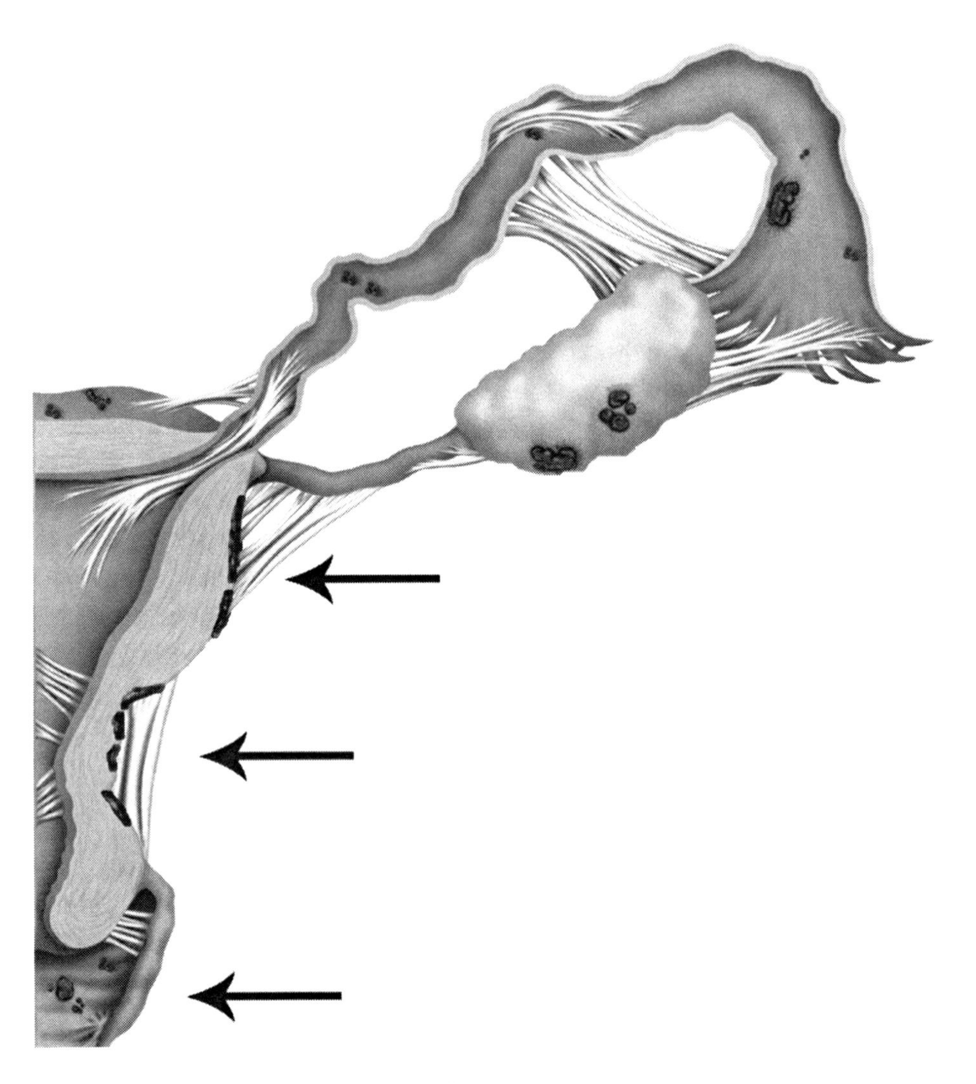

Endometrial adhesions cause tissues to contract, causing spasm or pain.

Treating Symptoms: A Major Problem with Modern Medicine

Until we stumbled upon and then expanded our work treating dyspareunia, modern medicine provided very few alternatives for women with intercourse pain. The most commonly prescribed modalities were:

- Pain killers (oral or topical)
- Desensitizing agents
- Psychological counseling
- Antidepressants
- Surgery

Pain medications and desensitizing agents have obvious drawbacks. Most women who are anticipating intercourse would like to be able to feel what's happening, especially if it is not painful. Pain killers and desensitizing agents remove the ability to feel in an area of the body that is very sensitive, and the most highly designed to experience physical pleasure.

Psychological counseling and antidepressants may help a woman cope with the fact that she cannot have intercourse without pain, but in most cases they do very little to actually decrease the physical pain. When there is a physical, mechanical reason for the pain, the best counseling or strongest antidepressant does not treat the cause of that biomechanical dysfunction. Thus, the condition persists as a permanent problem in the life of (literally) millions of women.

In rare cases, physicians find a reason to believe that surgery may help. We have found that surgery is a possibility for deep pain at the tailbone, such as coccydynia (tailbone pain), and some patients have told us that they received good relief after having the coccyx removed. However we have also treated many patients who underwent surgery for tailbone pain with terrible results. These patients came to us with much more debilitating pain than they had ever experienced prior to surgery. Most of these patients were on heavy doses of daily pain medications, including ibuprofen, narcotics, or morphine, when they arrived at our door. Some of them couldn't even get out of bed without experiencing severe and debilitating pain.

In other areas of the vagina or cervix, surgery can certainly cut adhesions. But scars left from surgery in this most sensitive area of a woman's body can leave a woman with debilitating, permanent pain. We have found that most gynecologists encourage women to try a more conservative option rather than opting for surgery for tailbone or intercourse pain.

Treating the Cause of the Pain

When we employ manual physical therapy to address sexual intercourse pain, we start with a thorough, physical evaluation of the external and internal vaginal tissues and structures. The examining team consists of two people — the therapist and the patient. Working together, slowly, gently, and with respect and sensitivity, the therapist first examines every centimeter of the opening of the vagina. We check the mobility in all directions, like the hands of a clock, examining the quality, mobility, and pain sensitivity of the structures.

> ***I had always thought the pain I experienced with intercourse was normal. I experienced a great reduction in intercourse pain (after CPT).***
>
> *– Sydney, mother of two after struggling with infertility and intercourse pain*

She notes any areas of pain, and together, they judge the amount of pain in each location on a scale of 0 to 10. We want to be certain that each patient leaves that evaluation with a thorough understanding of the precise areas causing her pain and the amount of pain each area elicits. As we proceed further into the examination we move deeper into the vagina if we are able to at that time, in order to check the cervix, pelvic floor, and pelvic wall muscles. If we are not, we will continue with deeper examination as we are able to during the next and subsequent sessions.

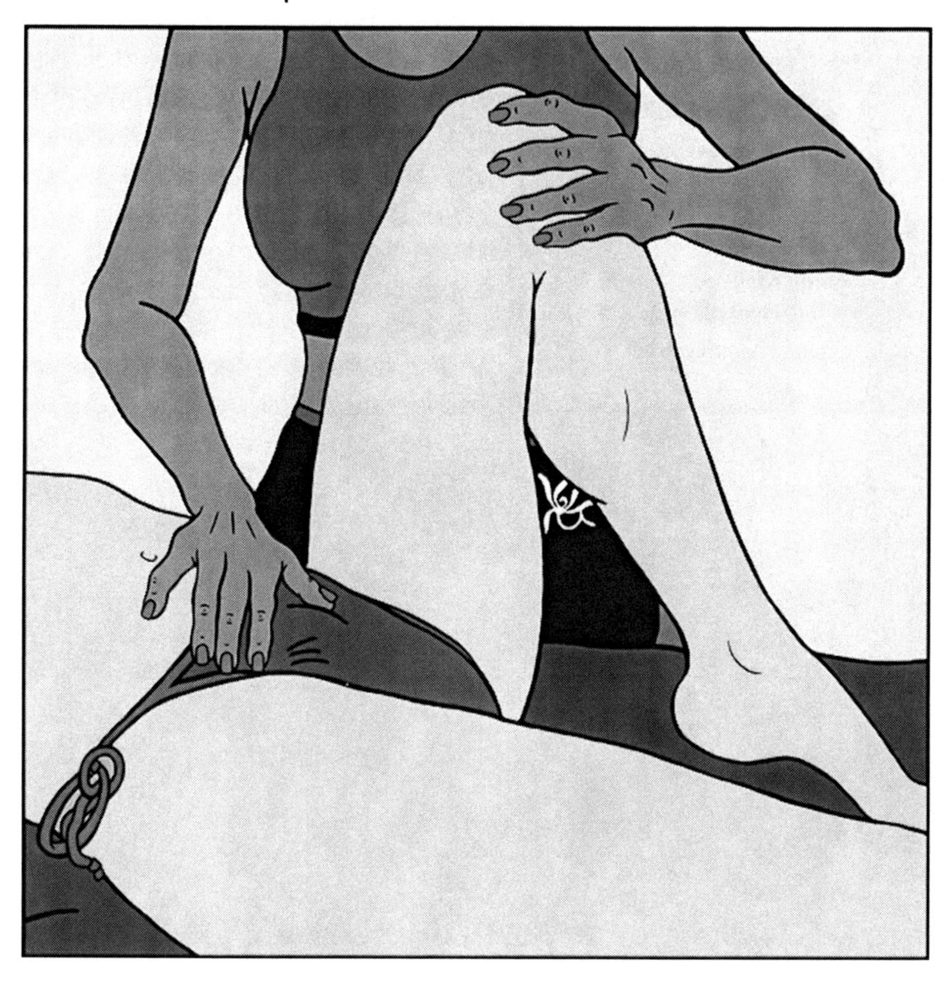

Thorough assessment and treatment of intercourse pain includes addressing all attachments into the medial pelvis.

We examine attachments into the legs, especially the adductors (the muscles on the inner thighs) which attach to the pubic symphysis (the bones at the front of the pubic mound). We have found that if a tear or trauma has occurred in this area earlier in life, it can create adverse consequences over time for the nearby vaginal and perineal tissues. When we examine this area, we note if any of the areas are tight, of if they replicate or increase the patient's pain. If they do, we know we must add that area to our focus of therapy. Thus, together with the patient, we thoroughly evaluate the full geography of the areas in and around the patient's vagina and perineum (crotch).

It didn't hurt anymore to go to the bathroom after therapy and sex was less painful.

– Kimberly, who struggled with chronic pain and endometriosis

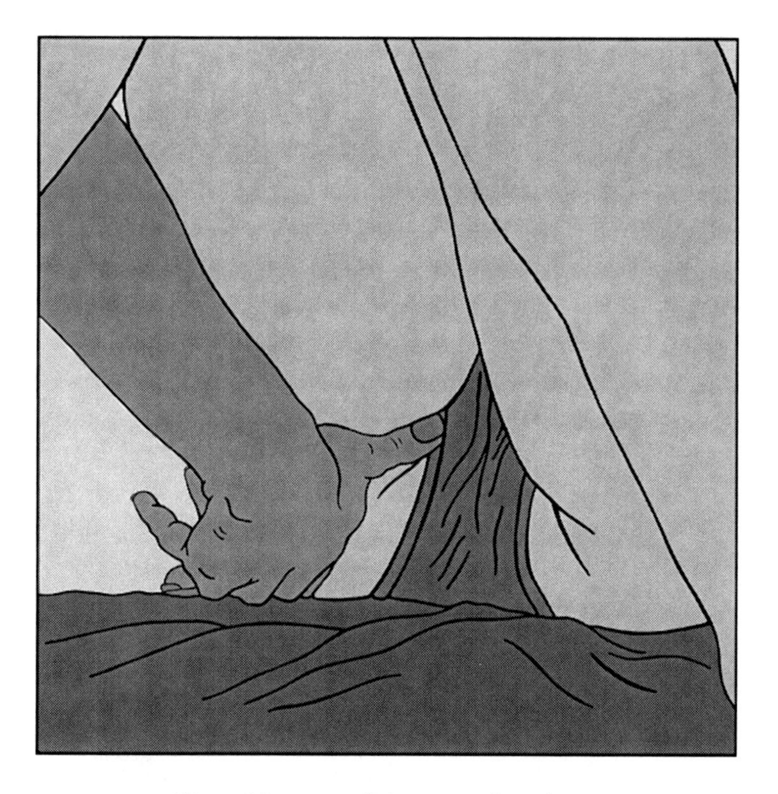

The adductors of the inner legs have strong fascial attachments into the urogenital area.

> **By the end of the week (at CPT), intercourse pain was completely gone – it was amazing!**
>
> - *Katrina, who struggled with chronic pain*

After assessing all of the adhered areas, we proceed slowly and gently into treatment. As we do, we detach adhesive cross-links, link by link. We describe what we are feeling in each area, and we ask our patient what she is feeling, "Is the pain right there where my hand is? Does it radiate to other parts of the body?

What is the quality of the pain (deep, piercing, sharp, burning, aching, etc.)? Now is it dissipating?"

Our published studies in this area have shown that the effects of this approach can be quite profound. Decreasing intercourse pain is definitely one of our highest areas for success. In fact, we have found that over the course of therapy, we have been able to decrease or eliminate intercourse pain in nearly every woman we treat. This encouraging outcome is supported by scientific data, published in highly respected medical journals. In fact, in two different studies, all but one patient received relief from intercourse pain after this therapy. [25]

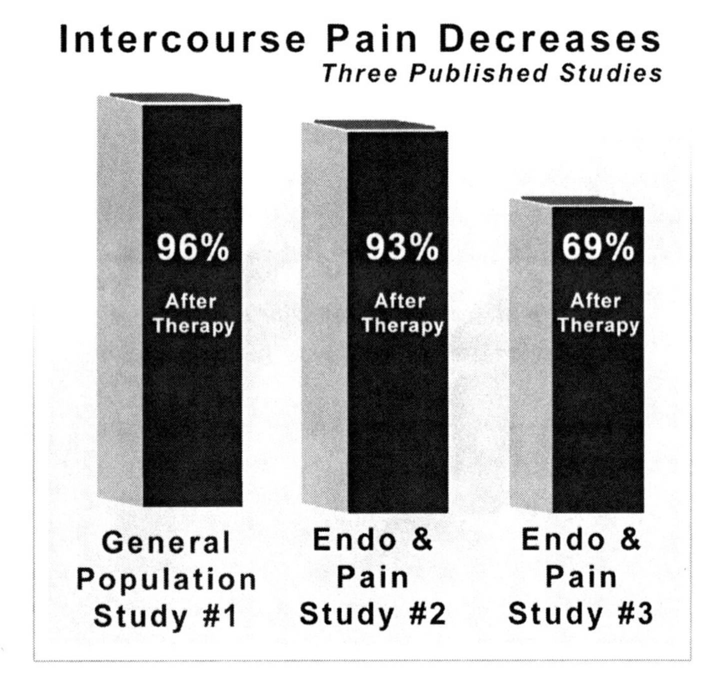

Three pioneering studies and citations examine our results treating intercourse pain. Medscape General Medicine (2004) and Fertility and Sterility (2006)

Unbearable Pain During Sex

- Emily's Story

When I was 27, I married my husband, Trevor. As a Christian, I had never had sex before I was married. I thought sex might be a bit painful the first couple of times, but on my wedding night and thereafter, it was awful! I felt like my husband was hitting a wall inside of me. I kept thinking, "We can work this out. If we can just push past the pain, it will be okay." However, he was just too nice to do that and he didn't want to hurt me.

Soon, the constant attempts and subsequent pain created a cycle. I would tense in anticipation of the pain to the point that it became both a physical and mental issue. I was so tight that at times he could not enter me at all.

It was awful! I felt like my husband was hitting a wall inside of me.

After a couple of years, I went to see my doctor. She gave me some small rubber dilators, but they did not help. At the time, I did not know other treatment options existed and I felt very discouraged.

About four years into our marriage, my husband and I decided we wanted to have children. However, he could not enter me fully and the pain was now almost unbearable. We tried to have sex more often, and the stress of trying to push past the pain was making my menstrual cycles irregular.

My doctor suggested I try Clomid, a prescription drug that aids ovulation. I knew that was just her way of trying to help me, even though the real problem was the painful intercourse.

After three months of Clomid and no pregnancy, she suggested I see a reproductive endocrinologist. I didn't think my doctor had evaluated me or truly listened to the heart of my problem to merit spending the money on a fertility specialist.

About that time, a friend at my church had returned from treatment at Clear Passage Therapies (CPT). Although they were treating her for endometriosis pain and infertility, she told me that the clinic also used manual physical therapy to relieve intercourse pain.

I was glad there was a place I could go to find help, but I didn't know what to expect. I decided to apply for a one-week intensive therapy regimen. My husband came with me for support.

The pain was 90% gone! It's been over six months since treatment now, and my libido and desire are still increasing.

I felt very comfortable at CPT, and in control of the treatment. At times, it was uncomfortable because they were treating a very pain-sensitive area, but I could tell the difference as the pain decreased with each session, morning and afternoon.

My husband and I had intercourse a few times that week, and I noticed that the pain was less. Once I returned home and the temporary soreness from treatment dissipated, my husband and I had sex again. He had no problems entering me and the pain was 90% gone! Before treatment he had never been able to enter me fully, and finally he was able to! No one knows but me, my husband, and God. What a miracle this is!

It's been over six months since treatment now, and my libido and desire are still increasing. My husband and I have been having sex more often and I am still amazed at the difference.

My menstrual cycles also became regular after therapy. Before treatment, sometimes I would go 40 days between cycles. After treatment, they went back to 26-28 days each month ... but that didn't last long. I thought I was five days late, so I took a pregnancy test and it showed I was pregnant! I took four more that weekend before returning to the doctor to confirm that I am indeed pregnant!

Although I could not get my doctors to listen to me, I always knew my "infertility" was due to the painful intercourse I experienced. I am glad I found a clinic that actually listened to me and offered a non-surgical solution.

Chapter Thirteen

Sexual Dysfunction

"I'm having orgasms like I've never had in my life."
- *Janet*

"I'm over 40 and I thought that part of my life would always be 'just okay.' Everything 'woke-up' after treatment; now my husband can hardly keep up with my new-found libido."
- *Carmen*

When we first started treating women with pelvic pain twenty years ago, we never considered that the work we were doing might affect female sexual function. Then in the early 1990s, a former patient, Regina, called Belinda two months after her treatment.

Regina began hesitantly, "Have any of your patients reported anything, uh, unusual after treatment?"

"Unusual, how do you mean?" Belinda asked her.

"Well, it's kind of embarrassing," Regina replied, hesitantly.

When Belinda pressed her for the reason for her call, Regina replied "Well quite frankly, since I've been home, I've been having orgasms like I've never had in my life. I mean, these are real toe-curlers!"

"I see," Belinda said. "So you're not having any problem with that?"

"Oh no," Regina stammered. "It's fine . . . I mean really r-e-a-l-l-y fine! I just wanted you to know, for the record, I mean. Other women might find this information very useful, Belinda. Honestly, I have never experienced anything like this ever — in my entire life!"

At the time, we found this information interesting but did not think much about it beyond that. We were content to know that pain was decreasing and that there were virtually no negative side effects to our treatment. Indeed, the only negative side effects we had ever heard of after treatment were temporary soreness or light spotting.

Over the next several months, however, we noted a trend developing in some of our patients. As we began to treat more women for fertility, more and more of our patients began calling in, reporting positive "side effects" of therapy that had more to do with sexual function than pain. The reports sometimes included dramatic increases in desire or lubrication, and increased or first-time-ever orgasms. We found the reports of interest because the aims of physical therapy are to decrease pain and increase function. For some of these women, their sexual function was apparently improving beyond anything they had ever experienced in their lives. This was totally unexpected, but welcome news.

We did know that when a woman has a deep orgasm, the vaginal walls narrow. The uterus becomes more vertically oriented and moves upward inside the pelvis. If any of these movements are restricted due to adhesions, orgasm will generally be diminished, or will not occur. It appeared that by freeing up all these restrictions and restoring normal mobility to the vagina and urogenital organs, orgasms were coming with greater frequency and intensity for many of our patients.

We stopped being totally surprised by unusual patient reports after we determined that we could actually open blocked fallopian tubes. But in this case, we were (once again) facing something very special. We knew of no medical or therapeutic technique that actually increased orgasms.

In what had become our usual protocol for examining surprise results, we allowed our patients' reports about their therapy to guide us into scientific studies. In this case, we had our eye on documenting and measuring any positive (or negative) changes our patients were having in sexual function.

Dr. King made us aware of the fact that physicians had very limited tools with which to treat sexual dysfunction. In fact, the studies that were published largely addressed the psychological component. Because of his encouragement and all the phone calls from patients who were excited about their new-found libidos, increased lubrication, and profound orgasms, we decided to create publishable science on this – yet another pioneering area of treatment. We did not know what results to expect, but based on the prevalence of the problem in the US, we felt it incumbent on us to investigate the possibility to return function (and pleasure) to women who found themselves burdened by these problems.

Sexual Function Restored

- Cher's Story

When the therapists at Clear Passage Therapies (CPT) told me that a common side effect of treatment was increased sexual function, I didn't know whether to believe them or laugh. I went to CPT in hopes of opening my blocked fallopian tubes and I never imagined they would be able to help me with my sex life.

Four years earlier, I learned I had 25 fibroids in my uterus, my left fallopian tube was blocked, and my right fallopian tube was filled with liquid (a hydrosalpinx). I underwent surgery to remove the fibroids and then IVF, but my husband and I were still unable to become pregnant.

I then learned of CPT from a dear friend in my bible study. She and her husband tried to get pregnant for five years and then went to CPT. Afterward, she became pregnant. She came to my house and shared her entire experience with me. I was overwhelmed with hope and immediately called the clinic and scheduled an intensive week of treatment.

When I arrived at CPT, I couldn't believe the attention and thorough evaluation my therapists gave me. They asked me so many questions and thoroughly listened to my responses. They were interested in every ache, pain, or sensation. My husband, Poppy, also attended my treatment. The therapists really made him feel a part of the team. They explained every technique they used and how it might benefit me.

After examining my tailbone, the therapists found that it was pulled forward. I shared with them that I had been molested as a child, which may have led to that injury. The therapists explained that a tailbone in a forward position could cause pain with deep penetration during sexual intercourse. I knew exactly what they were talking about. Whenever my husband tried to push deeper during sex, it felt like he was hitting something. I was never able to enjoy sex. After being told my entire life to wait until I was married, it was such a disappointment to not enjoy intercourse with my husband. I still tried to participate, but it always felt dry, tight, and painful.

The therapists gently worked to tilt my tailbone back into place and restore its natural mobility. I noticed that pressure in my back was relieved as the therapists moved my tailbone. When my husband and I had sex later that night, I couldn't believe the difference. My husband was able to enter me entirely without the same feeling of tightness, pain, and obstruction. I couldn't believe how good it felt. I started to cry and Poppy, my husband, asked me what was wrong. I told him I was crying because of what was finally right! My orgasm was incredible – toe-curling! It was the best I had ever had. I finally felt like a real woman - a woman in love with her husband who could enjoy the full experience of marriage.

I have noticed that my libido continues to increase. Before, I seldom wanted sex. But now, I think, "Yes, baby, I'm in the mood, too!" I actually have arousal and desire. I feel like I am 25 again!

My orgasm was incredible – toe-curling! Before, I seldom wanted sex. But now, I think, "Yes, baby, I'm in the mood, too!" I feel like I am 25 again!

In addition to the incredible changes in our sex life, my husband and I are now filled with hope. We left CPT knowing I was healed and ready for our new journey together as parents. The day my therapist worked on my fallopian tubes, I noticed a clear discharge – which I believe was the fluid clearing from my tube! I have my follow-up test in one month to see if my tubes are open and my husband and I are very optimistic.

I have also noticed a change in my menstrual cycle. I used to experience pain two days before my cycle and then severe pain the first day of menstruation. During my last period, I had no pain at all! Just a dull pressure – I didn't even need pain medication! This change fills me with hope that my body is ready for a pregnancy.

Before I went to CPT, I just wanted a baby. I had no idea that treatment at CPT would enable me to be healed in so many ways. I was finally able to put my past behind – both physically and emotionally. The changes in my sexual function alone made the treatment worth every penny! And my husband certainly agrees!

The Six Domains of Sexual Function

Over the years, physicians and scientists have divided and defined the various areas of sexual function into domains. While some schools teach slightly different domains than others, most include some form of the following:

- Desire (libido)
- Arousal
- Lubrication
- Orgasm
- Satisfaction
- Pain

When we searched the medical literature looking for information on other treatments for sexual dysfunction, we were surprised to discover (as Dr. King had intimated) that we could find no other therapy, drug, or medical procedure that addressed the entirety of sexual function. Psychological counseling was prescribed for depression and coping; pain relievers and "desensitizing agents" were used to address painful intercourse. So while some agents were used to address a single symptom, nothing else we could find addressed the cause or presented a long-term solution for most of the various domains of sexual function. Drugs could lessen the pain, but the drugs only worked while they were being taken. Lubricants and desensitizing agents could sometimes help lessen the pain, but we could find nothing else (except the work we were doing) that increased desire, arousal, lubrication, and orgasm — and also decreased pain. For something that started out as a side effect of therapy (increased orgasms), this was pretty neat, we thought!

An Unknown Cause of Sexual Dysfunction

The cause of sexual dysfunction was becoming increasingly apparent to us. Adhesions were not only causing the pain in our patients, they were apparently causing decreased desire, arousal, lubrication, and orgasm. We knew this because when we used the therapy on our patients, sexual function improved dramatically in most cases in which there was a prior problem.

We were surprised that our "discovery" was not common knowledge among gynecologists. While perhaps adhesions were suspected by some, physicians were ill-equipped to treat the cause of the problem.

The vagina is an area that does not respond well to surgery. Further, drugs have their limitations for these conditions, as noted above. A few physical therapists were brave enough to treat in this private area, but clearly, none of them were doing what we were doing.

In this light, the primary side effect of our therapy — increased orgasms — turned into several published studies, and a breath of hope for women who suffer needlessly.

We have our patients to thank for this particular discovery. If they had not cared enough to contact us and tell us of the dramatic turnarounds they were experiencing, we would never have known to investigate this area, which will become an important contribution to women's health and benefit many women in need, for years to come.

Our research into the previously published medical literature also yielded a very valuable assessment tool: a scientifically validated test, called the Female Sexual Function Index (FSFI)[26]. This test provides a scientifically validated method to measure the various domains of female sexual function, and to create publishable results.

Now excited about the implications of creating yet another pioneering study, we gathered our physicians and researchers together to design a study to test and quantify any success we might have in the various domains of sexual dysfunction.

With her expertise in "Tests and Measurements," Dr. Eugenia Scharf brought our project to the attention of Jonathan Shuster, PhD, a nationally-recognized expert in biostatistics. Dr. Shuster taught biostatistics at the nearby University of Florida medical school and had published over 200 studies in prestigious journals, including the *New England Journal of Medicine* and *Lancet: The British Journal of Surgery*.

Dr. Shuster had advised us on previous studies, and when we approached him about this project, he readily agreed to participate. Part of his task was to tell us how many patients we needed to test in order to create statistically significant results.

Dr. King provided medical oversight as usual, to help assure the safety of the patients, and to advise us of considerations that would be important to physicians.

Together, our team designed a controlled study in which we took measurements pre- and post-therapy in the six measurable aspects of female sexual function: desire, arousal, lubrication, orgasm, satisfaction, and pain.[27]

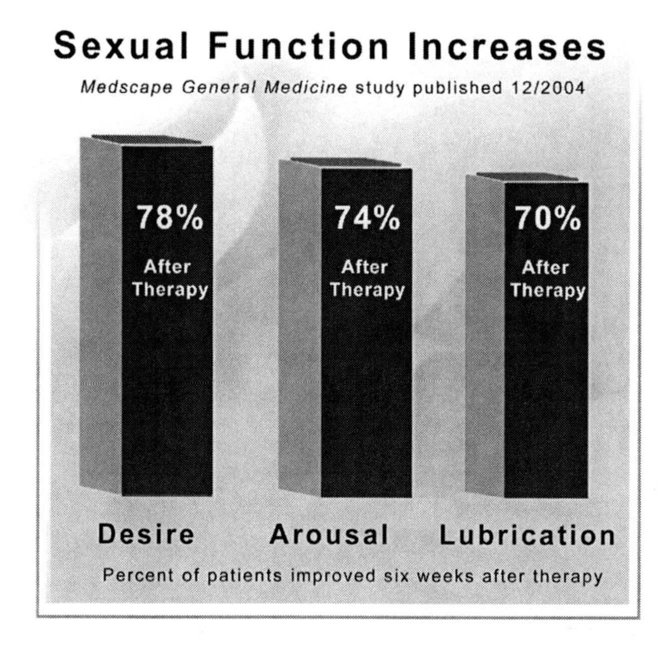

Improvements were noted in some surprising areas, measured six weeks after therapy

In the end, our study results were downright exciting! Desire (libido) increased in 78% of our patients and orgasms increased in 56%. In addition, lubrication, satisfaction and arousal were all up significantly – in well over 70% of patients.

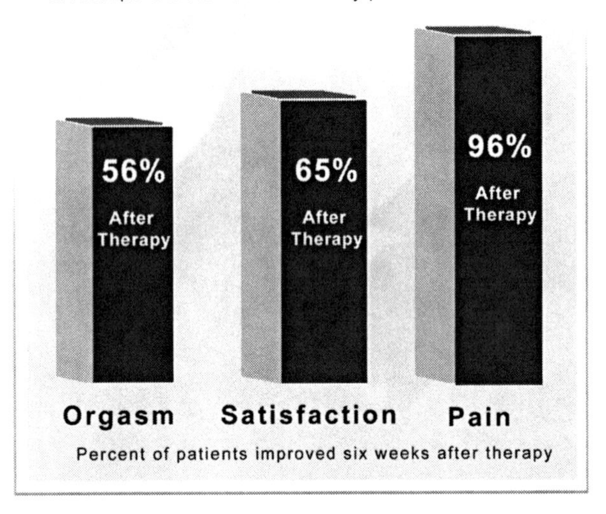

Published results showed pleasure increased for most women. Pain decreased significantly, for nearly all of them.

Our most dramatic change was in decreasing pain levels. As mentioned earlier, pain levels were decreased or eliminated in all but one patient. This equated to a 96% success rate of decreasing or eliminating intercourse pain. Considering that no other treatment existed to effectively address intercourse pain and its causes, this data made us feel terrific!

As one scientist told us, "In scientific studies, we are looking for improvements of 3% to 5%. If we show a 5% improvement at the end of a three-year study, generally we feel that we've really accomplished something. Sometimes, you work for years and see no improvement. But in our work, we were seeing improvements of 56%, 78%, and even 96%

Scientifically, we can only speculate on the exact mechanisms of why our therapy increased desire, arousal, lubrication, orgasm, and satisfaction in our study patients. However, we believe that treating adhesions is really the key that unlocks the mystery of sexual pain and dysfunction.

The women we treat with these complaints generally have a history indicative of adhesion formation, such as prior infection, surgery, trauma, or inflammation in the vagina or nearby structures. When we inquire, then palpate and treat the adhered, tightened tissues in these areas, pain generally decreases significantly, and sexual function improves markedly — as evidenced by this and other studies.[25]

Treating Near the G-spot

In many cases, we find tissues of an unusual texture on the front (interior) of the vaginal wall, in the vicinity of the Grafenberg area, or G-spot. While the G-spot has been referred to as tissue that surrounds the internal urethra, we note a bit broader geography as our area of interest.

You or your partner can check for yourselves to see if this area is adhered. To find the area that we find most affected, imagine the clitoris is a tree. The area we are feeling for is the root of that tree on the inside front of the vaginal wall. Simply place a finger inside your vagina to a comfortable depth, and curl it up. Then, allow your finger to sweep back and forth like a slow windshield wiper. As you do, notice the texture of the tissues. Is the tissue perfectly smooth and mobile? If so you may not have adhesions in that area.

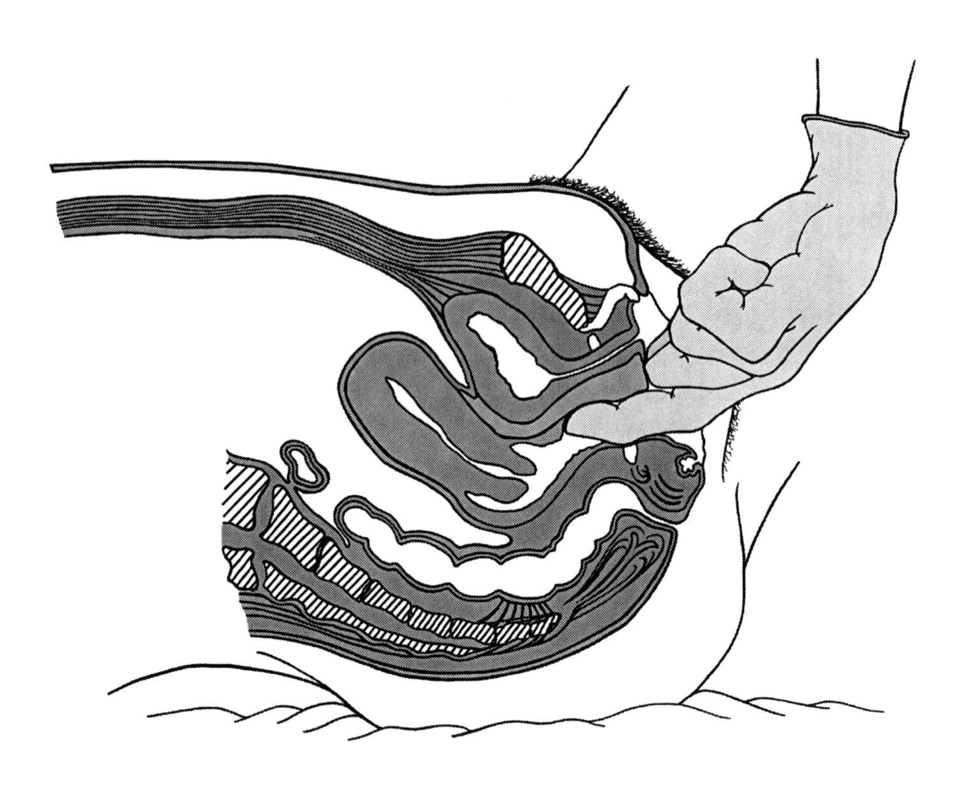

Tissues near the G-spot are involved in sexual dysfunction for many of our patients

On the other hand, if you notice bumps, wiriness at the surface, something that feels like corduroy, a stocking, a hairnet, or on any surface but smooth tissue, then you are feeling tissues that may have been compromised by an adhesive process that is likely decreasing your sexual pleasure and function, or causing your pain, or both.

We believe that adhesions can blanket this area, desensitizing it or pulling the tissues taut. When you lay a blanket over a sensitive structure, you cannot feel very well through it. We believe that it is this blanketing, tightening, or pulling sensation on and within the various areas of the vaginal wall that decreases desire, lubrication, arousal, and orgasms in women with decreased sexual function.

This is one area we generally cover thoroughly during treatment. When we treat this area (always with patient permission, keeping good communication), women may find the treatment somewhat uncomfortable. But we know for a fact, supported by published literature, that when we treat women who arrive at our clinics with diminished sexual function in any of the categories listed above, we tend to increase these functions for most of them.

New Hope: Sexual Dysfunction

The future is starting to brighten for women with dyspareunia (intercourse pain) and sexual dysfunction. Through clinical trials and published research conducted at CPT clinics, we are beginning to understand that adhesions cause glue-like bonds on and within the vaginal walls, at the entrance, or deep within the vagina or cervix. Wherever they form (and they can form anywhere) they appear to glue down delicate or pain-sensitive structures.

This new knowledge represents a major step forward in the understanding of intercourse pain and sexual dysfunction. Further, we found that we can actually treat adhesions on the vaginal walls without drugs or surgery. We can palpate their location and their effects, in concert with feedback from each patient. Finally, we can measure our success scientifically when treating these conditions. These discoveries, along with the published studies, are proving to be a boon to many women, their spouses, and their referring gynecologists.

Chapter Fourteen

Early Surgery and Trauma

It is heart-rending to us that children sometimes undergo abdominopelvic surgery or trauma during infancy or early youth. The physical scars that form in the body of a child do not always grow with the rest of the body. Thus, early healing events can create extremely tight, restricted, or adhered areas in children. The internal and external scars that form during youth can cause moderate to severe pain and significant dysfunction as the child grows through adolescence into adulthood, and attempts to participate in normal adult activities.

Early scars bind nearby structures together and prevent tissues from performing the way they would without the restrictive adhesive bonds. These scars often tend to cause other problems, such as infertility, digestive dysfunction and decreased range of motion as the child matures.

As these children compare their bodies to their "perfectly formed" friends, deep psychological scars may form as well. While mental health counselors can address the psychological pain and confusion, we have found great value in addressing, mobilizing, and freeing the physical scars that have bound these patients for most of their lives. A few specific examples follow.

Female Genital Mutilation (FGM)

The problem of early childhood scarring was first brought to our clinic from an unlikely source: tribal Africa. Several years ago, a number of women applied for therapy from their homes in equatorial Africa. While their initial goal was to improve their fertility, it quickly became obvious to us that most of them shared other problems, such as severe intercourse pain and diminished or absent sexual function (e.g., desire, lubrication, orgasm).

When these women presented at our clinics, even our most seasoned physical therapists were shocked and dismayed to see the results of the ritual surgeries that were performed on these women when they were children — some as early as the age of eight days old. In cases of infibulation (near-total closing of the outer labia), women who had actually been able to conceive were cut open for childbirth and then closed again, surgically.

In some parts of the world, children are surgically altered by tribal leaders or elders in accordance with beliefs or customs of that tribe. While some tribal surgeries are touted as benefiting the child (e.g., if the clitoris is removed, she will be less likely to get into trouble), others are clearly designed to benefit their families or future spouses — such as young girls and women who are cut and "tightened" for the eventual pleasure of the man who will become her husband. In an ironic twist of fate, one study of post-infibulation found that husbands of women who had undergone this extreme form of FGM were often injured when they tried to have intercourse with their spouses; the majority of them reported difficult penetration, wounds, infections and psychological problems. In fact, after marriage, most of the men said they preferred to marry a woman without a history of FGM. [29A]

According to WHO, 100 to 140 million girls and women worldwide are currently living with the consequences of FGM, and three million more girls are at risk every year.[30]

FGM reflects a deep-rooted inequality between the sexes, and constitutes an extreme form of discrimination against women. It is nearly always carried out on minors and is thus a violation of the rights of children. The practice also violates a person's rights to health, security, life, physical integrity, and freedom from torture and cruel, inhuman, or degrading treatment.

While procedures vary somewhat, all involve the partial or total excision of the external female genitals, and may include other surgical alterations. It is commonly performed during adolescence (typically before age 12), and may occur as early as infancy.

While sometimes performed by doctors, FGM is often performed in a non-sterile environment without anesthesia. In such cases, the "surgical instruments" used may include broken glass, tin can lids, scissors, or other items not designed for surgical procedures. The procedure can be fatal if the child goes into shock, hemorrhages, or becomes septic with infection.

Depending on the degree and severity of the procedure chosen for the girl, she may experience a lifetime of chronic pain, infertility, or sexual dysfunction associated with the trauma of the event and the scarring that occurs as the survivor heals. Because it is often done to several girls at a time using the same cutting implement in a ritual setting, FGM can contribute to the spread of HIV in its victims.

The Four Types of Female Genital Mutilation (FGM)

Amnesty International and WHO specify four main types of female circumcision or genital mutilation.

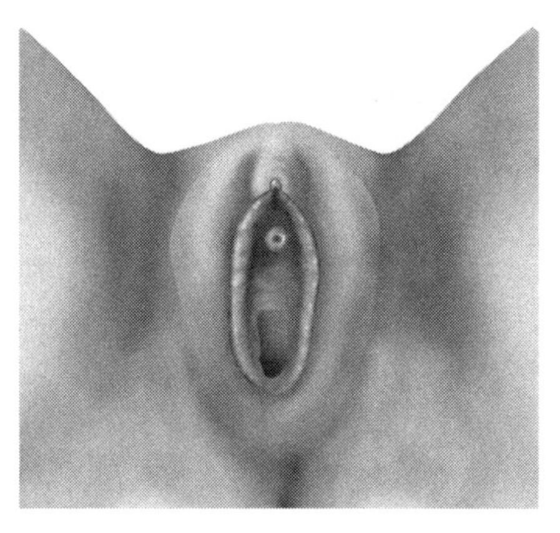

Normal external female genitalia

In a clitorectomy (type I) shown below, the clitoris is removed (partially or completely).

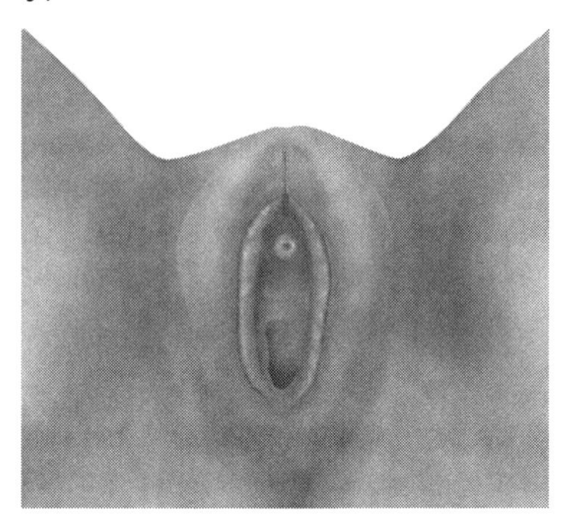

Type I mutilation: the clitoris is partially or totally removed

If an excision (type II) is performed (below), the clitoris and the labia minora (inner lips of the vagina) are removed.

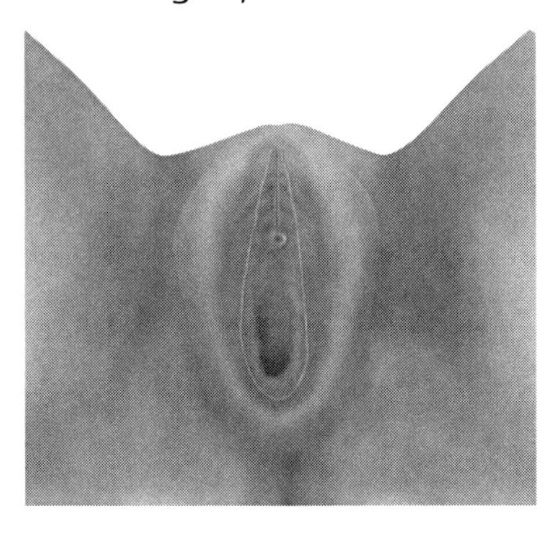

Type II mutilation: both clitoris and labia minora are removed

Type III refers to an infibulation, in which the vaginal opening is narrowed generally by stitching the outer labia together, often with the creation of a covering seal, leaving only a small hole for urine and menstral fluid to pass through. As noted earlier, this "operation" is often repeated in adulthood, after a woman is surgically reopened to give birth to her own child.

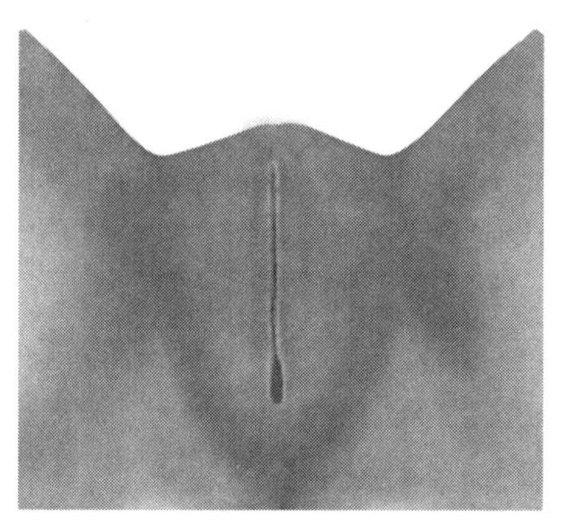

Type III mutilation showing the external labia sewn together, leaving only a small opening at the bottom for urination, menstruation or intercourse

Type IV FGM refers to a combination of any of the above, and any other harmful procedures to the female genitalia for non-medical purposes, e.g. pricking, piercing, incising, scraping, and cauterizing the genital area.

Restoring fertility and a fruitful sex life after FGM

Clearly, the scarring from such practices can be massive. We have treated women who were mutilated as early as eight days old. The scars that formed from these "surgeries" prevented the normal growth and function of the urogenital area in these women, dooming many of them to a lifetime of pain and dysfunction unless they could find someone knowledgeable enough to decrease their scarring and return mobility to the area.

One of the first women to come to us with a history of FGM arrived seeking help with her fertility. However, upon questioning during her initial evaluation, she revealed that she had "number ten (out of ten) screaming pain" whenever she attempted intercourse with her spouse.

When we examined her vaginal tissues, the adhesions were severe. She told us that they had been there since she was an infant. The poor lady was so bound down by vaginal adhesions that we could barely touch her.

Using a gloved hand, we gently and slowly examined her introitus — the entrance to her vagina. Although we were unable to place a single finger into her vagina at that time, we were able to evaluate the opening.

With a delicate touch, we began to evaluate and treat every centimeter of her vaginal opening. In some of her worst areas, we were only able to use what felt like a feather touch. In some areas we could apply more normal pressure, but even moderate pressure would elicit searing pain. We also moved on to her legs and nearby tissues that pulled into her scarred areas.

Tediously and meticulously, we palpated and treated every centimeter of her introitus for two days — the first eight hours of her anticipated twenty hour regime. By day three, we were able to access the deeper reaches of her tissues, and by the end of that day, we were at full depth inside her vagina. There, we found the cervix stiff and retroverted, pulled back towards her tailbone by thick internal adhesions.

By the end of her five days of therapy, we were able to access and deeply palpate all of her vaginal tissues without eliciting any pain at all. Basically, her pain was gone at the end of therapy.

We and our patient were both very pleased that we were able to make such huge gains for her within a week. (Actually, she was thrilled, unaware that anything could be done for her painful intercourse.) We feel confident that she will now be able to have a more normal life with her husband, and hopefully create the family of her dreams.

We are stunned and dismayed at the prevalence of the debilitating pain and dysfunction that comes from the brutal procedure known as female genital mutilation, or female circumcision. There is no good reason we can find for this surgery that causes so much pain and misery to so many women each year.

Physical and Sexual Abuse: Lasting Scars

Medical science recognizes that physical and sexual abuse can create deep psychological scars in its victims. Sound counseling can help victims come to grips with the confusing and conflicting emotions so often associated with abuse. Generally, the perpetrator was stronger, older, or otherwise overpowering — and may no longer be present as an object for venting unresolved feelings our patient may have. In many cases, conflicting experiences of pain and pleasure mixed into the setting of being with a family member or "friend" led to underlying emotions of guilt, mixed with anger, resentment, and helplessness.

In addition to the emotional scarring, many victims also experience physical pain or dysfunction after the abuse. Palpable physical scars can exist deep within the body's tissues for decades after the abuse has ended. These scars can endure a lifetime if left untreated. We have found that therapy can greatly help locate, treat, and eliminate the physical scarring, pain, and dysfunction associated with the abuse. In many cases, freeing the body from its physical scars has proven to be a valuable factor in unlocking a lifetime of psychological scarring associated with the trauma(s).

Reclaiming a pain-free and enjoyable sex life

Adhered areas can form on the surface and deep within the body as a response to the physical trauma of abuse. These scars can cause longstanding pain, tightness, or dysfunction. They often seem to create a physical space that houses the psychological trauma.

In some instances, our patients have experienced their trauma as a direct force, such as being struck or subjected to one or more forced sexual or physical encounters.

In other instances, the trauma may manifest more slowly. For example, when a person enlists a protective mechanism that must always be "on guard" against a recurrent perpetrator, the ongoing muscle spasm can cause physical adhesions to occur slowly over time (as naturally as they do from a direct strike). For example, we have treated some adhesions and pain in the neck or shoulders of patients who were bracing against repeat aggression by an abusive parent, spouse, or sibling. Thus in a very real sense, trauma creates internal adhesive straight-jackets that can immobilize body tissues, whether from a single devastating incident or from a series of traumatic events.

We understand the deep scarring that occurs from physical and sexual abuse and have successfully treated many severe patient cases. We treat the scars and adhesions that form within our patients as a result of the abuse. Like tiny but very strong, straight-jackets with a tensile strength of nearly 2,000 pounds per square inch, adhesions form wherever the body heals, binding down tissues that should be able to move freely, as they do for people who have not suffered abuse.

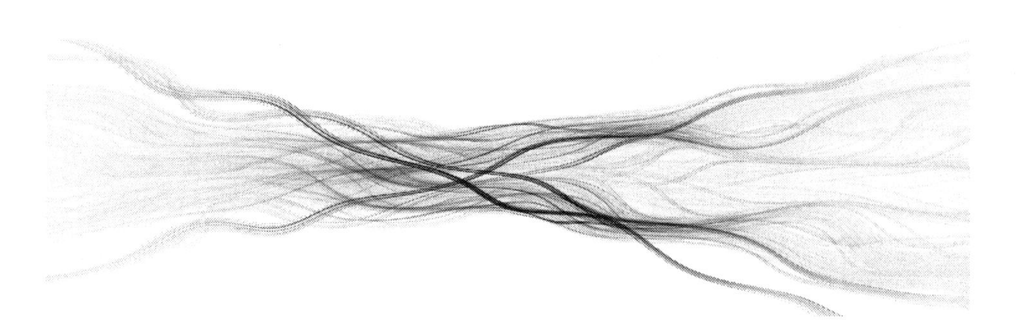

Like the small strands that comprise a nylon rope, microscopic cross-links join to create larger adhesive structures.

When we are able to physically free these adhesive straight-jackets using a manual soft-tissue therapy, patients report a dramatic reduction or resolution of their symptoms. Their bodies become much more mobile and pain-free.

Many have found that the process of freeing these internal physical bonds also opens the door to help heal the psyche and spirit, paving the way for greater resolution of their issues, so they can move on, less hindered by the shadows of the past.

Over the years, we have treated the physical aspect of scarring from physical or sexual abuse for many women. Some of our patients had developed multiple personalities as their only available defense against an untenable situation. Several of these women have told us that the physical release of adhesions opened a door to a deeper level of psychological healing. Some felt that the very act of being touched by caring hands, sensitive to direction and permission from the patient, contributed to their overcoming earlier barriers to intimacy.

It is perhaps unfortunate that psychologists are precluded from touching their patients. We have found that for many victims of abuse, the process of learning that touch can be caring, nurturing, and appropriate is an important component of their rehabilitation.

Along with that, we make certain that each of our patients understands that she (or he) retains the right to give (or rescind) permission for that touch at all times. Reflecting the views of a civilized democratic society, we feel the therapy room must provide a healthy, self-empowered setting where each person retains control over her body, and gives permission for each step of therapy. Along with that, each patient should understand that she is in a safe place, free from judgment or pressure to achieve anyone's goal except her own.

Prior Sexual Abuse

- Kelly's Story

I went to Clear Passage Therapies (CPT) for help with problems caused by sexual abuse which had occurred almost twenty years ago. I had a feeling that the therapy would help me resolve the pain and inflexibility in my vaginal area which had resulted in sexual dysfunction.

My manual physical therapist did a terrific job, the therapy worked beautifully, and I have had no pain since the treatment.

Tight hips, chronic constipation, and pain and stiffness in my hands, shoulders, and neck. Somehow, all of the problems were interrelated.

What I did not realize was that there were many other problems that would also be resolved — tight hips, chronic constipation, and pain and stiffness in my hands, shoulders, and neck. Somehow, all of the problems were interrelated. In the months following therapy, I discovered I had an entirely new body, which was flexible, strong, and ready to get back to work! I now run regularly, enjoy going to the gym, and I've lost about ten pounds through my healthier lifestyle.

Finally, and most mysteriously, I notice I'm less stressed-out these days. In the past, even when everything was OK in my life, I was always a little nervous. I had trouble sitting quietly, just doing nothing. The tension disappeared immediately after treatment and hasn't returned. Perhaps it was my body trying to tell me something was wrong. In any case, I've become a calmer and happier person.

Early Medical Surgery

Surgeries performed by physicians on infants and young children are designed to save lives, improve the child's appearance or quality of life, or for health or religious reasons. The scarring that is the near-inevitable by-product of most surgeries (see Chapter Sixteen) occurs in children with a few added complications.

One complication of early post-surgical scarring is that pre-verbal children cannot easily communicate any pain, pulling, or other sensation that follows surgery. A more lasting complication is that scars and adhesions bind tissues together. As the child grows, the scars from an early surgery generally do not grow at the same rate as the natural underlying structures. The body attempts to grow around the adhered tissues, but the constant strong pull from the surgical repair causes a dysfunctional state of growth. The affected tissues, whether muscles, organs, nerves, or connective tissues are unable to develop normally, since they are glued down by powerful adhesions in one or more places. This can cause pain or dysfunction in the child that can persist, and even become worse, as the child enters adolescence and adulthood.

To illustrate this phenomenon, let's consider a subset of early surgeries that are frequently performed on infants and young children.

Congenital Adrenal Hyperplasia (CAH) and Reconstructive Surgery

Congenital adrenal hyperplasia (CAH) refers to a family of inherited disorders associated with an inability or deficiency in the ability to produce cortisol, a hormone made by the adrenal glands. In affected individuals, the disease begins early in gestation and leads to conditions that may become obvious or visible at birth.

In some females, congenital adrenal hyperplasia causes an excess of androgen, a hormone that stimulates the development and maintenance of masculine characteristics. This often comes to medical attention due to physical anomalies in the female infant's urogenital and reproductive structures when she is born.

Classical congenital adrenal hyperplasia (CCAH) is considered a relatively common condition in Europe and North America, affecting one in 15,000 newborns. Overproduction of androgen hormones in classical CAH can cause the clitoris to become enlarged in the female infant to the point that it may look like a small penis. Further, the labial folds may join to resemble a scrotum.

These external anomalies do not affect the function of the internal female reproductive organs, which remain intact. However, the visual appearance of the anomaly may be so great that the female infant may initially be misidentified as a male.

In addition to medical (hormonal) treatment, parents of affected infant girls often want to save their daughter from a lifetime of embarrassment due to her visible anomaly. Thus, many parents of infant girls with classical congenital adrenal hyperplasia schedule the child for one or more reconstructive genital surgeries. These may begin as early as infancy.

While the early surgery may help the child look more "normal," these surgeries can leave scarring and adhesions that can cause pain and dysfunction during their youth.

At whatever age surgery is performed, it can cause severe scarring and adhesions at the delicate tissues of the vagina, perineum, clitoris, labia or vulva. The adhesions which formed at such an early age may result in significant problems later in life, such as painful intercourse, inability to have normal intercourse, or other types of sexual dysfunction, (e.g., decreased or absent desire, lubrication, and orgasm).

Creating a Pain-free, Functional Life

Children are delicate, and most do not understand why they received debilitating or ugly scars, when all their friends seem "perfect." Like the cases of CAH or FGM surgeries cited in this chapter, the early scars of genital surgeries formed in the most delicate and private areas of the body.

Over the years, we have come to understand well the physical scars that occur at and around the reproductive organs. In fact, we have been treating post-surgical vaginal adhesions for two decades. Our work in this area began over 20 years ago, when Belinda began her search for relief from her own post-surgical vaginal and pelvic adhesions. We have treated pelvic and vaginal adhesions in hundreds of complex patient cases since that time.

While we find it is best to treat post-surgical scars early (optimal is to start 8 to 12 weeks after surgery), that opportunity has generally long passed by the time a patient is referred to us. Perhaps this is for the best in children, since adults are better able to understand why we are touching their scars in intimate areas. Early surgical adhesion patients tend to come for therapy from adolescence to adulthood.

Parents of minor children are welcomed to inquire, and required to attend all therapy sessions with their child, in all of our clinics.

A therapist must understand the need to treat these delicate tissues in a "safe place," with the dignity and sensitivity each unique situation requires. While our work is physical, we also understand the psychological issues that can naturally accompany a lifetime of pain, dysfunction, or simply knowing that you are somehow different from everyone else. A physical therapist should always be available to consult and work with physicians or counselors before, during, or after therapy.

In therapy, we use our hands to slowly peel apart adhered tissues, working with respect for the patient's comfort and tolerance levels. Like meticulously breaking apart a nylon rope composed of hundreds of tiny strands, we work to detach the adhesions from structures that are causing pain, tightness, or dysfunction.

We have found that this manual focus on adhesions can open doors of mobility which have not existed in the body for years — or decades in most cases. Most post-surgical patients find that when we free them of adhesions that formed so many years ago, their bodies become mobile and pain-free in ways they have never before experienced. This paves the way for them to move on in their lives, no longer hindered by the powerful physical scars, pain, and dysfunction that have been their unwanted companions for a lifetime.

Section Four

Chronic and Recurring Pain

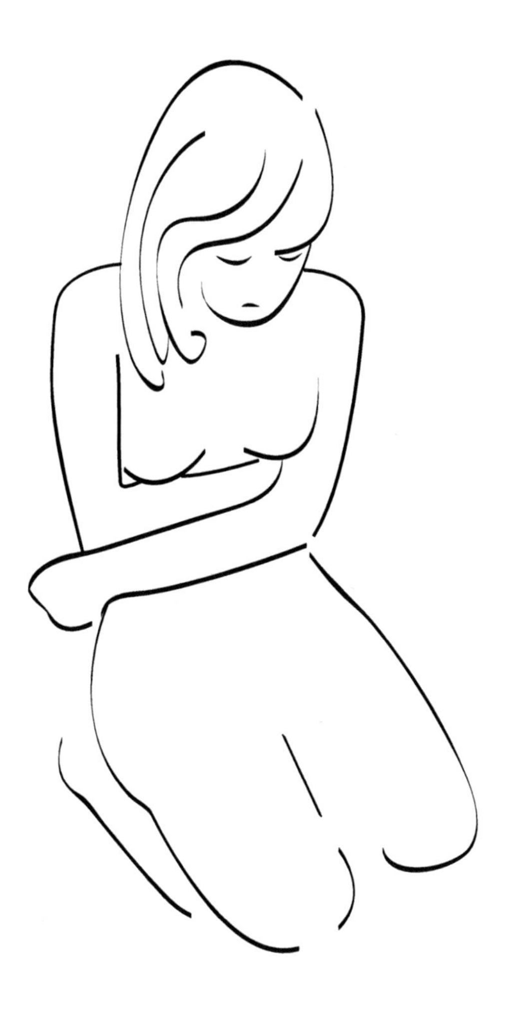

Nearly a year after Belinda received the best and most current medical treatment available (surgery and radiation) to cure her cancer, she started to experience pain at and near her surgical sites. Over time, the pain spread and new pains began to appear in other locations in her body — far from the site of the surgery (such as her pelvis, lower and mid-back). In short, Belinda began to experience chronic pain throughout her body, leaving her unable to work or move without pain.

That pain started our quest, and we learned about the adhesions that form whenever and wherever we heal. We attended so many continuing education courses that the folder that held our diplomas finally split from the weight. Over time, we synthesized the best teachings from all of our professors and refined them while we were treating Belinda's chronic pain. That work would eventually become the Wurn Technique®.

Eventually, we were able to help Belinda become functional and largely free of the pain that had been so debilitating that she could not work. It did not take long to realize that we were not alone; we found there were thousands of people who faced the same trials Belinda had undergone.

Understanding the principles of fascia and adhesion formation, and feeling that we could unwrap or unravel the adhesive bonds that had bound Belinda's tissues from their ugly grasp, we offered our services to local physicians and their patients who suffered from chronic pain.

We were actually stunned by the response. Apparently patients weren't the only ones struggling to find pain relief. Physicians started sending us their chronic pain patients first by the handful, then by the dozen. As we unraveled adhesions within patients who had been in pain for years or even decades, they returned to their physicians asking, "Why didn't you send me there years ago?"

Encouraged by the response, doctors sent more and more chronic pain patients until we had to open another clinic and then another. In the end, we had five busy physical therapy clinics with 650 referring physicians sending us their most challenging and complicated pain patients.

Treating chronic pain is still dear to our hearts. Following are some of the stories from those years in the clinic, the conditions we continue to treat, and a deeper look at the processes that adhered our patients and our theories of why our treatment relieved so much of their pain and suffering.

Chapter Fifteen

Chronic Pain

Chronic pain robs people of their quality of life. As it becomes more debilitating, it can reduce the strongest person to a state of depression or hopelessness. Even when the pain is not severe, the fact that it is always present in the foreground or background makes people begin to identify themselves as "a person with pain."

Pain that is caused or exacerbated by adhesions can bring new levels of frustration for several reasons. To start, adhesions are difficult to diagnose and challenging to treat. Unless they are massive, adhesions do not show up on most diagnostic tests (x-ray, CT scan, and MRI). Thus, people in pain become frustrated when their doctors say, "There's nothing there," or "I don't see anything." In some cases, they give their patient the totally disempowering, "It's all in your head," or "You'll just have to learn to live with it." As we have come to realize, the smallest adhesion can pull on pain-sensitive structures within the body with great strength, and create pain which is called "unexplained" because its cause is impossible to visualize using traditional medical diagnostic tests.

Adhesions pain is considered a soft tissue injury, yet there is no visible sign that the patient has an injury. The victim is not wearing a cast and doesn't have a neck brace (in most cases), and yet the patient is in a state of nearly constant pain.

If your physicians cannot see your adhesions, it is even more difficult for family, friends, and coworkers to understand why you complain about your pain. Many of our patients say, "My spouse thinks I'm a hypochondriac," or, "My boss is tired of making special concessions for me," or, "I feel like I am complaining all the time — what's wrong with me?"

Pain levels may be greater or less day to day, but some people cannot escape thinking of themselves as a "person for whom pain is always present." However invisible it is to others, pain is a fact of life for them.

Learning to Treat Chronic Pain

After Belinda's experiences with rushed and insensitive medical care, we wanted to provide a lovely venue where people might find total relief from their chronic pain at last. We knew that most physical therapy protocols involved exercises, ice, hot packs, ultrasound, electrical stimulation, and a few minutes of light massage. While these techniques seemed to do fine for some people, especially those with recent injuries, we felt there was a large population of patients who were basically unserved — those with chronic recurring pain symptoms.

We spoke with local doctors and suggested they send patients with chronic pain to our clinics. The general reaction was: "Are you kidding? I have dozens of those! I'd be glad to send them to you, but I will tell you that you are asking for a heap of frustration." True to their words, they sent us patients experiencing chronic pain. By the time we had visited three physicians, our books were full and we were scheduling waiting lists, booking patients two months ahead.

Early on, Belinda and I would notice that so many of these patients had a variety of seemingly unrelated symptoms. A typical patient reported chronic low back pain, severe headaches at the base of the skull and top of the head, and a pulling down one leg with occasional numbness or tingling. In addition the patient had irritable bowel syndrome and poor digestion, as well as painful intercourse.

Prior to coming to our clinic, the patient was typically sent to physical therapy for back and leg pain, to internal medicine for irritable bowel syndrome, to a gynecologist or urologist for painful intercourse, and to a neurologist or neurosurgeon for the chronic headaches. If no relief was found, s/he was sent to an anesthesiologist with a specialized chronic pain clinic to consider anesthetizing whatever area could be accessed with a pain reliever or nerve blocker. In that case, pain relief would last as long as the medication, but never effectively addressed the cause.

By the time this patient arrived in our clinic, s/he was confused and disheartened by the multiple diagnoses from specialists. Often, our patients were exhausted from trying to follow up on the schedule and regimen of physician appointments, diagnostic tests, referrals to other specialists, medications to address symptoms, traditional physical therapy, and possibly surgery, only to be left with ongoing pain or dysfunction.

When each patient arrived at our door, we viewed that patient's body as a whole. Trying to "connect the dots" of our patients' various symptoms, we found it helpful and often necessary to take a full body view. We quickly ascertained the importance of understanding the patient's lifetime history of traumas, surgeries, infections, and inflammations — conditions that cause adhesions to form.

We knew that whenever the body healed from any tissue trauma or the body compensated for an injury (e.g. shoulders lifting, limping, etc.), adhesive cross-links often formed within this fascia along lines of tension or physical compensation. As they formed, they pulled the fascial sweater of the body out of its normal alignment with tensile strengths of nearly 2,000 pounds per square inch.

We often found that a trauma or a healing event had started the process that led to the pain. The example below is a compilation of the type of stories we hear every week:

Pain after Childhood Injury

- Ellen's Story

Ellen had fallen off a horse at the age of 14 and landed on her left hip and buttocks. When we palpated the site of the trauma, we felt very thick adhesions running down both sides of her sacrum and down into her tailbone. Above the injury, adhesions were running up the left side of her low back, thickening the quadratus lumborum or "hip-hiker" muscle between her ribs and low back. When we questioned her further, we discovered that she had landed in a position in which her right leg was pulled back, over-stretching her psoas muscle and the hip flexors, at the front of her right thigh. The psoas muscle neighbors the fallopian tube, ovary and kidneys, so any inflammation of the psoas could affect those structures. In fact, upon palpation, her digestive system apparently received and absorbed some of the force of the trauma, as did her right kidney.

The adhesive healing process spread into the nearby bowels, causing inflammation there. The force of the fall also pushed her tailbone forward, creating a physical barrier to her descending colon, causing constipation. Thus, the original injury caused inflammation to spread to various areas of the abdomen, pelvis, hip, and low back. Intercourse pain with deep penetration was a direct result of her partner hitting her tailbone, which had been pushed forward by the fall. Thus the tailbone created a physical block whenever she attempted to have intercourse with her husband and contributed to constipation, as it created a physical barrier at her descending colon. She also complained of neck and TMJ (jaw) pain, which we felt was exacerbated by an unstable pelvis.

Having thus surmised the history and progression of the injuries and symptoms our patient experienced, we were able to see, treat, and deal with the wide range of symptoms as a whole-body approach.

Our next challenge was to ask ourselves, "Where do we begin and where do we take this next?"

Like taking apart nylon rope one strand at a time, we began to palpate, detach, and free the major adhered tissues and structures from each other, one by one. To us it feels like we are pulling out the run in a three-dimensional sweater. As we free restricted areas, we move on throughout the body, following the "run" wherever it goes.

Like taking apart nylon rope one strand at a time, we began to palpate, detach, and free the major adhered tissues and structures from each other.

As the strong collagenous bonds began to slowly release, symptoms dissipated and normal range of motion returned. As entrapped nerves were freed, Ellen's pain decreased. As the pelvis and low back were freed, we were able to return symmetry to the spine so her neck and TMJ symptoms could resolve at last. Direct treatment at her tailbone and nearby structures resolved her constipation and intercourse pain.

Helping patients became a marvelous adventure for us. We would first uncover the cause of our patients' pain, and then unravel adhered structures and soft tissues in the fascia, freeing them from the adhesive straight-jackets that caused pain and dysfunction in various bodily systems.

Over the course of therapy, patients reported relief in seemingly unrelated areas, "I can breathe deeply!" patients told us, "I don't have headaches anymore;" "My gait has changed, I feel stable again;" "There is mobility where I felt stuck;" "I can take longer steps."

Severe Fall, Subsequent Pain and Headaches

- Michael's Story

As a 24-year-old construction worker, Michael suffered a severe fall on the worksite, landing on the right side of his buttocks and tailbone. Over the course of four years, Michael had been to over a dozen physicians and had attended virtually every physical therapy and rehabilitation clinic in our medically-oriented town. By the time he arrived in our clinic, he was still in a debilitated state.

During our initial evaluation, Michael's left shoulder was severely elevated in constant spasm, rising up toward his neck. He did not have the strength to grasp objects with either hand. In addition, he was dragging his right foot behind him so badly that the front inside of his shoe had worn out. He had significant neurological symptoms: his left hand shook constantly, and his legs shook frequently. He reported severe daily headaches that started a few days after his fall, and had gradually become worse over time.

We hardly knew where to start with this young man, but we knew that we were probably his last chance to regain some semblance of a life. Emotionally, he was remarkably stable for all he had been through; he was in constant pain in so many places, and he just wanted to get his life back.

Michael had been to over a dozen physicians and had attended virtually every physical therapy and rehabilitation clinic in our highly medically-oriented town.

We described adhesions, fascia, and the inner structure of his body to him so he could act as an informed member of the team that was trying to help him regain his life. Trying to envision the adhesive pattern that had formed in him since his fall, and noting that he had severe impingement on nerves in many areas, we asked him to tell us what techniques felt better and which ones did not help, or made him feel worse.

As we palpated different tissues, we described the inner structure of his body to him. We asked him to tell us where he was feeling sensations when we touched various areas. Often, Michael would identify relationships that physicians would tell us do not exist in modern medicine — such as a pull from his shoulder into his opposite leg. Yet when we treated that shoulder, he would feel relief in his opposite leg. And after a session of treating that shoulder, we noted that his gait improved markedly. The complex adhesive pattern that was created within him after his fall was starting to unravel.

Over the course of his therapy sessions, both of his shoulders became level. Eventually, he was able to walk normally, swing his arms, and lift objects again. He returned to work on light, then moderate duty.

Toward the end of treatment, he still experienced daily headaches that were often severe and debilitating. Since the rest of his body was doing so well, this remained a great mystery for us.

Then one day, we had an experience with Michael that knocked our blinders off. In fact, it would have significant ramifications for our headache, pelvic pain, and infertility patients for years to come.

One day, we had an experience with Michael that knocked our blinders off.

While Larry was treating Michael's neck, he noted severe tightness at the base of his skull. Clinically, we had noticed that this is often an area associated with headaches, and the area felt totally jammed. In fact, as he tractioned his head, it felt as if the tissues of his neck and the base of his skull were anchored much further down his spine.

Larry mentioned this "anchoring sensation" to Belinda that evening. She asked, "Do you suppose that when Michael fell at the worksite, he may have pushed his coccyx (tailbone) forward and it got stuck in that position as it healed?"

As we talked, we decided that this was not only possible but likely. We also knew that one of the primary fascial attachments at the sacrum and coccyx is the dura — which is the thick, fascial covering of the brain and spinal cord. The dura starts at the tailbone, attaches to the sacrum, climbs the spinal cord, and has strong attachments at the base of the skull. Then it continues up into the cranium to surround and infuse with the tissues of the brain, divide the brain into left and right sections, and create the floor of the brain.

"Do you think that when that happened, it pulled down on his dura, and that the anchor I was feeling at his head was the pull coming from the coccyx?" Larry asked.

"Sounds reasonable to me," Belinda said. "Anatomically, it makes sense, but in that case, what are we going to do about it?"

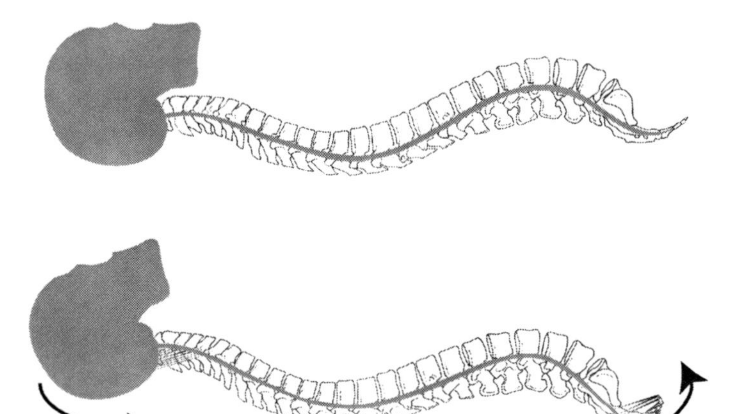

A tailbone pushed forward in a fall, or pulled by pelvic surgery scars can pull the spinal cord down, exerting pressure into the skull.

"What about this," Larry suggested. "What if one of us decompresses (pulls back) the joint at his coccyx (internally) while the other tractions his head? Do you think that might work?"

"Mechanically, that sounds reasonable. I really can't think of a better way to do that," she said.

We told Michael what we were thinking. "There are no guarantees, of course, and we would never push anyone into something they do not want to do," we said. "Frankly, it may be pretty uncomfortable for a few minutes. But we have tried so many things; mechanically, this makes sense to both of us. We think it could be the key that unlocks the door to your chronic headaches."

"Well," he said, "you have done more in the course of therapy than anyone else has been able to do in several years. If you think it'll help, let's just go on and do it."

We treated Michael the way we described and hoped he would find relief. Michael had an appointment set with his physician three days later.

"They did *what*?" the doctor exclaimed when Michael told him about our treatment.

"Yeah doc, they sure did. They said they released the pull of my dura. I don't understand it much, but the headaches I have had daily for over three years are completely gone now! I haven't had one since they did that!"

It was a matter of simple biomechanics, and our treatment with Michael was a clear and dramatic demonstration of how listening deeply to patients and thinking of the body's mechanics from a "whole body" perspective could lead to profound results.

The physician called us amazed and promptly began sending his most complicated tailbone and headache patients.

Decreasing and Eliminating Chronic Pain

Pain can interfere with all aspects of a person's life and impact the lives of families and friends. Pain or dysfunction which persists for more than 12 weeks is considered chronic.

Adhesions present several problems for medical science:

- They are very difficult to detect, making a definitive diagnosis difficult. They do not show up on most x-rays, MRIs, or CT scans.
- They can be so small that they are virtually undetectable, even during surgery.
- Surgery can cut or burn some adhesions, but others are difficult or risky to access due to their proximity to delicate tissues.
- No matter how skilled the surgeon, it is very difficult to perform surgery without creating more adhesions.

In the following sections, we discuss how adhesions can directly cause multiple conditions. We also explain how treatment can return a patient to a pain-free life.

Abdominal pain

Abdominal pain and dysfunction affects millions of people. When pain is not due to disease, we begin to suspect mechanical causes.

Adhesions are a major cause of mechanical abdominal dysfunction, due to the inflammatory process.

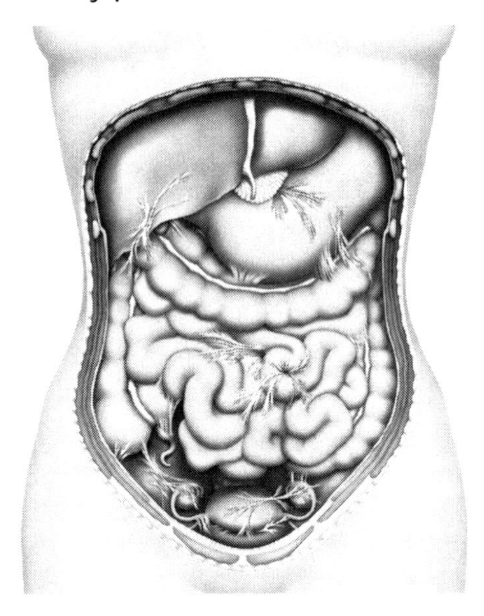

Adhesions may occur anywhere the body has healed from trauma, infection, inflammation, or surgery.

Adhesions may occur in any of the abdominal organs as a natural by-product of healing. Abdominal adhesions may initially form as a response to disease, inflammation, accident, surgery, or radiation therapy. Surgery is a common cause of abdominal pain and adhesions, as internal structures glue down during the healing process that follows surgery. Diseases of organs are also known to cause adhesions and subsequent pain.

Unexplained abdominal pain can be extremely frustrating as the patient goes from specialist to specialist in search of a diagnosis. When no organic cause (such as disease) can be found, or when concurrent symptoms occur in nearby areas (such as low back pain or digestive problems), we begin to suspect a mechanical cause of the pain , generally adhesions.

Unexplained Abdominal Pain

- Rae's Story

My two weeks in Gainesville, Florida were a turning point for me. I don't think I will ever be able to put into words what they did for me, my health, my approach to good health, and my outlook on life.

I have been no stranger to the acronym "ICI" (Invisible Chronic Illnesses), and had a plethora of TLAs (three letter acronyms) as diagnoses for my various levels of ill health, pain, and inability to "have a life." What brought me to Clear Passage Therapies (CPT) was the four years of fighting stomach pain, a pain that made all other pain issues pale in comparison.

I don't think I will ever be able to put into words what they did for me.

I developed stomach "clutches" that literally doubled me over and brought me to my knees. Having pain issues from FMS (Fibromyalgia Syndrome) and MPS (Myofascial Pain Syndrome) did not prepare me for this sharp and focused wave of pain. It hurt so badly, the pain would make me throw up whatever was in my stomach, and then for the next "n" number of hours (sometimes days) heave pure bile. That was my cue to go to the emergency room (ER).

After my third visit there, one physician decided that gallstones were the issue. He admitted me, and I waited three days until the surgeon was available. I was afraid of surgery, my health not the best to begin with, but the knowledge that this would end the cycle of excruciating pain was what kept me strong.

Recuperating from the surgery was no picnic, but I was free of the stomach issue, or so I was told. All it took was one roughage full meal to have me dialing 911, and awaiting the ambulance. It was so frightening and disheartening, but I hadn't put two and two together yet; even worse, neither had the doctors. They all believed this was all part of the "recovery process" from the surgery, and my system trying to handle the digestion process without the gallbladder to do its job breaking food down with enzymes and directing it into my intestines.

I hadn't put two and two together yet; even worse, neither had the doctors.

Much later, it became apparent to all of us that my stomach issue was not resolved by surgery. In fact, the surgery had exacerbated my problem (origin still unknown).

I then went to multiple GI specialists, "la crème de la crème," who all were adamant that I had an issue, but no one could diagnose it. I soon found myself chasing pain clinics, and having tests of pure discomfort. I had MRIs and CT scans with and without dye; I swallowed markers to track my digestive system by x-ray, and swallowed other nasty stuff to clean my system the night before. I underwent all of these tests and procedures to show the medical folk how my digestive tract worked, how fast it moved, what path it took, and other arcane data. I had endoscopies and colonoscopies. And still, I had to go to the ER again and again with the pain. The ER doctors took so many x-rays of my entire torso that I am surprised I don't glow in the dark!

So between tests, specialists, and pain clinics, I kept having to find relief in the ER. They would insert an N/G (nasal gastric) tube into my stomach, give me enemas, experiment with intravenous medicines, inject Atropine... After a while, they'd create any concoction or cocktail they could think of. They too were frustrated, and also "suspicious," since the relief inevitably came when they finally gave me the injection of a narcotic, along with anti-nausea medicine.

I went to multiple specialists... who all were adamant that I had an issue, but no one could diagnose it.

Sometimes they used an IV, and they'd maybe add something to hydrate me, but inevitably, excruciating pain in my stomach recurred. Depending on what they saw, they would either calm my pain with drugs, or admit me due to a bowel obstruction, or "ileus."

My ER visits eventually became even more frequent. My primary care physician kept suggesting exploratory surgery as the only way to figure out what was wrong. He put me on narcotics to try to keep me home and help me to minimize going to the ER over and over again for pain relief. There were weeks when broth and Jell-o were my only fare — I

My ER visits eventually became even more frequent.

remember being so excited when I could add some food to my Jell-o. There are not nearly enough Jell-o flavors available!

As my pain, bloating, and digestion problems continued, along with trips to the ER, including admission to the hospital, my doctor became more insistent on the need for exploratory surgery. He assured me that if there were the expected adhesions from my prior (unnecessary) surgery, the way to eliminate them was more surgery.

I started to attack the Internet for information. I found CPT.

After reading horror stories about adhesions being compounded by multiple surgeries that attempted to release previous adhesions (which sounded both scary and logical to me) I approached my MD about going to CPT. His feeling was that it would not harm me, and at most it would only cost me some time and money. He felt it was worth a shot — he was supportive of my efforts.

I can't tell you how warm and welcoming everyone at CPT was. I filled my form out very, very completely, and I have a long and complicated health history, as I alluded to earlier. I held nothing back. I spoke to a therapist on the phone, and she soon became my new best friend and confidante. Despite my weight, CPT was willing to work with me, as long as my expectations were realigned to recognize that it might impact the level of my success.

My therapist did not hold back, or "weasel-word" what I was in for and what to expect. She was a professional always, but with such heart. I went to Florida, where their team of therapists worked together to create a plan for me. Every step of the way I found caring, smiling, people who listened to me and encouraged me while the therapists worked; rather WE worked together — I had to be actively involved, mind and body. The rest of the staff always smiled, answered questions, suggested places to visit, and accommodated my schedule needs.

By the end of two weeks, I had made new friends, really more like sisters: a family of my choice. I was so sad to leave them, but it was time to "graduate" and say goodbye. They gave me resources, paperwork, cheat-sheets of exercises, and more to continue the process at home.

After I returned home, it was eleven long, lovely MONTHS before I ever hit the ER with a stomach issue again. Now almost 7 months later, I've not gone to the ER since. Compared to my schedule of multiple ER trips every year, this feels like magic (albeit based on their science, intuition, training, and heart). I never imagined this could be my reality!

I am now on the brink of getting off of the narcotics which, at one time, were the only things that kept me from being in the hospital 24/7. I admit I'm anxious about this step, but excited too. This could never have been possible without my time at CPT.

Western physicians often spent their energy and my dime treating my pain symptoms, and seeking a label for my illness(es) and pain— rather than really treating me.

Another benefit from my CPT experience is that

my pursuit of health has broadened the scope of professionals I seek. In retrospect, I see that in my case(es), "western" physicians often spent their energy and my dime, treating my pain symptoms and seeking a label for my illness(es) and pain — rather than really treating me. They tossed western pharmaceuticals at me, but those always seemed to have side effects. In fact, some side effects required a different medicine to balance them out, ad nauseum (pun intended here). Ultimately, they gave me a "waste-basket diagnosis" (a label) when they couldn't find the cause. Some even dismissed me as some "hysterical woman" whose pain and symptoms were "all in my head," a more modern version of "the vapors."

I've since turned to more "alternative health" options that see "me" in my entirety, and try to treat the whole person, not find a label to pigeonhole me. My path towards the quest for health has changed, and I try to keep open-minded regarding my well-being, combining both alternative eastern and western modalities.

CPT opened a new world to explore, one with options and hope. I'm not there yet, but what an opportunity they offered me! As CPT knows, I am willing to speak about my experience, and answer any questions about my personal experience.

Certainly everyone gets their own unique help and lessons from CPT. As they say, YMMV (your mileage may vary). But know this, I cannot thank Clear Passage enough for their work with me, and their taking a chance, inviting such a "complicated" case into their care, and helping turn my life around.

Back pain

Chronic back pain can be physically and emotionally debilitating, affecting virtually all aspects of a person's life. Back pain that has persisted for more than three months is considered chronic. Symptoms may include back or leg pain with certain movements, when standing, walking, sitting, or prolonged morning stiffness. Even when the pain is bearable, the persistent or recurring nature of the pain can be so frustrating that life loses quality as the patient loses hope for recovery.

Two important elements in low back pain are biomechanical and soft tissue dysfunctions of the sacroiliac joints. The sacrum and pelvis are the body's center of gravity and stability, simultaneously negotiating forces transferred from above and below.

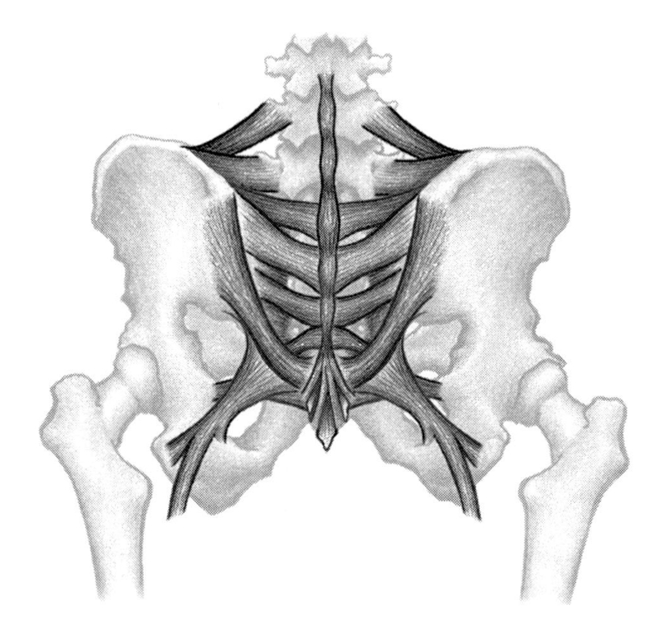

The bones of the pelvis are held together by strong ligaments to create a foundation for the torso, neck, and head above.

A complex series of ligaments attach the sacrum to the two large pelvic bones (the ilia) at the sacroiliac joints. In doing so, they help provide a stable transition between the upper and lower body. The sacrum also forms a joint with the fifth lumbar vertebra, the lumbosacral junction at the base of the spine.

> **"Before treatment, I had chronic pain in my back that would flare up after walking or shopping for an hour. I thought it was a normal part of aging. But after treatment, that pain vanished."**
>
> *– Christine, mother of one after struggling with chronic pain and infertility*

The ligaments of the sacroiliac joints contribute significantly to the stability of the low back, while the lumbosacral junction contributes to low back stability and mobility. Together, these joints and ligaments support the entire body above the pelvis.

If the pelvis, sacrum, or low back are out of alignment and this misalignment persists long-term, adhesions tend to form, perpetuating the dysfunction, and further pulling these structural elements out of their normal balance. Instability and pain are the near-inevitable result.

Trauma, injury, surgery, or years of poor posture can cause inflammation in the body, which creates additional collagen cross-links as a response. These cross-links form even more glue-like adhesions, further binding structures that should be mobile. Once the inflammation has passed, these adhesions remain in the body as a permanent by-product of healing, freezing the dysfunctional posture in space.

When adhesions form, the pelvic or lumbosacral joints become increasingly fixed in a dysfunctional or asymmetrical orientation. Any asymmetry in this area can create compensatory responses in struc-

The therapists also resolved back pain I had for years. I had even seen several physical therapists before and one of them told me, "You will need surgery by the time you are 40." But after CPT, I had no pain.

– Sydney, mother of two after struggling with chronic pain and infertility

tures above (upper back, shoulders, neck, head, and TMJ) or below (hips, knees, and feet). This asymmetry may be relieved by a knowledgeable chiropractor or structural body worker.

However, if symptoms persist or recur, we find it is often because the chiropractor or structural body worker has addressed the bones of these joints and not the collagenous cross-links that pull bones out of their natural symmetric relationship. Once we have addressed these adhesions, the bones of this region generally return to a symmetric state.

Fibromyalgia

Fibromyalgia (FM) is one of the three most common conditions seen by rheumatologists. It is a complex, chronic condition of unknown cause affecting an estimated three to six million Americans. It is ten times more common in women than in men, and most patients are women between the ages of 30 and 60.[31]

Patients with FM often complain that muscles and joints ache throughout their bodies. A large number of other symptoms may be present, including fatigue or pain that ranges from a dull aching, flu-like feelings to more severe discomfort. Other symptoms may include body stiffness in the morning, after prolonged sitting or standing in one position, or with changes in temperature or relative humidity. When patients with FM adjust their postures to try to avoid pain, they can complicate the condition by developing unnatural compensatory patterns of movement.

Patients may complain of sleep disturbances or cognitive difficulties such as difficulty concentrating, "spaciness," memory lapses, and becoming mentally overwhelmed easily. Some patients develop irritable bowel or bladder, digestive disturbances, abdominal pain, bloating, constipation, and/or diarrhea. It is not unusual to have swelling, numbness or tingling of fingers or toes, cold hands or feet, and itchy, dry, or blotchy skin. Patients may experience headaches, TMJ or facial pain, depression, or anxiety.

FM has been called soft-tissue rheumatism because it primarily affects the fascia and muscles. Unlike arthritis, FM does not cause pain or swelling in the joints. Rather, it produces pain in the soft tissues, and within the fascia. Severity of pain varies from day to day and can change location. Pain may become more severe in parts of the body that are used the most (e.g., the neck, shoulders, and feet). In some people, the pain can be intense enough to interfere with daily tasks, while in others it causes only mild discomfort.

It has been suggested that the pain of FM is related to micro-trauma in deconditioned muscles and that exercise helps by conditioning these muscles.[32] However, some tender points are not over muscles or tendons, such as those over the inside fat pad of the knees.[33] Further, many FM sufferers are frustrated by the fact that even mild exercise exacerbates their symptoms.

It has also been suggested that FM may be due to non-restorative deep sleep.[34] Patients with FM often report insomnia, trouble staying asleep, or light sleep, with an increase in symptoms after disturbed sleep.[35] Despite sufficient amounts of sleep some nights, FM patients may awaken feeling unrefreshed, as if they have barely slept. Controlled research trials have confirmed the value of aerobic exercise in the treatment of FM.[36] Exercise appears to increase time spent in deep sleep, which may be a mechanism for its therapeutic effect in some FM patients.[37]

Development of the syndrome may involve a predisposing (possibly inherited) factor. There may also be a precipitating factor, such as trauma (accident, fall or injury), illness, disease, infection, emotional stress or sleep disruption that acts as a trigger.

In our own experience, FM appears to represent a tightening or pulling of the entire fascial sweater toward the spine. As the fascia tightens, pain may appear in any part of the body. As a patient with FM undergoes his/her various activities of daily living, the tightened fascias can pull on remote areas, often eliciting pain in different locations.

Through clinical observation, we have come to believe that the tightening of the fascial sweater throughout the body and the pull in toward the spine and spinal cord accounts for some of the cognitive problems faced by many patients with FM. We have come to feel that the spinal cord may be squeezed by the tiny straight-jackets of the tightened fascia. When this happens, function may decrease throughout the body as the brain is literally squeezed and the head is pulled forward and down, pulling the base of the skull down onto the vertebrae at the top of the cervical spine. This pull can affect the normal flow of blood and nerve impulses into and out of the brain, and cause concurrent headaches at the attachments of the dura.

Patients with FM tend to respond well to the Wurn Technique®, or other deep connective tissue therapy such as myofascial release. While some patients flare up with increased symptoms for a day or two after therapy, our intent is to open, loosen, and increase mobility of the entire fascial sweater, from the base of the skull and the spinal cord out to the extremities (arms and legs). Patients with FM generally note a significant reduction in their symptoms after therapy.

Headaches

Roughly 45 million people in the United States live with chronic headaches, according to the National Women's Health Information Center (NWHIC), and ten million visited a physician's office for headaches, according to a National Hospital Ambulatory Medical Care Survey published in 2001.

Headaches appear to have affected humankind from the dawn of civilization. During the Stone Age, pieces of a headache sufferer's skull were cut away with flint instruments to relieve pain. Another unpleasant remedy used in the British Isles around the ninth century involved drinking "the juice of elder seed, cow's brain, and goat's dung dissolved in vinegar," according to the National Center for Neurological Disorders and Strokes — a branch of NIH that focuses on the neurology of the brain. We have to assume that headaches were a major problem for these patients to go to such extremes in search of a cure.

Most researchers categorize headaches into three types: cluster, migraine, and tension. According to the Mayo Clinic, even though tension headache is the most common type of headache, it is not well understood. Mayo states, "A tension headache generally produces a diffuse mild to moderate pain over your head. Many people liken the feeling to having a tight band around their head. A tension headache may also cause pain in the back of your neck at the base of your skull."

Clinically, we see this pattern quite often. In most cases, the headaches are relieved with therapy, which leads us to believe that there is a strong mechanical component to many of the chronic headaches of patients we treat.

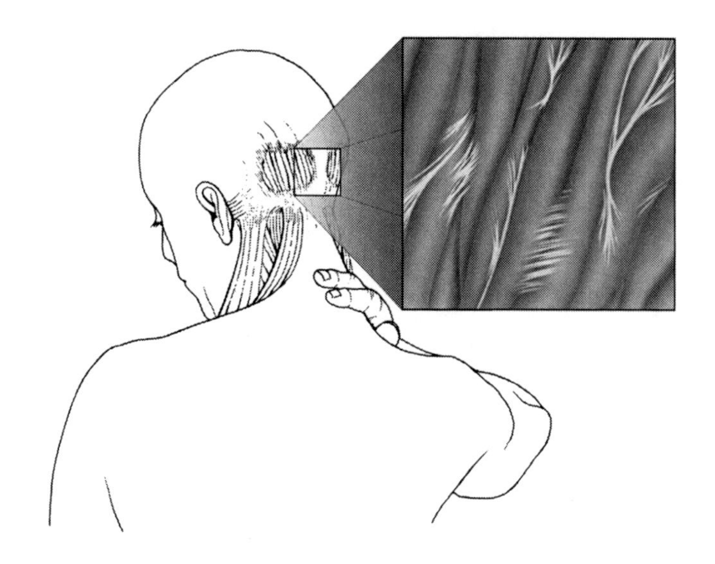

Muscles in the neck and base of the skull tend to become thickened by adhesive processes, as we age.

We believe that adhesions caused by inflammation at the head, neck, or related structures are a direct or perpetuating cause of many headaches, as strong glue-like bonds pull on pain-sensitive structures at the base of the skull, and/or into structures located deeper within the head. Muscles in spasm may impair circulation within the head and neck due to their pressure on nerves or blood vessels, causing pain.

Compression of blood vessels at the base of the skull due to forward head posture or a downward pull of the spinal cord can increase pressure in the head, as blood flow is slowed from leaving the enclosed skull through the foramen magnum — the silver-dollar sized hole at the base of the skull. The spinal cord enters the head through this passage, as do many blood vessels. When patients complain of chronic headaches, we often note moderate to severe tightness in this area. The thickened tissue feels to us like other adhered tissues of the body.

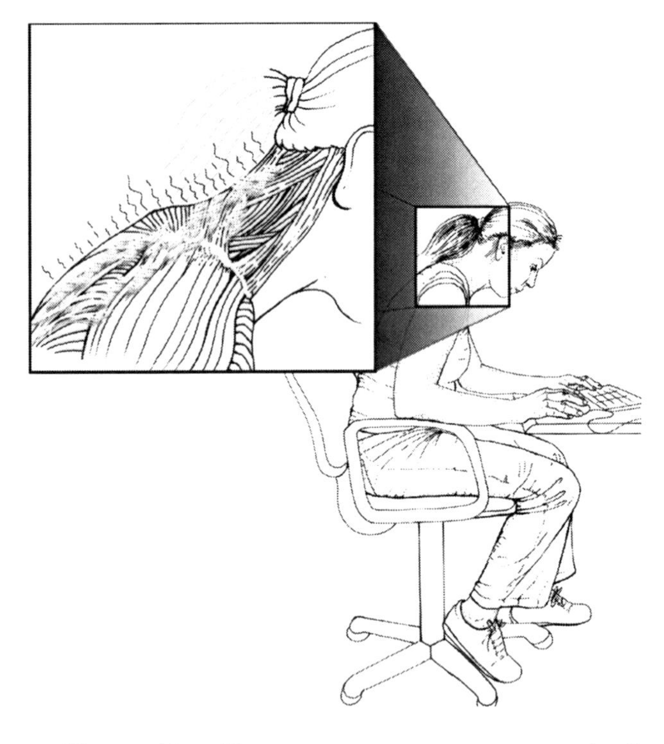

Chronic "forward head" posture can cause spasm and adhesive repair, thickening the tissues at the base of the skull, and sometimes causing chronic headaches.

The patients we treat with chronic headaches often work in chronic "forward head" work posture. This position can result in spasm, inflammation, and adhesions in the neck, shoulders, or upper back.

Patients with mechanical headache pain often report that they feel a place in their head or neck "where my headache starts, or resides." We generally find this patient feedback to be geographically accurate and important, as it so often points to a specific biomechanical cause, such as adhered tissue or a nerve compressed by spasm or adhesions. Patient feedback helps us find and test the specific mechanical forces that cause and exacerbate chronic headaches, and also opens the door to address these areas and attain permanent relief.

One "missing link" in chronic headache diagnosis and treatment is the pull on delicate bones and nerves of the skull from thickened fascia, further down the body.

As noted in the early chapters of this book, the significant weave of the body's fascial sweater extends from the top of the head to the bottom of the feet. Thickened tissues in the mid-back, shoulders, and neck can exert tremendous force on attachments in the head, especially at the base of the skull.

While this area (the cranial base) is a keystone in unlocking the mystery of so many chronic headaches we treat, we find that limiting therapy to this area alone generally does not bring permanent relief. It is necessary to follow and treat the adhered tissues throughout the entire myofascial (muscle and fascia) complex, dissolving or dissipating collagenous attachments wherever they exist below the cranium. Only then can we find lasting relief from chronic head pain, for most of our patients with severe recurring headaches.

Severe Pain and Chronic Headaches after Car Accident

- Barbara's Story

(Full Story Featured in Chapter Six)

In 1986, 10 months into my marriage, I had a severe car accident. For years I had sought help from physical therapy, orthopedic doctors, and chiropractors in Colorado. Now, in Florida, I had continued this process. I was still experiencing pain and severe headaches on a daily basis when my chiropractor recommended I see Belinda Wurn, head of a new physical therapy clinic that had recently opened. At first, I was skeptical, but I was told that she had a new physical therapy technique and, as a massage therapist, I knew her manual treatment could only help.

I started attending treatment with Belinda and my body improved greatly. Over time, my one lingering complaint was severe headaches. Belinda explained that the dura runs from the base of the skull all the way to the tailbone. She felt that my car accident caused my dura to be pulled, leading to constriction and headaches at the base of the skull. She wanted to loosen the scar tissue around my sacrum and tailbone to see if it would help reduce my headaches.

After her explanation, I agreed and she performed the techniques to reduce scar tissue. Because I was a massage therapist, she also showed me how to perform some of the techniques myself.

Within eight to ten treatment sessions, my headaches disappeared.

Myofascial Pain Syndrome (MPS)

Millions of Americans have musculoskeletal pain. An estimated 10 million American adults (5% of the US population) suffer from either myofascial pain syndrome (MPS) or fibromyalgia (FM).[38] While they have much in common, these conditions are now recognized to be two distinct syndromes. MPS is a localized disorder, and FM is a systemic disorder.

Janet Travell, MD, a pioneering researcher in the field of MPS, describes this syndrome as "a regional muscle pain disorder that is characterized by tender spots in taut bands of muscle that refer pain to areas overlying or distant to the tenderness.[39] Some patients develop MPS following trauma, although they may not be aware of the connection since the trauma can precede the onset of pain by weeks, or even months. Besides trauma, other potential causes or perpetuating factors for MPS include muscle strain and frequent exposure to cold, overwork, and fatigue.

Some mechanical problems within the structure of the body are also thought to be possible causes of MPS. These may include a short leg, an asymmetrical pelvis, a long second toe in the foot, and dental abnormalities. Other factors that are thought to lead to MPS are overly tight bra straps, as well as compression of the hamstring muscles (on the back of the thigh) by the edge of a seat. The typical sitting posture of today's office worker at a desk or computer terminal, forward head and slumped body posture, has also been linked with the increased prevalence of MPS in recent years. We view most of these abnormalities to be intimately related to cross-link formation.

We find that the mechanism of adhesion formation in the fascias of our patients with (regional) MPS are similar to our patients with the broader condition of fibromyalgia (FM). Thus, our therapy for MPS is similar to therapy for FM. After taking a thorough history, we evaluate the patient's entire body and conduct extensive palpation of the tissues. The therapist will note any areas of tightness, tenderness, heat, or decreased mobility, as well as any distal areas to which palpation elicits pain. During this evaluation, the physical therapist will also check range of motion to note any deceases from the norm.

As the therapist allows her/his hands to sink deeply into the tissues, our intent is to find thickened, adhered areas and to break or detach collagenous cross-links that formed during a healing process.

We generally follow soft tissue therapies with a stretching and strengthening program focused on the core of the body as well as the areas of prior pain, dysfunction, or decreased range of motion.

Pelvic imbalance

Chronic imbalances of the bones of the pelvis are common. These can create far-reaching mechanical and soft tissue dysfunction within the body systems. Because the pelvic bones are the foundation and base of support for the upper body (the back, spinal column, chest, shoulder girdles, neck, head, and jaw) asymmetry in bones or joints of the pelvis often causes pain and imbalances in any of the areas above.

The pelvis is also the transition point of weight between the legs and the upper body. Anatomically, a single column of central weight (the spinal column, trunk, and head) must be structurally transferred into two columns (the legs) with every step we take. This transfer occurs at the sacroiliac region of the pelvis. Nature designed this area to be highly stable to promote the even transfer of weight from one column into either of the other two. The sacrum (in French *os sacre* or "sacred bone") is also the body's center of gravity. If the pelvis is not stable, the body begins to compensate above or below. Thus, compensatory patterns of adhesions, pain, or dysfunction may occur in almost any area of the body.

Similarly, we find that treating in this core area of the body often brings lasting relief from chronic pain or dysfunction.

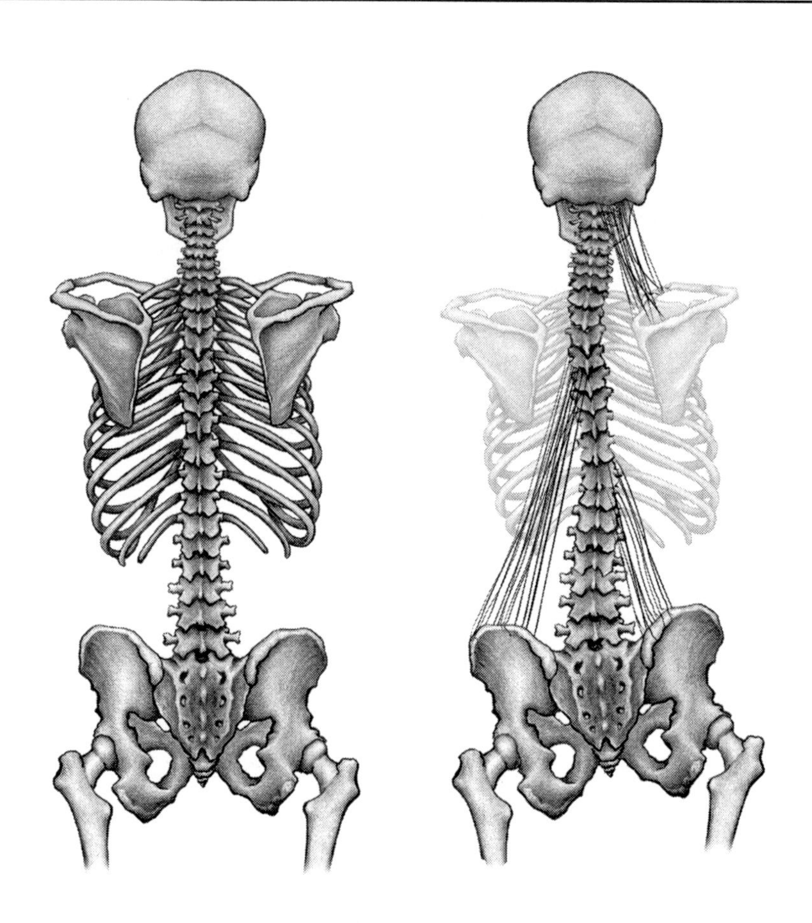

As the foundation of our upper body, an unbalanced pelvis can create symptoms up the spine and into the head.

An unstable pelvis creates a spine that tilts to one side or the other as it rises from the pelvis to support structures above it. For example, due to pelvic imbalance, the lower spine may initially veer off to the left (as shown above). When it does, the muscles of the right low back and right waist must tighten to keep the torso balanced above the body. Once these muscles have tightened, muscles at the left thoracic spine (near the shoulder blades) tighten to keep the shoulders centered over the pelvic foundation. Finally, muscles on the right side of the neck and shoulder girdle tighten to keep the eyes, ears, and their semicircular canals (which monitor our balance) level.

Thus, an unstable pelvis can initiate a scoliosis-like pattern in the body that can precipitate pain into the lower or upper back, shoulder blades, shoulder girdle, neck, head, or temporomandibular joints (TMJ). This same asymmetric patterning may also occur (often to a lesser degree) in the lower body. In that case, one leg may become shorter than the other leg as it is pulled into the hip by compensatory adhesions. The feeling is a bit like walking with one foot on a curb and the other down on the street, or with a heel lift in one shoe. In this case, the longer leg receives the greater share of the trauma with each stride. This can cause consequent pain in the ankle, knee, hip, or low back. Over time, the longer leg on one side perpetuates the imbalance of the pelvis.

One focus of our therapy is to restore leg and pelvic symmetry to create a stable foundation for the entire body. Patients generally find that once their pelvic symmetry is regained and a properly aligned foundation of support is restored, pain subsides.

Pelvic organ pain

Conditions such as endometriosis, sexually transmitted diseases, pelvic inflammatory disease (PID), and vaginal, bladder, and yeast infections can cause pelvic pain. Tiny adhesions form during the healing process and remain in the body after healing. Thus, these conditions may cause symptoms long after the inflammation has passed.

A bladder infection can generally be cured with a course of antibiotics. But after the infection has passed, the adhesions that formed as a response to the original infection often remain within the bladder or outside the bladder, on its support ligaments. There, they may cause pain or a tightening at the bladder, increasing the frequency of urination and sometimes causing spasm or pain. Due to the bladder's proximity to the uterus, we believe that those adhesions can interfere with embryo implantation, as well.

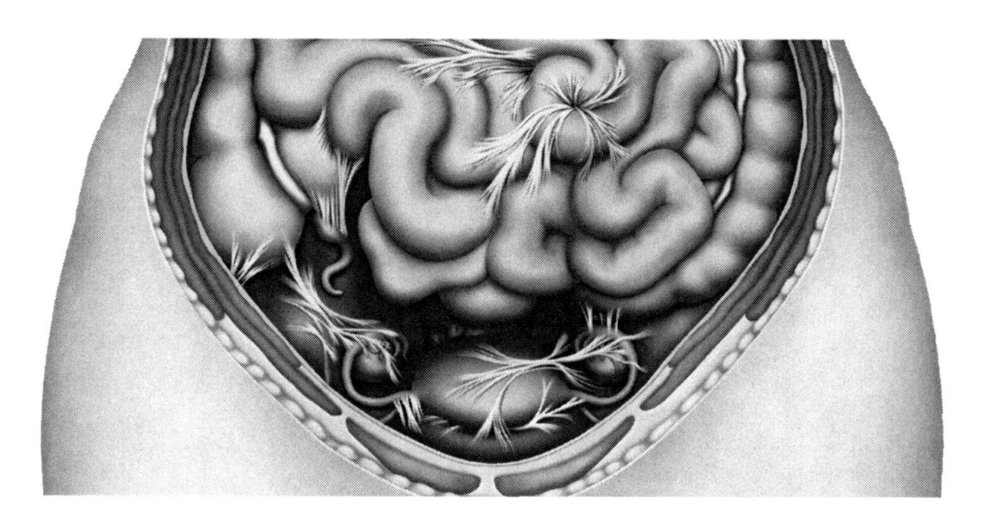

Adhesions from a bladder infection can spread to neighboring areas.

The same process that adheres the bladder can also take place within the uterus or vagina with farther reaching effects. Inflammation or infection in these and nearby structures can cause significant adhesions to form as a response to pelvic inflammatory disease, vaginal infection, abortion, poorly lubricated sex, and physical or sexual abuse.

While the uterus and nearby structures may heal, adhesions that formed as a part of the healing process can remain in the uterus for years (or a lifetime) after healing. There, they may form on the uterine wall creating pain, spasm, or changing the surface to one that is less hospitable to implantation by a fertilized egg.

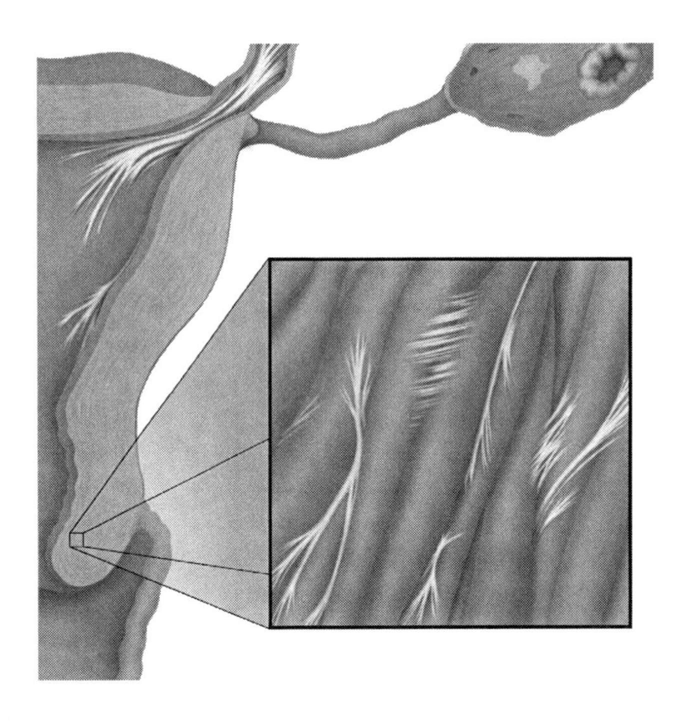

Tiny cross-links can form between muscle cells of the cervix, causing pain with some activities, and with deep intercourse.

Tiny, but strong adhesions can even form between muscle cells, deep within the uterus or cervix. This can cause tightening of the cervix and pain with deep intercourse, as the man's penis pushes a cervix that used to be supple and mobile, but has now become adhered, inflamed, or stiffened by collagenous bonds.

Adhesions that develop in the uterus may cause a state of ongoing inflammation due to their constant pull on that organ or nearby structures. This inflammation and its consequent adhesions may advance into the fallopian tubes, blocking those delicate structures or causing pain.

Severe Pelvic Pain after C-section

- Marcella's Story

Before I attended Clear Passage Therapies (CPT), I had been to 11 different doctors and health practitioners, trying to figure out why I was having so much pain in my pelvic area. Sex was also close to impossible. I had a C-section in 2007 and when I tried to have sex afterward, I knew something was wrong.

However, I continued to be passed off from one specialist to another, none of them giving me a clear diagnosis, much less a treatment option.

I continued to be passed off from one specialist to another, none of them giving me a clear diagnosis, much less a treatment option.

When my doctor told me I would have to have a hysterectomy, because he didn't know what else to do, I knew I had to keep searching on my own. I knew that I wasn't crazy, and that I needed someone to step back and look at the whole picture.

The day I stumbled upon the CPT website, I was completely filled with hope and with relief. For the first time, I saw something that made perfectly logical sense, described everything that I felt was wrong with me, and gave me the hope that one day I really could be out of pain. I scheduled myself as soon as possible.

During the time I spent there, it felt like all of the puzzle pieces finally fit together. Everything finally made sense! Not only the actual treatment, but through their care, acceptance and warmth, I made more progress in healing my body in five days than I had done in the past 12 years! It was as if I had finally found the answer to what my body had been begging for.

All of the puzzle pieces finally fit together. Everything finally made sense!

I am now 100% out of pain. When I was ready to have sex again, I was so nervous! But, everything worked beautifully and I had zero pain or discomfort. I can honestly say that the results I have experienced from my treatment had only been a dream before.

Fourteen months have passed since treatment, and I am still completely pain-free and have been able to use what I learned about my body and how I got into the chronic pain situation to make adjustments in my life to take care of myself and my body. Not only am I pain-free, I have lost weight and feel great about myself again.

Poor digestion and elimination

If stomach mobility is restricted due to adhesions, the patient may experience symptoms such as heartburn, gas, acid reflux, heaviness, bloating, difficulty wearing a belt, or lying prone (face down).

Restricted mobility of the small intestine can cause symptoms such as a feeling of unease and pulling under the navel (especially three to four hours after a meal), difficulty wearing belts or tight trousers, lower abdominal pain, pressure, or tightness after prolonged standing, and breathing difficulty when standing which is improved upon lying down.

Symptoms associated with restricted mobility of the colon may include constipation, spastic colon or irritable bowel syndrome, kidney or right ovary pain or dysfunction, hip or knee problems (due to muscles and nerves these areas share with the colon), impotence, and sciatica. In some cases, adhesions may create partial or total blockage of the small intestines — a life-threatening condition. To learn more about our treatment for this serious condition, please see our section on bowel obstruction in Chapter Sixteen.

By treating adhesions that restrict various areas of the digestive tract, patients find their symptoms are greatly reduced.

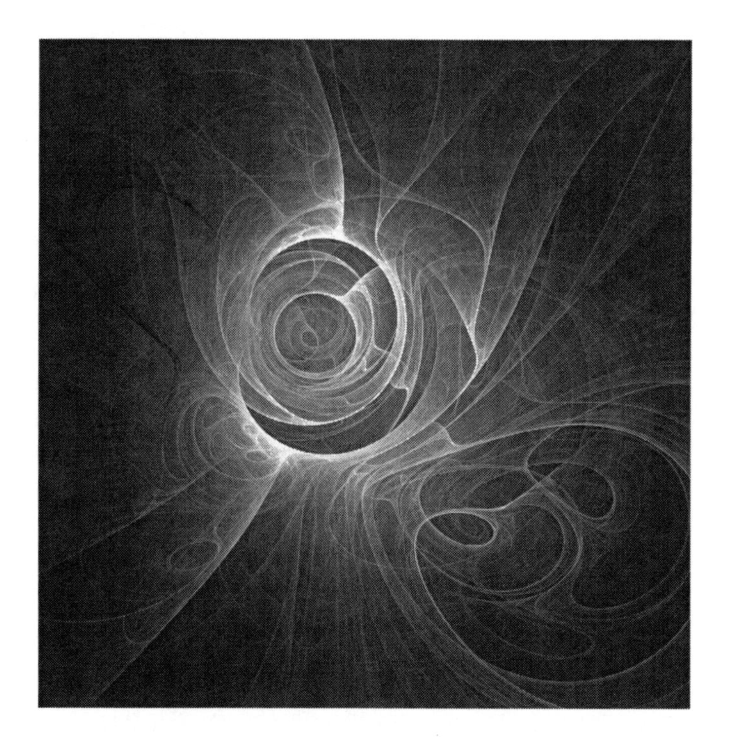

An artist's rendering mimics adhesions forming inside and outside the intestinal walls.

Tailbone pain

The coccyx (tailbone) is a small bone situated at the lowest point of the sacrum. Its position in the body leaves it vulnerable to trauma from falls onto the buttocks, car accidents, childbirth (especially difficult deliveries), and scarring from abdominal surgeries such as a hysterectomy or episiotomy. Physical or sexual abuse and chronic slumped sitting posture are other causes or contributors to tailbone pain.

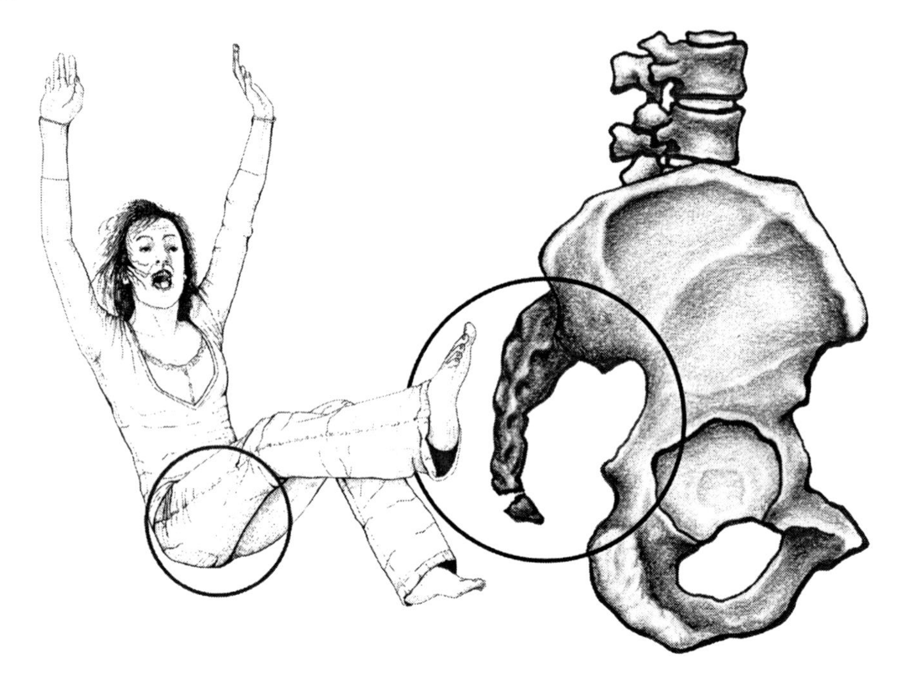

A fall onto the buttocks can create adhesions with pain appearing or increasing over several years.

In any of these situations, the coccyx may be pushed or pulled into an awkward angle, usually forward, occasionally side-bent, and rarely bent backwards. The result may be moderate to debilitating tailbone pain, often spreading into the low back, hip, or neighboring structures. Reproductive function can also be adversely affected by this

> ***I experienced some immediate improvements; I no longer experienced the tailbone pain that occurred after my second pregnancy.***
>
> *– Madeline, mother of two after struggling with secondary infertility and tailbone pain*

mechanism as inflammation spreads to nearby structures.

Tailbone pain that has persisted for more than three months is considered chronic. Symptoms may include difficulty sitting for long periods, pain with deep penetration during sexual intercourse (for women), constipation, pain with bowel movements, and headaches at the base of the skull, temples, or top of the head (due to attachments of the dura that runs from the tailbone to the base and inside surfaces of the skull). Many people also report concurrent low back or sacroiliac pain.

In many of these cases, we find that adhesions have formed on the ligaments that run from the tailbone to the hips or "sit bones" of the pelvis. These tightened ligaments tend to fix the coccyx in a malaligned position, causing a state of near or total immobility. Fixed in place, the tailbone creates inflammation and pain when moving, trying to have intercourse or bowel movements, or even when sitting. Once we clear the area of adhesions in a non-surgical manner and restore normal tailbone alignment and mobility, pain generally decreases significantly, or totally.

> ***Sex no longer hurt in that position, my appendectomy scar felt completely different, and my tailbone was more properly aligned.***
>
> *– Ashley, mother of one after struggling with infertility and pain*

TMJ, facial pain, ear ringing (tinnitus)

The temporomandibular joint (TMJ) attaches the jaw to the skull just below each ear on both sides of the skull. This area is a major source of discomfort and pain for many people.

While most patients first see a dentist about TMJ symptoms, we generally find this is actually an orthopedic problem more than a dental condition. Patients who have had their teeth ground down or built up by their dentists but are still having problems need to look further down the structure into the neck, back and pelvis. If the structures below (legs and pelvis) do not create a level foundation to support the trunk, neck, and ultimately the TM joints, the effect of the asymmetry below will cause compensatory asymmetry at both sides of the jaw.

TMJ symptoms may include headaches, dizziness, and pain or pressure in the upper back, upper shoulders, upper neck, base of the skull, pain around the eyes, cheeks, face, or at the jaw joint(s). Patients may experience popping or clicking when opening or closing the mouth, inability to open the mouth fully, ringing in the ears (tinnitus), stuffy ears or ear pain, tender neck and upper back muscles, fatigue, clenching and grinding of the teeth (bruxing) at night or when stressed, or pain during or after eating.

Symptoms sometimes begin after whiplash from a motor vehicle accident or fall, or after wisdom teeth or back molars are removed. They may also follow years of thumb sucking, breathing through the mouth (rather than nose breathing), or an overbite.

Many people experience chronic pain that originates in or around these joints. The pain can be disabling and can affect nutrition, lifestyle, and interpersonal relationships. This can become the site of arthritis and other degenerative problems, which compounds the actual joint dysfunction. As noted above, the pain can also originate from asymmetries below the jaw, such as a neck or pelvis that is out of alignment.

In the case of TMJ pain and related symptoms, we have found that we need to treat the whole body to correct asymmetries and adhesive tensions in the structures below the jaw (legs, pelvis, back, chest, and neck) if we are to achieve lasting results treating this area. Thus, while we treat tissues at this joint, we find that lasting results generally require that we treat and balance all of these body structures.

Relief at Last

When chronic pain patients come to our clinic for treatment, we review their histories extensively with them, then palpate their entire bodies to check for adhesive restrictions that might be causing their pain. As we discussed earlier, adhesions tend to form after surgery, trauma, infection, inflammation, or chronic postures over time. Patients are frequently unaware that these adhesions attach structures to one another or cause pulling in one area that may affect another area of their body. As we manually deform, dissipate, or detach these adhesions during our treatment, patients generally find that their chronic pain decreases and function improves.

I have had no pain since treatment. What I did not realize was that other problems would be resolved: tight hips, chronic constipation, pain and stiffness in my hands, shoulders, and neck. Somehow, all of the problems were interrelated.

– Kelly, who experienced chronic pain after sexual abuse

Chronic Pain after Multiple Traumas

- Trudy's Story

I arrived at the clinic with a great deal of hope. Not only was I feeling desperate to become a mother, but I had searched for years for someone to release my body from intense physical pain. After the first morning's treatment, an image became clear in my mind, and a vision of what this therapy was going to do.

I saw a very old, run down ship, almost like a pirate ship from the early 18th century. It was falling apart and could no longer sail as it was built to do. It was permanently anchored. It had obviously been abused and had never been given the loving attention it needed to return it to its original glory. The picture was in sepia tones, devoid of life and vibrancy. As I lay with this image I knew this was a metaphor for my body. It had been abused over the years through multiple traumas including four car accidents, and many falls onto back, tailbone and hip during sports or other intense activities. After years of searching for relief, I had resigned myself that no treatment would be able to return my body to its original state of glory – pain-free and functional.

I had searched for years for someone to release my body from intense physical pain

During the week of therapy, I was delighted to find that the image began to change. Color returned to the picture and the ship started to take on its original magnificence. It looked anew again as if it had gone back in time and returned to a fully functional ship, able to sail through even the toughest of storms. Then I realized that this was what was happening to my body. The treatment was like going back in time for my body, back to a state when my entire body functioned healthily. I was becoming the vessel that could carry my future children into this world. I felt an enormous burden being lifted and a rising hope coming from within.

The treatment was like going back in time for my body, back to a state when my entire body functioned healthily.

This metaphor was a vision that carried me through the amazing experience that I had during my week at Clear Passage. Now, for the first time in 16 years since my first motor vehicle accident, a therapist acknowledged and treated the underlying causes of my immense physical pain. I felt a renewed hope and excitement for the future.

Being a physical therapist myself, I have been trained to think scientifically regarding treatment types and efficacy. Simply stated, the Wurn Technique makes sense, both anatomically and physiologically. The treatment is not rocket science to understand. It is simply a multitude of differ-

Being a physical therapist, I have been trained to think scientifically regarding treatment types and efficacy.

ent manual techniques combined in such a way as to "unglue" the areas that became adhered over a lifetime of healing. Once all individual parts of the body have freedom of movement, they begin to function better individually. Hence, each organ, system, and part can begin to synchronize and work in harmony. During the course of therapy, I felt my entire body begin to regain mobility and function – in various areas.

I have been home for only two weeks, but I am already feeling so different it is almost hard to describe. The constant pain in my mid and lower back, that I had previously learned to live with, has improved immensely, and certain areas feel completely pain-free (an amazing statement for me). I used to awaken every morning and the first thing I felt was pain. Now I awaken and can start my day in a positive mental and emotional state, without the heavy burden of chronic pain. My entire abdomen is softer and more mobile, and I can breathe more deeply than I ever knew was possible. My balance is remarkably better, and my range of motion is greatly increased in almost every joint of my body. In addition, my digestion has greatly improved, and my overall functional level has increased immensely.

My overall functional level has increased immensely.

I no longer think of my body as my enemy. Now it is the vessel that is allowing me to travel more easily, and experience a high quality of life again.

The gratefulness I have for the therapists at Clear Passage is truly boundless. The therapists are amazing, warm hearted individuals who work from a heart space of love and compassion. Their innovative, time intensive treatments give results in areas way beyond the scope of reproductive health. They have helped bring my body back in time to an overall healthier state where bodily systems work better, and with better communication.

I also feel that my body is now healthy and strong enough to be the vessel for our children. I finally have been able to accept the help I so desperately needed – and I did it for me, so that I can live a healthy, active life. Becoming a mother will be a much welcomed result, but even before that, the treatment I received at CPT was the best investment I have ever made, a true investment in me.

Chapter Sixteen

Surgical Adhesions, Bowel Obstructions

Surgeries save lives and improve function for thousands of people each year. The surgical processes of modern medicine have proven to be miraculous healing procedures for people in need of internal repair. However, surgeries carry risks and can create unwanted side effects.

No matter how skilled the surgeon, the surgical process may leave its recipient with scarring and adhesions. Cross-link formation which occurs in tissues that have been cut or burned during surgery is simply a part of the healing process.

Many patients' bodies seem to easily tolerate the tightening of tissues that occurs in areas where adhesions bind and draw structures together after surgery. But in some people, the scarring and adhesions which originally helped them heal from the surgery continue to lay down in a pattern that causes pain or dysfunction later in life. Depending on how we heal, whether or not we have adhesive problems after surgery, is a bit "the luck of the draw."

Why Adhesions Form After Surgery

Post-surgical adhesions help us heal

Whenever a surgical instrument enters the body, it slices through living human tissue. Then, surgeons may cut or burn other living tissue to perform their intended procedures.

After the surgery, the tissues must recover from the exploration and any repair. Collagenous cross-links lay down to form adhesions or scar tissue as the first step in the healing process. In doing so, they form adhesive blankets or bonds on structures that were cut or burned during the surgery. These primary healing adhesions remain within the body for life, performing a vital function in the repair mechanics of healing.

Surgical adhesions draw structures together

As adhesions form to help the body heal, they sometimes draw nearby structures into their glue-like network. In most cases, the pliability and extensibility of the human body allows for this pull. The muscles, organs, or connective tissues may be pulled toward the area of surgical repair, but for most people, the body is able to accept surgical intervention with relatively few side effects.

In some cases, this drawing together of adhesions can decrease function or cause pain. As these patients heal, they may notice tightness or a pulling sensation in areas near the surgical site that did not exist before. Clinically, we have found that appendectomies, stomach or intestinal surgeries, hysterectomy, gall bladder removal, and back, hip, and other major surgical interventions may create pain and sensations in areas near the surgical site. We find that these tensions are often created by secondary adhesions, pulling structures far away from the scar toward the site of the surgery.

Adhesions sometimes cause inflammation

Months or even years after surgery, inflammation can occur due to the trauma of the original surgery or as a result of direct or indirect pulls into the site of surgical repair.

The body's response to inflammation is to lay down collagenous cross-links, the building blocks of adhesions. The result can include different types or configurations of adhesions. But whether filmy, blanketing, or cord-like, these adhesive formations can attach to nearby structures. When they do, adhesions may cause pain or decrease function, due to the bonds they create between neighboring structures.

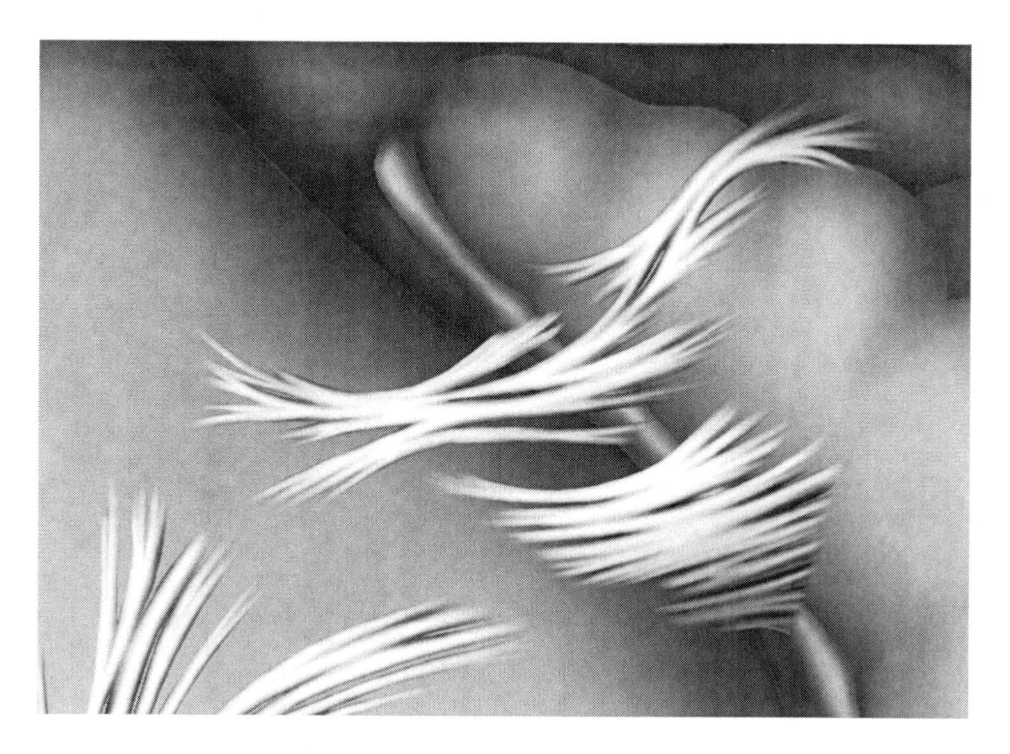

Adhesions can cause inflammation due to their attachments between structures.

Adhesions adjust to posture along lines of tension

After years of palpating our patients, we frequently notice adhesions that appear to be compensatory in structure. This is what we feel happens: As a patient heals from a surgery, certain areas of the body become tightened by surgical scarring. Then compensatory postures form along internal strain patterns as the post-surgical patients stand and move in awkward postures, to avoid the pulling or pain.

Over time, the decreased mobility in some areas coupled with the need to conduct activities of life in unusual postures appears to create an adhesive pattern in the three-dimensional weave of fascia that is arguably the primary structural element of the body. We have found that compensatory adhesions can form wherever one or more muscles have been required to hold static or awkward tension patterns for weeks, months, or years in the case of long-standing chronic pain cases.

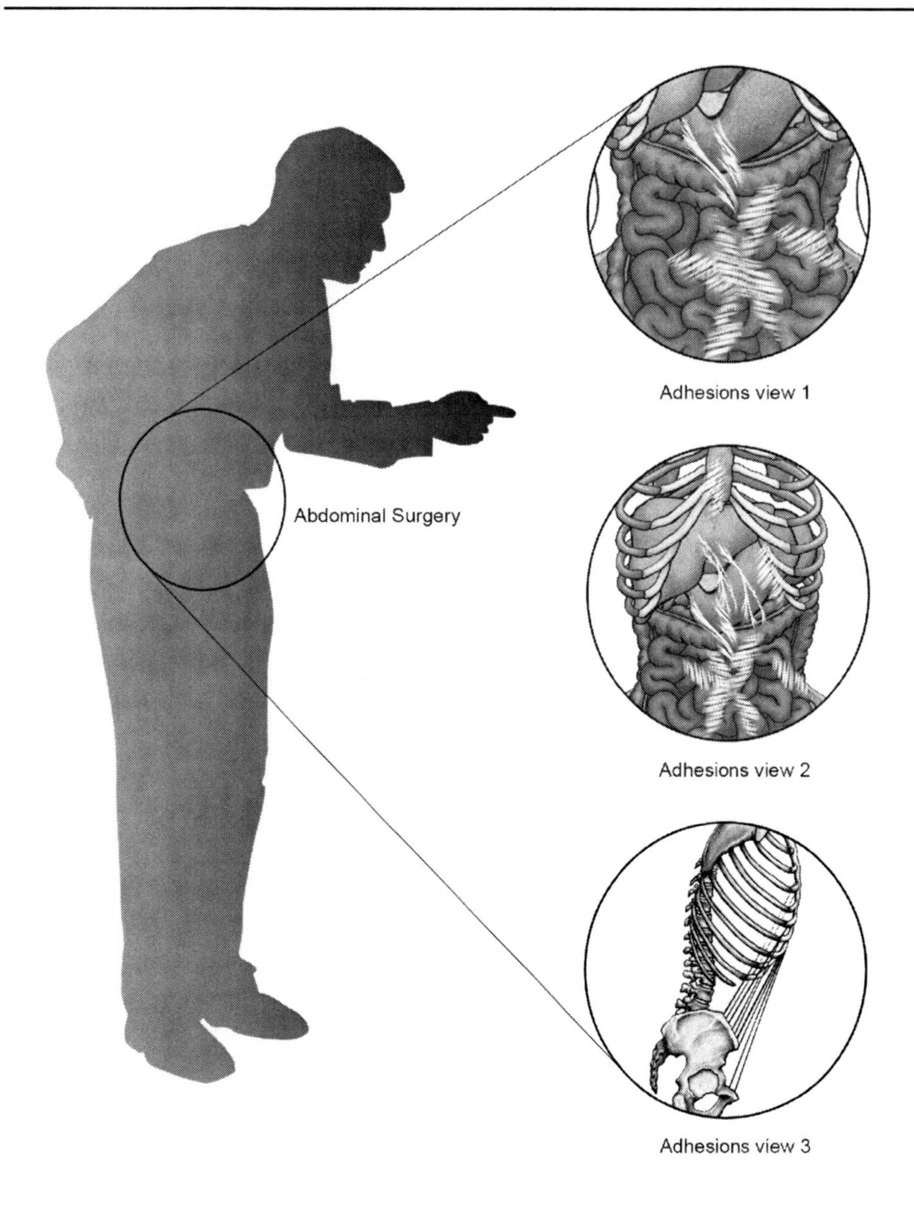

Post-surgical adhesions can bend us forward over time, causing pain in the back as we struggle to stay upright.

After surgery to the abdomen or pelvis, adhesions on the front of the body can bend a patient forward. After weeks in a forward-bent posture, the adhesions from the surgical scars can grow to emulate the position the patient takes. This can perpetuate the forward posture by creating more cross-links up into the chest or down into the pelvis or the front of the legs — or both. At the same time, the back fights to keep the patient vertical in space as the head looks forward.

Thus, many post-surgical patients tend to develop adhered tissues at the top and back of the shoulders, the back of the neck, and the base of the skull, due to these muscles firing in a near constant state.

Compensatory adhesions may form slowly over time and build up over the course of our lives. Unless this process is reversed and the adhesions are broken down, the adhesive pattern will spread. Thus the compensatory adhesions that form in our body are often found far from the original site of the surgery. They form to assist muscles to help us maintain functional postures after our tissues have been compromised by surgery.

How Surgical Adhesions Can Lead to Pain

Surgical pain generally passes within the first days or weeks after a surgery. In the most invasive surgeries, pain may take two or three weeks to dissipate. When pain persists several weeks or more after surgery, we suspect that post-surgical adhesions may be causing the symptoms.

Chronic pain caused by adhesions is generally noticed within the first 6 to 12 months after surgery. In some cases, patients notice a pulling immediately after surgery, a pull that never goes away. In other cases, the pull of surgical and secondary adhesions may cause pain weeks or months after surgery. In other instances, the slow formation of compensatory adhesions in the body causes inflammation that begins two or more years after a surgery. These compensatory adhesions can create pain that increases or spreads geographically over time.

In some cases, pain occurs as a direct response to adhesions attaching to nerves. This is generally experienced as a sharp or piercing pain. In other cases, adhesions can create a pull into broad areas or larger pain-sensitive structures, such as muscles, organs, and their support tissues. In this case, pain may come with certain movements or body positions. This pain may be specific, but is usually duller than with adhesions that have attached more directly to nerves.

Post-surgical adhesion symptoms can range from confusing and annoying to totally debilitating. In the digestive tract, they can decrease the ability to move or digest food. In the case of bowel obstructions, they can become life-threatening. They can close intestines, squeeze arteries and veins, impose upon muscles, nerves, and supporting ligaments. In short, they can glue tissues down, from the strongest to the most delicate structures in the body.

Pain may also radiate into a broad area, or into other areas of the body. When this happens, the pain pattern that evolves can be confusing to the patient and the physician. Patients with post-surgical pain may be sent to specialist after specialist to try to determine the cause of the pain. The tragedy is that beyond the confusion, this steals time and valuable quality of life from the patient who is searching for relief of pain, but cannot even find the cause.

When the Cure is the Cause: Surgery and Adhesions

The usual medical solution to post-surgical adhesions is to first administer pharmaceuticals to decrease inflammation, ease the pain, or improve function. If drugs fail to adequately address the symptoms, the physician may suggest a "second look" surgery to help determine the exact cause of the pain. If the surgeon finds more adhesions, the usual response would be to cut the ones which are accessible.

There are several challenges for the surgeon, namely;

- a conscientious surgeon will avoid adhesions on delicate structures that might be damaged by surgery, such as certain parts of the fallopian tube or ovary,
- the surgeon will also avoid areas where cutting might harm the patient, such as parts of the bowel where too deep a cut could spill intestinal contents into the abdomen or pelvis (causing peritonitis), and
- as noted earlier, even the most skilled physician cannot prevent the body's natural healing response from creating additional adhesions, as a natural part of healing after surgery.

Adhesions have always been a big problem for surgeons and their patients. A study published in *Lancet: The British Journal of Surgery* showed that a third of all patients who received open surgery returned for repeat surgery to address adhesions within two years after the original surgery.[40] As shocking as this statistic is, a large number of these people then went on to have subsequent adhesion removal surgeries over the next several years.

A study in *Digestive Surgery* showed that between 55% and 100% of women who undergo major pelvic surgery develop adhesions, and adhesions occur in more than 90% of patients after abdominal surgery. The study went on to say, "Small-bowel obstruction, infertility, chronic abdominal and pelvic pain, and difficult reoperative surgery are the most common consequences of (the) adhesions."[41]

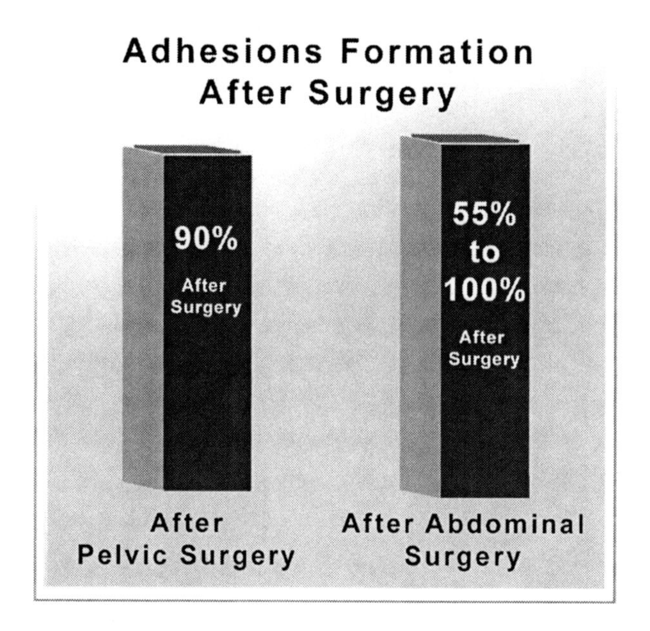

Adhesions form at a high rate after surgery, causing pain, bowel obstruction, infertility, and often reoperative surgery.

In our professional careers, we have met people who have undergone 17, 19, even (in one case) 47 surgeries in their lives — most of which were designed to address post-operative adhesions. In other cases, patients have told us, "I tend to grow a lot of adhesions; I generally have about one surgery a year to help clear out the adhesions that have formed in me." While this may sound to some like madness, it has too often been the only answer that medical science has been able to offer patients with adhesions that cause pain and dysfunction.

Eight Prior Surgeries

- Ginny's Story

After eight surgeries and two serious falls, my body had become severely adhered and I was in nearly constant pain. The adhesions were so strong that they began to affect my posture; they caused my back and neck to ache and the pain made life very difficult. Adhesions in my abdominal cavity were closing my bowels, preventing waste from moving. After eating, I would be curled up in a ball in severe pain. It was humiliating and extremely painful.

I (was) in a vicious cycle of pain and hospitalization. I needed surgery to reduce the adhesions and relieve my pain, but the surgeries would cause more adhesions to form.

I had already undergone a resection surgery to remove bowel obstructions (essentially adhesions) by cutting, then rejoining my intestines. I soon found myself in a vicious cycle of pain and hospitalizations. I needed surgery to reduce the adhesions and relieve my pain, but the surgeries would cause more adhesions to form, necessitating more surgeries. So I had to find a more non-invasive way to solve this problem.

I began desperately to search for other treatment options. I worked at an acupuncture clinic at the time, and one of our patients told me that she was receiving treatment to reduce adhesions at a physical therapy clinic called Clear Passage Therapies (CPT). I spoke with my gastroenterologist about the therapy and he told me, "It can't hurt to try it." I scheduled an appointment immediately.

By the time I found CPT, my health was plummeting. At my initial evaluation, my therapist told me there was very little mobility in my abdominal organs. She was also concerned that I was becoming adhered in the muscles and support structures on the front of my body.

I attended treatment for an hour at a time twice a week and found that my pain reduced markedly. Before long, I stopped experiencing pain in my bowels, neck, and back. Things in life that most people take for granted, but that had been denied to me for so long, slowly began to return. I can still remember the first day I was finally able to have a bowel movement without pain or laxatives, and the first time I was finally able to eat without pain. It was amazing.

(Functions) that most people take for granted, but that had been denied to me for so long, slowly began to return.

At one point, my insurance decided it would no longer cover the cost of my treatment, and I was forced to stop attending. I worked relentlessly with my insurance company until they finally agreed to continue covering my treatment, but it was too late. Adhesions had formed again and blocked my intestines. I was back in the hospital with an obstructed bowel for 13 days. I knew I had to return to CPT if I didn't want another surgery. They helped my body recover and broke down other adhesions that had formed.

Over the time I have attended therapy at CPT, I have met many patients. After therapy, most people tell me that their pain is relieved, their adhesions are reduced, and they never have to return again.

My body, on the other hand, is different from most. For one reason or another, my body continually forms adhesions. My doctor says my body is an "adhesion factory."

Because my body continually produces adhesions, I choose to return to CPT for treatment. The therapists not only help reduce any pain I experience, they also prevent other adhesions from forming by increasing the mobility and flexibility of my organs and tissues. I know that if I didn't have CPT, I would end up back in the hospital.

I cannot say enough about CPT. I would recommend them 250%. I even had my husband attend after a serious car accident. He was in so much pain that it hurt for him to even be touched. But today, he's out working in the garden.

If they were able to help someone described as an "adhesion factory," I know they will be able to help others who experience pain or adhesion formation as a normal response to healing.

Twenty Years of Surgeries after Partial Hysterectomy

- Katrina's Story

Some women have experienced so many surgeries in their lifetimes that their bodies continue to form adhesions, even years after the surgeries end. Ginny shared her personal journey through years of surgeries and the subsequent pain and dysfunction she experienced. Because her body was so traumatized by her surgeries, her doctor said that her body continues to form adhesions.

Katrina, one of our former patients, is much like Ginny. In fact, when Katrina called our clinic to see if treatment would be appropriate for her, we discussed former patients like Ginny, who had experienced similar problems.

After speaking with a CPT therapist, Katrina knew she wanted to come for treatment. Although she felt she was coming on blind faith, Katrina had high hopes that this alternative option for the breakdown of her adhesions would work, and she was very optimistic.

> ***It gets to the point where it never goes away and the pain overrides your thoughts.***

Her pain and dysfunction had started almost 20 years earlier. After a partial hysterectomy, Katrina began experiencing pain and had to undergo a subsequent surgery to remove her ovaries and a partial bowel obstruction.

Just two years later, she had to have another surgery to remove adhesions that formed beneath her previous incision, causing her bowel to become partially obstructed again.

Over the next 14 years, Katrina endured eight more surgeries and procedures to treat adhesions, bowel obstructions, and numerous other dysfunctions that had resulted from her devastating cycle of surgeries.

Katrina told us, "I was in a lot of pain during those years, but I had to keep working. You just take as little pain medication as you can and deal with the pain until it becomes too much, and you need another surgery."

Over the next 14 years, Katrina endured eight more surgeries and procedures to treat adhesions, bowel obstructions, and numerous other dysfunctions.

After surgery to remove adhesions in May of 2004, Katrina knew she needed to find another option. As each week progressed, she experienced more and more pain. "It's hard to explain the pain unless you have had it," Katrina told us. "You get a lot of abdominal swelling and localized pain in certain spots. The swelling gets really bad and your clothes don't fit. At night, your body throbs. It just gets to the point where it never goes away and the pain overrides your thoughts. You can't even walk properly because you are in so much pain and you feel your body drawing up."

It was out of her pain and desperation that Katrina searched for other options on the Internet and found our clinic.

Katrina noticed changes almost immediately after treatment with us and told us, "The therapists worked on my rectum one time and the next day I had a normal bowel movement! By the end of the week, intercourse pain was completely gone — it was amazing. Some of the scars felt thinner or had disappeared."

Once her treatment was finished, we explained to Katrina that her body would make adjustments over the following months as her organs and systems learned to function without the adhesions. Katrina was happy to find that her body kept improving over time and told us, "I had more energy and people told me I looked healthier."

As time passed though, Katrina began to notice some pain gradually increasing in her body. Although our treatment successfully reduced many of the adhesions that existed in her body, we could not prevent her body's natural process of building more adhesions.

The majority of the people we treat never have to return to us for treatment. However, there are some, like Katrina and Ginny, whose bodies continue to form adhesions. Although patients who need ongoing care with us are rare, we can at least provide them with an alternative to cyclical surgery.

When Katrina's body started to produce more adhesions again, she was faced with a choice: either more surgery or returning to us for treatment. She was happy to return to us for a natural treatment. We were once again able to reduce the new adhesions that formed and reduce the pain and symptoms she was experiencing.

Although we genuinely hope that Katrina will not have to return again, we cannot control how her body produces adhesions. If she needs us again, we will be here as a safe and natural alternative to surgery.

The Formation of Bowel Obstructions

Once food has passed through the stomach and duodenum, it proceeds to the small intestines, or "bowel". This long tubular organ fills the lower abdomen in a sinuous course over its 7½ to 12 foot length.[42]

Since it is not located within the rib cage which encases or partially protects many of the upper abdominal organs (stomach, pancreas, and spleen), the bowel is more exposed to trauma than many other organs. Whether it receives the blow of a steering wheel or air bag in a car accident, or a more indirect trauma, such as absorbing the shock of a fall, the bowel may be more susceptible to trauma than neighboring organs above it.

The bowel is also close to and adjacent to the pelvic organs. These structures are even more susceptible to tissue damage from infections, inflammation, and surgery. These organs are often deeply involved in cases of endometriosis, infections such as Chlamydia and pelvic inflammatory disease, and traumas such as a fall onto the back, hip or tailbone.

Finally, the bowels themselves are often diagnosed with inflammatory conditions such as diverticulitis, appendicitis, irritable bowel syndrome, and Crohn's disease.

Any and all of these conditions may cause an adhesive response, as the body sends out thousands of tiny but powerful collagenous cross-links to begin the healing process. Adhesions begin to form first at the site of greatest tissue damage, and then at other areas of inflammation.

In the best event, adhesions confine themselves to a small area on the surface of a single organ, the tissues below heal, and the body returns to normal function.

But when the geography of healing is more extensive, adhesions may spread more deeply into the organ, to support structures, or to neighboring organs. The subtle geographical shift between structures can set up a pattern of increased adhesion growth that may become problematic. The pull between structures tends to cause additional inflammation as the body participates in the activities of life. The inflammation begets more adhesions, and new adhesions can cause further inflammation. This can create a spiral of adhesion formation within the delicate folds of the bowels.

These adhesions can create a weave of occlusion within the bowel, constricting its inner walls. slowly decreasing its ability to allow food and nutrients to pass. Adhesions may be found on the outer walls of the bowel, kinking them like a garden hose or binding them to other structures in the abdomen or pelvis. The recurrent build-up of adhesions can lead to a partial or total bowel occlusion (or obstruction). Adhesions may also form within the tube-like bowel, much as they do in fallopian tubes.

Total Bowel Obstructions

Bowel adhesions or spasm can become so severe that they totally block the small intestines in a life-threatening condition called total small bowel obstruction (SBO). We became all too familiar with this when 20 years after Belinda's pelvic surgery and radiation therapy, she suffered a total bowel obstruction on her 53rd birthday.

The onset was unexpected, sudden, and severe. She began vomiting and couldn't keep food down. She also could not have any bowel movements. We rushed her to the hospital where physicians inserted an NG (nasogastric) tube through her nose into her stomach to relieve pressure in the digestive tract. They hoped that by doing so the bowel would untwist, allowing food to pass. They also inserted IV (intravenous) tubes into her arms to give her nutrients because without them she would literally starve to death, and fluids so she would not become dehydrated. This is standard procedure for women and men with small bowel obstruction.

Belinda waited in the hospital bed for three days, rolling back and forth, with Larry treating her as he could. Unfortunately, the damage to her bowels from the over-spray of radiation therapy had apparently finally collapsed part of her small intestine. The same radiation therapy had made her tissues friable – which means they could fall apart and bleed easily with deep touch, thus limiting the amount of manual therapy she could receive. Once again her early cancer treatment was coming back to haunt us in an unexpected way — 20 years later.

In the end, her physician cut Belinda's gut in an open surgery (laparotomy). The surgeon removed 30 inches of her small bowel, and resected (re-attached) the two ends of the bowel that remained.

During the recovery process, we had the opportunity to ask the surgeon about the amount of adhesions present in Belinda's bowel. She told us that when she opened Belinda's abdominal cavity, there were no adhesions, although moderate to severe tissue damage from the radiation therapy was evident throughout the bowels, abdomen and pelvis. When the doctor inquired further about Belinda's history, we related the extent of radiation therapy she had received.

The surgeon shook her head, "It's amazing," she said. "You received so much radiation therapy 20 years ago, and yet your abdomen was essentially free of adhesions when I opened you up. Given your history, I would have expected massive adhesions and a bowel obstruction within two years of your radiation therapy."

Unfortunately the healing process did not go well. Either because of a spill from her bowel or other contamination during surgery, a deep internal infection (peritonitis) followed the surgery. The physicians re-opened the surgical site by removing two-thirds of the stitches, inserted a drainage tube, then left the site open, so it would "heal from the inside out", the doctor said.

Naturally, the scarring and adhesions from this surgery, subsequent infection and open healing were massive.

Thinking back, we wish we would have spent more time treating Belinda's small bowels, because the radiation therapy had a "spill-over" effect which destroyed the integrity of much of those organs. Twenty years ago, our sole focus was on her pelvis (below her navel) where Belinda was experiencing so much pain. But twenty years ago, we were just starting on this quest, and just beginning to understand the "whole body" nature of fascia and adhesion formation. At the time, our exploration into treating Belinda was solely focused on her areas of pain. We had since learned to look further in our patients' bodies, but had never considered that spill-over radiation might have damaged Belinda's bowels, which were relatively far from the focus of her original surgery and radiation, at her cervix (in her pelvis).

This proved to be an expensive lesson for the both of us, one written in Belinda's body. This lesson reconfirmed the need to assess and treat the whole body with every patient.

The physician's decision to leave the surgical site open to help reverse the post-surgical infection left massive adhesions in Belinda's abdomen. She nursed that open wound for eight weeks and was given several antibiotics (intravenous and oral) to try to cure the infection. Slowly, the wound healed, but the infection never totally resolved – a fact we were to discover on a delayed honeymoon trip to India, six months later.

Emergency Bowel Surgery in India

- Belinda's Ongoing Story

(told by Larry)

Although we had been married twenty years, we never had the time to take the honeymoon I had promised my bride two decades earlier. Belinda wanted to visit India and Nepal, countries I had visited in my 20's courtesy of a photo and book assignment I had done for an art museum.

Nepal was presently inaccessible to Westerners due to a heavy-handed Chinese invasion and resulting instability in the capital city, Kathmandu. Instead, we visited nearby Bhutan (a country dubbed "Shangri-La" due to its mountainous vistas and it's King's avowed focus on "Gross National Happiness" over "Gross National Product.")

After a week in Bhutan, we moved down into India. It had always been Belinda's dream to see the Taj Mahal, so after a short visit to Delhi, we drove down to Agra, the site of that magnificent edifice. The four hours of traffic surrounded us with every method of transport imaginable: ancient, hand carved ox-carts, camels, elephants, cows and monkeys wandered among the cars, tractor-trailer trucks, and three wheeled vehicles of every description; it was both slow-moving and remarkable. Belinda and I have always enjoyed expanding our minds by immersing ourselves in either nature, or in totally different cultures from our own, from time to time. We find the experience both challenging and enriching to our bodies, minds and souls. Along the way, we passed numerous medical clinics.

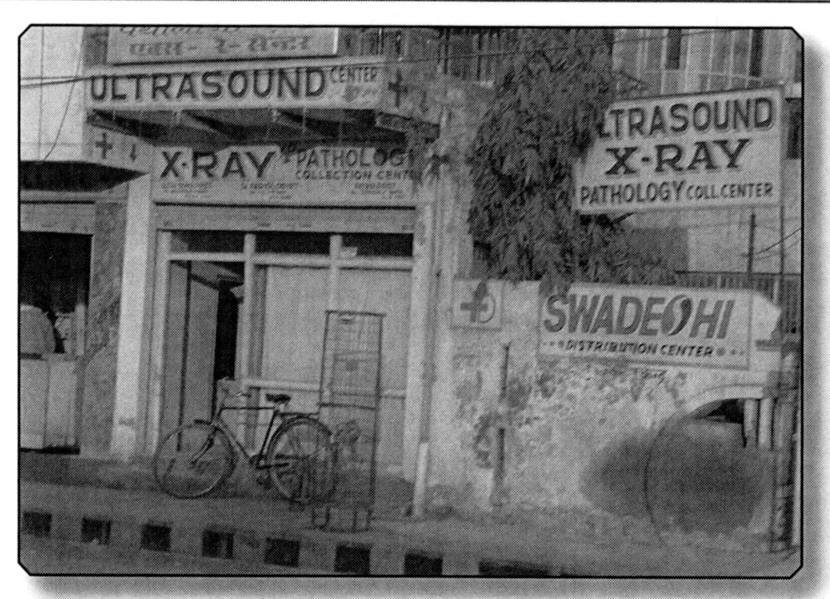

Medical clinics along the road
felt a bit primitive

Unfortunately, that night brought problems. Belinda found herself unable to eat or pass foods — both classic signs of another total bowel obstruction. A physician who came to our hotel room inserted an NG tube into her stomach through her nose, then hooked her up to intravenous feeding, fluids and pain medication. Belinda rolled back and forth trying to get food to pass through. I treated her, but this time things went very differently. During treatment both of my hands were being pulled toward a single point in her intestines that felt hard, and hot; it felt like an infection.

This presented a major problem. While we felt our work might help open a bowel obstruction, our therapy is contraindicated in cases of active infection. Since we are treating fascia that includes the interstitial spaces (between muscles and organs), we avoid treating infected areas, lest we create an opportunity for the infection to spread.

Belinda lay there for three days, hoping that the occlusion might just be a spasm that would release, allowing food to pass. With each day, she was becoming weaker. Finally, we made the decision to move her to a hospital.

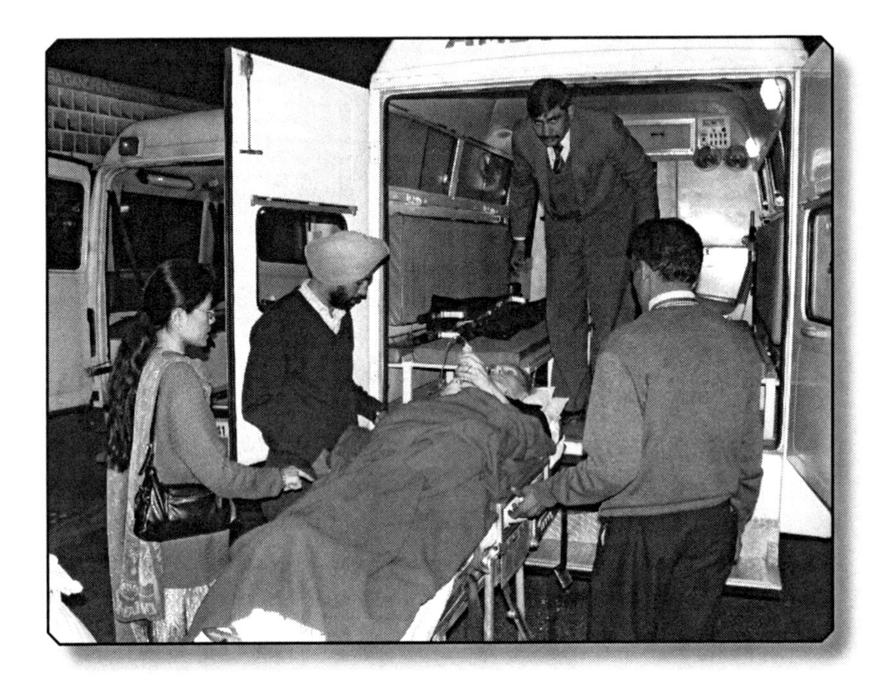

Our honeymoon was not going exactly as planned

We made the decision to life-flight Belinda to Delhi, where we hoped to find a modern hospital. Agra did not have a facility to handle her complex situation.

On the way to the airport, the ambulance driver was kind enough to divert his route to a promontory across the river from the Taj Mahal so Belinda could fulfill part of her childhood dream to see this lovely edifice – a testament to another husband's deep love for his wife centuries ago. I began to softly cry thinking of our life journey and the love that has persisted through all of the trials and traumas of our lifetime adventure. With all of the traumas Belinda has undergone, we both still feel very blessed by the gift of our lives, the therapists, patients, physicians, and scientists we worked with – so many of whom have become friends, or touched our lives deeply, as we have touched theirs.

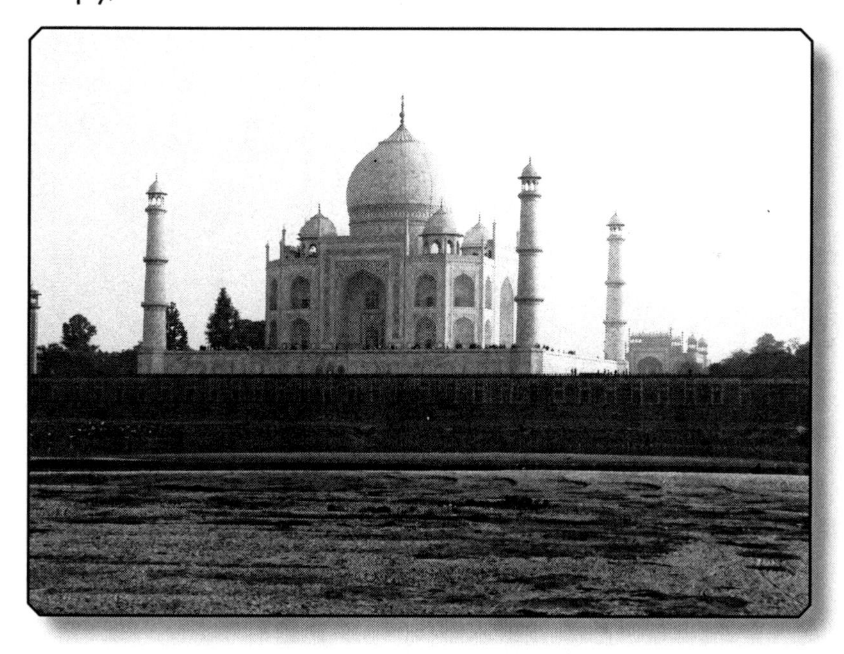

The ambulance stopped across the river so we could see theTaj Mahal, one man's testament to his love of his wife

The flight helped us avoid the elephants, camels, ox-carts, and large potholes in the road between Agra and Delhi. Still, the physician who accompanied us had the pilot maintain a low altitude "so your wife doesn't explode from the low pressure at high altitudes," she said. That was when we realized that this particular situation would resolve in India – not at home with our own physicians and modern hospitals.

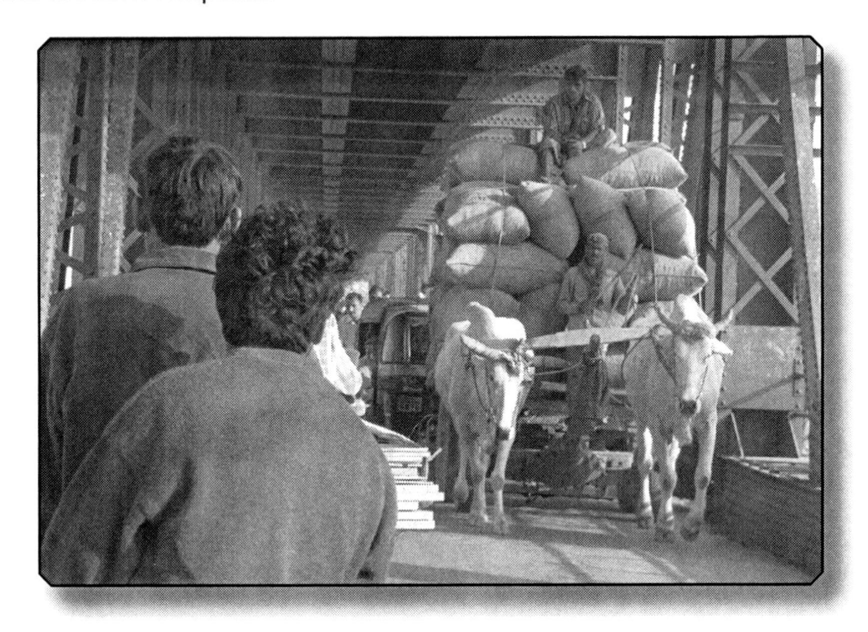

The drive to Belinda's life-flight was hampered by the usual traffic

After the emergency flight to Delhi, we were transported to a disgusting and filthy facility that was reported to have excellent physicians. I moved Belinda to the Apollo Hospital, which was much cleaner and more modern. The Boston-trained physician was aware of our work, and was patient as I continued to try to clear the blockage. Still, we continued to feel a single site with increased temperature. Remembering Belinda's difficulty with the previous post-surgical infection, it made sense that the culprit was likely a persistent infection from that surgery. In the end, Belinda elected to undergo her second bowel resection surgery.

They took Belinda to the operating room at 5:30 in the morning. I was not allowed to join her, but at 8:30, an orderly came in to fetch me. He spoke only Hindi, even though English is the common language that unites India, but he was very animated, gesturing for me to follow him. His only explanation (and apparently his only English) was "come sir."

The trip downstairs was other-worldly and sometimes nightmarish. As we arrived at the ground floor, we kept following two arrow signs, always going in the same direction. One read "Surgery;" the other read "Morgue."

As we finally reached a very long corridor, they were wheeling a dead body from the area, covered by a sheet. Part of me wanted to lift the sheet to see if it was Belinda; another part of me didn't want to know...

Like being in an "Alice in Wonderland" dream, we passed a small wing of the hospital whose entrance sign read: "Test Tube Baby Unit." I am sure they have good doctors there, but the wording of the sign and the feelings it evoked in me seemed strange to my western mind.

At last, we arrived at the end of the hall where we faced the (now familiar) two signs, now giving very different directions. The "Surgery" sign pointed to the left and the "Morgue" sign to the right.

My guide picked this moment to stop, breathe, and catch his breath from our long trek. It was the longest moment of my life...

At last, he stepped to the right, turned and put out his hand indicating that I should go left, into the surgical suite. I began to breathe again.

He had me scrub in, put on a surgical cap, gown, and booties, and enter the main surgery room. The room was wide open, about 30 feet square with eight people being operated on simultaneously. Looking around at this scene in awe, I saw someone gesturing to me from the third table on the right. It was Belinda's surgeon.

Slowly I approached the table. There was my love, totally anesthetized on her back, with a mound of bright red intestines piled up on her rib cage. The doctor started moving her bowels around with his hands to show me what he found. "See," he said, "No adhesions. You did your job well. But this, here is the culprit."

He lifted a section of the intestines for me to see. There, like a wedding band or the gold label on a cigar, a tight infected band encircled her intestines in a vice-like grasp, decreasing the 1½ inch diameter of her intestines to a tightly banded closure about a half-inch in diameter. The yellow-green color of the band indicated a state of severe infection.

"Good we operated now," the surgeon told me. "Otherwise this would have burst, causing infection to spread throughout the abdomen and pelvis." He proceeded to cut out the infected area and rejoin the cut sections.

As it happened, Belinda's physician was an excellent surgeon. She healed without infection this time, despite the proximity of seven other open surgeries of various types that surrounded us.

When Belinda and I met with the surgeon afterwards, he offered some words of wisdom. "There is nothing you could have done to treat the infection, but you really did a remarkable job clearing adhesions in Belinda's abdomen and pelvis. The fact that you could clear all of the adhesions that must have been there considering her history, leads me to believe that you can delay or prevent surgery in people with partial bowel obstructions. I encourage you to explore that area; you may be able to relieve much suffering and hardship."

Post-script to the story:

After spending a couple of weeks recovering in the hospital, and having totally missed most of our delayed honeymoon, Belinda and I asked permission to move to a different hospital. "We'd like to be near a historic site, or a beach," we said. "Do you have a sister hospital to which we could move for our final days in India before our flight home?"

"Oh yes," the Administrator said. "We have an affiliate hospital on the Southeast coast, in Chennai. I could move you there Monday." It was Friday night, Christmas eve. Christmas was coming Saturday, and there was no flight Sunday so we arranged for the first flight out to Chennai, on Monday morning.

Sunday (the day before our flight), the Tsunami hit India, making its greatest landfall at Chennai. I would have been on the beach when it hit at 9:30 that morning, since I always rise early and go to the beach when we are near one. Belinda would have become a very low priority patient among the survivors of the 53,000 people who died there, that day.

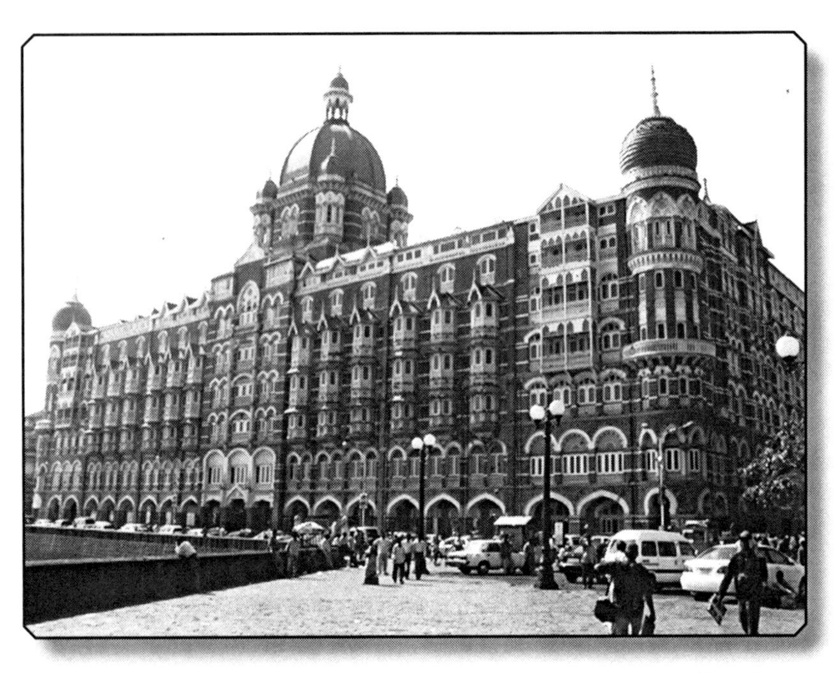

We escaped the Tsunami and moved to a nice hotel in Mumbai, a few years before terrorists attacked western tourists there.

Blessed as we were to avoid that massive tragedy, a catastrophy of global proportions, we moved on to the city of our departure, Mumbai. After having Belinda in the hospital for over three weeks, I splurged and got us a room at the Taj Mahal Hotel in Mumbai. This hotel was a magnificent edifice — one that was recently attacked and burned as a target of terrorists using automatic weapons and hand grenades. Over 200 people died in the Mumbai attacks, which targeted western tourists.

I guess you just have to live your life each day knowing that "this is it." The moments that we spend in life are all that we have, each of us. Each of us needs to make the best of the time we have here on earth. Life is not a dress rehearsal.

As noted earlier, adhesion formation is a process that occurs over time, and can continue for months, years, or even decades. Surgery to decrease abdominal adhesions can create an immediate improvement, but nearly always causes more adhesions to form. Thus for many patients, that first surgery begins a cycle of surgeries and adhesions. These are followed by more surgeries and more adhesions in a process that continues for a lifetime, for many people.

Unfortunatelly, surgery has been the only effective procedure to treat abdominal adhesions or small bowel obstruction, until we started using and testing the Wurn Technique®.

We first discovered the effectiveness of this manual therapy when we started opening fallopian tubes blocked by adhesions, using only our hands. Once we realized that we could open the spaghetti-thin fallopian tubes in the deepest part of the pelvis, we knew we could help open intestines which are larger and generally much more accessible to our hands.

We knew the results of our therapy on fallopian tubes lasted for years; many of our patients had experienced successive full-term pregnancies several years after we opened their tubes. How logical was it then, and how wonderful to think that we could reverse a threatened bowel occlusion in patients with partial intestinal obstruction?

The principles are the same, the therapy is the same, and the affected organs are larger and more accessible.

Breast Surgery, Inguinal Surgery and Six Abdominal Surgeries

- Reese's Story

I am sure it was destiny that I would speak to Belinda; I just "knew" that wherever this woman was, was where I was headed. We instantly connected and I felt as if I had known her all my life.

Besides that, I had never met anyone who could really understand what I was going through, the pain and agony I had felt, and the despair that I was facing. I was at my wit's end and had given up on finding some way to defeat these ever persistent abdominal adhesions that had taken hold of my poor weakening body.

> ***I left his office more broken than I had ever felt in my life.***

Eight days before heading to Clear Passages Therapies (CPT), I had learned from my surgeon that abdominal adhesions had grown back for the 7th time. He wanted to put a tube into my stomach to help release some pressure and evaluate my situation. I chose not to be hospitalized and left his office more broken than I had ever felt in my life.

I could not understand why my body was doing this! I just had surgery to save my life not 12 weeks before and at that time, the adhesions were strangulating my stomach in half and I had eight to ten adhered kinks in my small intestine. The adhesions also devastated my female organs, which had to be removed.

Thank God, I had found Sanoviv Medical Institute in Rosario, Mexico. For the last year they treated me integratively, cleansing mycoplasma from my body. This saved me from having parts of my organs removed during my surgery in July of 2008. Although Sanoviv was awesome and helped me greatly, they could not stop the adhesions from taking me over after surgery.

Needless to say, I was devastated and sat in my car and cried my eyes out. How could I tell my husband? What would become of the quality of my life?

How could I tell my husband? What would become of the quality of my life?

Talking with Belinda that day changed my life forever. But, I am getting ahead of myself so, let's start with some facts.

I was a typical tomboy and have all the scars to prove it. I have had many falls, accidents and illnesses. Just to name a few; I was bit by a brown recluse spider twice, developed SLE (Lupus) because of it, suffered several miscarriages, I was rear-ended with severe whiplash and chest bruising, swallowed a fish bone and had throat surgery to remove it, had malignant breast surgery – and then all hell broke loose with my abdominal adhesions. I had to close my business and stop my professional singing career.

Within two weeks of the breast surgery in June 2006, my abdomen swelled up like I was eight months pregnant. I was hospitalized and no tests of any kind showed anything was wrong. After six days of suffering in the hospital, I had exploratory surgery. The surgeons found adhesions, cysts, and tumors growing out of control.

I had no idea that my life had been at risk until I awoke in the hospital with tubes coming out of me, and I could not move. It was a wonder I did not pop from all the pressure. But, I really did pop as tissues tore in my abdominal wall and both inguinal walls (in my groin) from all the pressure inside of me.

To shorten a long torturous story, I had six full abdominal surgeries, appendicitis, a 6x8 patch holding my intestines in, one left breast surgery, and a double inguinal hernia repair with two 4x4 patches holding my lower abdomen wall together, all in the course of two and a half years.

Now, once more, I was facing yet another surgery; the scariest part was these abdominal adhesions were growing back faster and faster… I just had surgery 12 weeks ago! How could this be?

I heard it from more doctors I can list that there is no cure… abdominal adhesions were killing me slowly and there was nothing I could do about it. I tried all the great hospitals and clinics that I could find in those two plus years to help me… they all said the same thing. "Your surgeon knows you best and our protocol are the same as his. Just go back home and have him surgically remove them again."

Abdominal adhesions were killing me slowly and there was nothing I could do about it.

I was horrified to think I would have to live this way. My surgeon saved my life more than once and I am so grateful for him, but I did NOT want to live this way, having surgery after surgery just to stay alive.

I was backed into a corner with no time to lose; the adhesions were clogging up my system, affecting my breathing, and strangulating my intestines so I could not eat any food and could barely drink liquids without throwing up. I knew my time was running out before I would need surgery to release the armored grip on my internal organs strangulating the life out of me.

My life was great outside of this disease. Awesome husband, a thriving antique/photography business, and a great singing career. I wasn't going to give it all up now! I was hell-bent on beating this disease but, I was so tired and weak and felt so defeated.

Then I got a return call from Belinda at Clear Passage Therapies (CPT). After that conversation, I knew what I had to do; I began to pack my bags and plan my recovery.

Before I knew it, I was on a plane heading to Gainesville, FL. I could barely get through the airport with my luggage in tow, cringing in pain and breathing heavily with each step I took. I was so determined and focused.

I will never forget limping into the clinic that first day, holding and rubbing my abdomen in so much pain.

I will never forget limping into the clinic that first day, holding and rubbing my abdomen in so much pain. But, from that moment on, as the day progressed, I knew I would be taken care of. Unlike most of the doctors I had been to, this place actually WANTED to hear of all my pains and aches and problems! They were gentle and loving and very considerate each step of the way. They explained every technique they performed and why it would help me. This place was like an oasis of hope in a desert of despair for me. Was this treatment for real? Why do I say that? Because two miracles happened to my body that first day of treatment.

Focusing on the most urgent of needs for me, they immediately went to work on my abdominal obstructions. The therapists, with their talented hands manually performing the Wurn Technique® movements released the strangulating, burning, and stabbing pain right below my diaphragm that I had suffered from since all this began – over two years ago! I could barely wrap my mind around what had happened. I could feel it happening deep inside my body, but could I dare to believe that this would work? I was fearful of jinxing it! But, as I took my walks and went through the day, I could barely believe how much better I felt. I was no longer near tears in pain with each breath and step I took! I had a total of five bowel movements that night and the next morning. I was beside myself! I literally felt my body give in and let go!

The second miracle happened when Larry worked the outside calf of my right leg. I had chronic stabbing pain that never went away and had been there since 1992 when I got the bit by the brown recluse spiders and had caused me to limp all those years. No doctors could ever tell me why I had it. They called it a "mystery pain" that I would just have to live with. Larry worked hard and released that burning, debilitating, deep painful pulling sensation that had bound me! I could feel him free the adhesions as he worked layer by layer. I was in total disbelief because I was not limping when I left that first day and have not limped since! That burning pain in my abdomen has not returned either.

Oh, I must mention this... I am a rock and roll singer and since having so many tubes down my throat, scar tissue had formed, causing my throat to close when I sang, and it felt horrible. Larry worked his magic all down the front and sides of my neck, voice box, and upper chest. I now can sing stronger and with more ease than I have in years. Larry gave me back my singing voice!

Session after session, day after day...my body was slowly and methodically worked on. As each hour passed, my body was loosening up and moving with less effort, and with less and less pain. I slowly began to eat soft foods and soups...no problem! My system was working just fine! On my fourth day of treatment, my 50th birthday, I enjoyed baked salmon and mashed potatoes! It was the best meal of my life!

I have shocked my surgeon! He wanted to know what was done and how it was done. He had tears in his eyes and was so happy for me. He truly did not want to cut into me again. My husband is just so happy to see me out of pain and to have his wife back. I am bouncing off the walls with energy and gratefulness. I truly feel like I had a full body renovation from the tip of my toes to

I have shocked my surgeon. He wanted to know what was done and how it was done.

the top of my head. Long gone are those migraines and waking up feeling 80 years old.

The only side effect was some tenderness in areas worked on and way too many positive effects to list. Imagine that? 95% less pain, ease of movement, better mobility, able to eat and drink with proper digestive health, loads of energy, no more migraines, a bounce in my walk, a smile on my face and hope and song in my heart. What more can a girl ask for? CPT manual physical therapy makes sense – and it works. It is as simple as that.

Complications and Bowel Obstruction after Abdominal Surgery

- Mae's Story

As a woman in my fifties, I love to feel good, embrace life and live it to its maximum. My great-grandfather rode his bicycle every day until he died in his nineties, and I'd like to do the same.

I have been extremely healthy and athletic throughout most of my life; in fact, I was a gymnast and ballerina during school, and a physical fitness devotee afterwards. I had some fleeting abdominal problems in my forties, which were diagnosed as probably Candida or ulcer related, but I was still going strong.

While visiting Italy three years ago, I began to experience serious complications with my health: I suddenly began to lose my breath, and then I lost consciousness. Later I discovered that my husband had first tried to wake me by pouring water over me. When that didn't work, he desperately slapped me and shook me until I finally came back to my senses.

When I fainted again four hours later, someone called an ambulance. Meanwhile, my husband frantically performed CPR and almost fractured a rib to revive me. That time, I was unconscious for almost four minutes.

I was hospitalized for tests for seven days, but all the tests came back negative or inconclusive. Suspecting a small bowel obstruction, the physicians would not allow me to eat solid food. My weight dropped to 98 pounds (I'm 5'2" and normally weigh about 110 or 112).

When I was finally released, I wondered if the cause of this unexplainable event was air pollution since, during this time, I had heard that several people had suddenly lost consciousness throughout Italy. Still, I had an early history of bowel problems, and I remembered the hospital physician restricting my food intake, due to his concerns about my bowels.

I suddenly began to lose my breath, then I lost consciousness.

Three years later, in September of 2008, I began experiencing something that felt similar to a bowel obstruction, with pressure on my rectum. As the month neared its end, I started to feel unusually weak. Then once again, I fainted, and again my husband forcefully revived me (this time with my son). My memory took me back to my terrifying experience in Italy; then fear set in. Because of the recurrence, I knew it had to be something serious.

I went to my doctor immediately, and requested a prescription for oxygen. In the past, oxygen enabled me to feel better when I knew I was close to fainting.

I could always tell when I was going to faint: I would get a terrible pain on my right side, by my colon, in the morning or evening. My legs and feet would become ice cold, I would feel extremely weak and have to lie down. Then my intestines would rumble and they would feel very weird, almost as if worms were slowly slithering through them. My abdomen would then distend and I would have to change into pants without a belt so that I could breathe better. Gradually, my breath would slowly slip away from me and my tongue would turn white. It wouldn't feel as if I were being strangled; it would feel as if my breath were going away, never to return. It was the worst feeling imaginable. It felt like imminent death.

My abdomen would distend and I would have to change into pants without a belt so that I could breathe better.

During these times, I was often unable to eliminate. I sought help by having a few colonics, visiting more doctors and completing more medical tests.

After I fainted another time, I decided to go to a different hospital where I hoped they might provide us with some answers.

After four days, a colonoscopy, a barium swallow test to see if my small intestines were working properly, and many other of tests, I was informed that I was perfectly healthy. The doctor never told me that adhesions cannot actually be seen by diagnostic tests – only by surgery.

It was the worst feeling imaginable. It felt like like imminent death.

Having no further reason to hold me in the hospital, the doctors became somewhat verbally disrespectful and treated me as if I were a hypochondriac. For example, when I awoke in the middle of the night feeling the onset of the symptoms that generally preceded my unconsciousness, I asked the nurses for oxygen. After numerous pleas, they very reluctantly gave it to me, at last. The next morning, the doctor was furious with me for "hassling" his nursing staff. I was "being ridiculous and needed to leave," he said to me. I think he truly believed I was just trying to fool them, for some reason. However, he allowed me to remain because it was the weekend, and I had the "right" to meet with the gastroenterologist to discuss my test on Monday.

In the meantime, my husband continued to research about small bowel obstructions online, and found valuable information. He learned there was a Catch-22 with bowel obstructions and surgery. Surgery could remove the obstruction, but it would often cause another one to form.

We shared this information with the gastroenterologist, and he agreed. He suggested I change to a liquid diet and start taking a mild laxative daily. I asked him if I could return to the healthy state my body was in before the obstruction, and I was dismayed to hear him say that would be impossible.

After all of these experiences, I was terrified to ingest anything but liquids, so I slowly became very weak. As my weight continued to decrease, I lived in fear of another fainting episode. I dreaded the night, scared to close my eyes. I didn't want to sleep. I wanted to stay awake and be vigilant of all of my symptoms. I felt absolutely helpless and couldn't imagine continuing my life this way.

Through lengthy research, my husband found Clear Passage Therapies (CPT) and, within a week, I flew to Florida. I had no strength, and I was scared, but it didn't matter. I had hope and faith that I was going to be well.

When the therapists examined me, they noticed that my initial bowel symptoms started after I had several bladder infections following an early appendectomy and (more recent) C-section surgeries. When they felt my pelvis and abdomen, they immediately found extensive adhesions in these areas. They told me that some of the adhesions at my surgical sites felt three inches thick.

I don't want to live thinking about death, or to deal with physicians who become abusive when they can't provide answers.

They slowly began peeling these adhesions apart, layer by layer. Though it felt uncomfortable and painful at times, I was happy to notice positive results, almost immediately. In the end, my adhesions were so extensive that I stayed at CPT for two weeks. At four hours a day, that was a very intense schedule, but I could feel the changes in my body. I felt that they were saving my life.

Over the course of therapy, I started to regain my strength. My belly went from feeling like an inflated ball of steel to feeling like soft skin again. A few days into therapy, I was finally able to have a bowel movement again – this time, without any pressure in my rectum. My body began to function better; my energy began to return.

I started eating solid foods again. In the weeks following therapy, I gained 12 pounds. It was incredible to eat something crunchy and fearlessly enjoy it.

When I left CPT, I told them they saved my life, for I really believe they did. I remember the feeling of helplessness before I went to CPT, and I never want to relive that again. I don't want to live thinking about death, or to deal with physicians who become abusive when they can't provide answers. I was given a healthy body to use and feel great. That body was slowly taken from me because of adhesions, but I now have it back.

Multiple Surgeries for Bowel Obstructions

- Teena's Story

When I woke after surgery and looked down at my stomach, I could see staples cinching my abdomen. Although I was only 19, I knew the staples meant my doctors had decided to perform a hysterectomy.

From the time I was 15, I had recurring ovarian cysts and severe pain. The pain became so awful that my doctors suspected I had endometriosis — a condition in which the lining of the uterus grows in places outside of the uterus. They told me that they would have to perform surgery to diagnose and remove the endometriosis. They also warned me that they would have to perform a hysterectomy if the endometriosis was severe.

So, at age 19, I underwent the surgery. As I stared at my stomach in disbelief, the doctor came in to inform me that the staples in my stomach were not from a hysterectomy. I breathed a sigh of relief. They told me that during the surgery, they discovered my bowels were almost completely blocked from adhesions. They removed the adhered area and were optimistic that my pain would decrease.

During the surgery, they discovered my bowels were almost completely blocked from adhesions.

However, not even a year later, I began vomiting regularly with severe pain. For nine months, I could barely keep food down. My doctors finally discovered I had appendicitis and I underwent surgery. The physicians suspected the chronic appendicitis had also created adhesions near my bowels, and they hoped that removing my appendix would prevent further adhesions.

I remained relatively pain- and symptom-free for a couple of years. I was even fortunate enough to become pregnant and deliver a beautiful son.

After his birth, I began experiencing pain in my uterus. Over the next few years, my pain increased and I started to have problems with constipation. Given my history, my doctors suspected I had another blockage and performed surgery. Sure enough, they found adhesions blocking my bowels.

Although the surgery relieved my constipation symptoms, a few months after surgery, my health decreased again and I found myself vomiting after meals. I had to undergo another surgery and they found that, yet again, adhesions had blocked my intestines. The doctors were puzzled; they couldn't understand why adhesions continued to form in my body.

I became pregnant later that year, and gave birth to a second son. Because I had experienced some pain after the birth of my first son, I knew to expect some pain after my second delivery. However, the pain was far more than I had imagined. My uterus was so swollen that it felt like it was going to fall out.

My doctors decided to perform a hysterectomy. During the surgery, they found that my uterus was covered in adhesions. They decided to only remove my uterus and leave my ovaries — in hopes of sparing me early menopause. But nine months later, they had to remove my ovaries as well, because they too were being strangled by adhesions.

Over the next four years, adhesions continued to form and I had to undergo two more surgeries for intestinal blockages. I was so familiar with the symptoms of intestinal blockage that I could even tell where the blockage was. If the blockage was lower, I had problems with constipation and feeling full all of the time. If the blockage was higher, I would uncontrollably vomit after I ate.

Over the next four years, adhesions continued to form. I had to undergo two more surgeries for intestinal blockages.

After all of these surgeries, my stomach looked like a war zone. Scars stretched across my stomach and I literally had skin hanging down. Because they had to cut through my abdominal muscles so many times, my stomach also seemed to just hang. The damage from the surgery was so extensive that my insurance agreed to cover the cost of surgery to repair the area.

I remained relatively free of symptoms for a number of years after that surgical repair, but then I began experiencing the tell-tale signs of intestinal blockage again. I spent eight to nine months trying to find any other treatment besides surgery. I was desperate to find a natural treatment that wouldn't cause more adhesions to form. However, nothing seemed to work.

My husband couldn't understand why I didn't just have the surgery and kept urging me to have it. On the other hand, I faced perplexed and confused doctors who did not want to touch me because of my extensive history. Furthermore, because adhesions do not show up on tests, they could not see the blockages before surgery. One doctor suggested I had irritable bowel syndrome, even though extensive testing had shown I did not have that condition. One doctor even surmised I was addicted to surgery!

I felt like I was being torn apart by the various opinions. My husband wanted me to have the surgery so he could have his wife back, but my doctors were hesitant to pursue another surgery. In the meantime, I continued to experience severe side effects. I had to reduce my eating to extremely small portions. All day long I would feel full and usually vomit in the middle of the night.

I finally underwent surgery and sure enough, I had adhesions blocking my bowels.

The physical, emotional, and psychological damage ran my body completely down.

As usual, my body remained symptom-free for a few months after surgery. I began seeing a nutritionist, and after reviewing my history, she casually mentioned a manual physical therapy clinic, Clear Passage Therapies (CPT), that treats adhesions. I was dumbfounded. After all the time I spent searching for a treatment option, she just casually mentioned the clinic like it was no big deal. I knew it was something to consider if my symptoms returned. Luckily though, I was able to stay on top of my health for a few years.

Then two years after my surgery, I was brutally raped. The physical, emotional, and psychological damage ran my body completely down. One of my doctors before had suggested that stress could cause adhesion formation. Although it has never been proven scientifically, I thought back about my life and realized that some of my adhesions had formed right after extremely stressful times.

Whether it was mere coincidence or a direct cause, about a year later, I started experiencing symptoms that I knew were indicative of adhesion formation. I first experienced spasms in my intestine, and then after a few months, I began vomiting again after meals.

I remembered the therapy my nutritionist had told me about and contacted CPT. I was cautious to get my hopes up and I certainly had my doubts, but I knew I had to try the therapy before another surgery.

I went for one week of intensive therapy. Each day, I was treated for four hours. Halfway through the week, I ate breakfast and I didn't get sick afterwards. I had lunch later and I didn't get sick either. I can't tell you how unusual that was — I virtually always got sick after eating when I had a blockage. I couldn't believe they had broken down the adhesions that had caused my blockage, but there it was — I could feel the results in my body!

By the end of treatment, it just felt like everything was the way it should be. Before CPT, the tightness in my abdomen pulled so much that sometimes I felt like I was being pulled over. After therapy, I could stand straight and everything felt looser.

It has been six months since my treatment at CPT and I am still symptom free. I don't know if adhesions will form again, but if they do, I know I will not have to pursue surgery again. I wish I had known a treatment like this existed long before I had so many surgeries.

We are naturally pleased to find that we have been able to reverse partial bowel obstruction for patients we have treated with this condition, and end the cycle of occlusion – surgery – occlusion for them. It is especially gratifying for our therapists to find they can delay or reverse a life-threatening condition.

Breaking the Cycle of Surgery-Adhesions-Surgery

Our non-surgical treatment of adhesions is proving to be a viable and appropriate answer for many women and men who have undergone multiple surgeries to remove adhesions.

The primary goals of the Wurn Technique® are to find the adhered areas of the body, places where the body has healed, then break the bonds that hold our patients in these organic straight-jackets.

As noted earlier, the structure of adhesions may be likened to strong nylon rope. At 2,000 pounds per square inch, naturally occurring adhesions can be strong enough to lift a horse. In fact, physicians often tell us that they have difficulty cutting through or burning some of these adhesions. How can manual physical therapy possibly address these?

In our example, the nylon rope is made of thousands of small strands, each of which is composed of even smaller fibers, running roughly parallel. The rope's incredible strength comes from all of these strands working together.

The tiniest fibers that compose a nylon rope are each individually detachable with very little effort. Like nylon strands, adhesions are made of very tiny, molecularly-bonded strands of collagen. When they attach to each other, these collagen fibers create a tremendous tensile strength.

With this manual therapy, we are apparently able to detach the fibers of this adhesive collagen rope strand by strand, then group by group. When we do so, the therapy seems to reduce and even eliminate very strong adhesions, without creating new ones.

As we treat, we can feel the groups of tiny collagenous cross-links that form adhesions begin to detach from their neighbors. As they detach, we believe these fibers simply fold into the collagen wall of the structure to which they are still attached (at the other end of the strand). Thus, they become a harmless part of the existing collagenous wall of that structure. No longer bound to its neighbors, the structure can move freely again, as it did earlier in life.

In a sense, it's like we are turning back time for that part of the body. As the adhesions that formed over years or decades begin to unravel, their collagen attachments release their grip on internal structures, leaving them more mobile, functional, and relieved from pain.

There is no question that surgery saves lives and lifestyles daily, and that surgical skills are among the miracles of modern medicine. Unfortunately, surgeons and patients are too often stymied by adhesion formation that occurs after surgery. This process occurs with many surgical patients throughout the U.S. and around the world, as surgeries generate adhesions time and again.

Results came fast. Within two days, Joseph and I began to see visible changes in (my surgical) scarring. My incision site began to flatten and I had a belly button ...wow!

– Gabriel, mother of one who struggled with infertility after surgery to remove an ectopic pregnancy

We hope and believe that non-surgical treatment for patients who are now sent to surgery (such as for extensive adhesions) will be a future treatment of choice. Happily, that treatment is becoming available now to those who do not wish to undergo another surgery, and for those who wish to break the cycle of adhesions-surgery-adhesions.

Chapter Seventeen

Endometriosis Pain

"Often, I pass out from the pain."

- Jane

"Between the endometriosis and the adhesions, I have already had seven surgeries."

- Gretel

"I double up from the pain; then my husband takes me to the emergency room."

- Ariel

"Sex is not even a consideration."

- Summer

"I'm having about one surgery a year."

- Alexandra

Initially, we were surprised to hear patient complaints like the ones above. While our physical therapy clinics were treating complex musculoskeletal and neurological symptoms (most of our earliest caseload consisted of chronic pain patients whose symptoms had not resolved at other facilities) patients with endometriosis presented new challenges for us. Truth be told, we knew very little about the causes of endometriosis pain. As we were to learn over the next few years, neither did anyone else — including medical experts in the field.

Once again, unexpected improvements in patients with unusual symptoms (this time, women with severe endometriosis) were to lead us into yet another path of investigation, using the Wurn Technique® to address the adhesions, and pain associated with this debilitating condition.

Searching for the Cause of Pain

Endometriosis is a common and often painful disorder. Estimates of the prevalence of endometriosis range from 2-4% of all women and girls to 10-15% of all women in their reproductive years.[43] Part of the confounding nature of these estimates is the fact that the diagnosis of endometriosis is often delayed or missed – sometimes for a decade or longer. In place of a diagnosis, many women and girls with endometriosis are told that their pain is normal, or imagined.

We do not believe that pain is normal anywhere in the body. To tell a patient that her pain is imagined seems to us to be a double insult: first, that she must endure the trauma of undiagnosed (often debilitating) physical pain, and second, that she and her family may begin to question her mental capacity because her physician cannot find a reason for her pain.

Endometriosis Stages

- **Stage One** - few endometrial implants, most often in the cul-de-sac (the space between the uterus and the rectum).
- **Stage Two** - mild to moderate levels of endometrial implants (usually with a few small areas of scar tissue or adhesions).
- **Stage Three** - moderate levels of superficial and deep endometrial implants in several reproductive areas (often with several areas of scar tissue or adhesions).
- **Stage Four** - widespread superficial and deep endometriosis implants often throughout the pelvic area (usually with large adhesions).

The overwhelming extent of this "inability to diagnose" was underlined by a large and important study which compiled data from over

7,000 confirmed cases of endometriosis. Results of the study showed that average time to diagnosis of endometriosis was *over nine years*. One conclusion of that study seems to be a significant understatement: "the impact of endometriosis, a disease that already produces intense symptoms, is worsened by a current lack of understanding of the disease"[44]

Endometriosis is associated with significant dysfunction and pain. It may be present in 30-50% of women with infertility[45] and in 69% of teenagers with chronic pelvic pain which does not respond to anti-inflammatory medication or birth control pills.[46]

In this condition, the tissue that lines the inside of the uterus, called the endometrium, is found outside of the uterus. Endometriosis is most commonly found on the structures of the lower pelvis (e.g., the reproductive organs, lower bowel, and bladder).

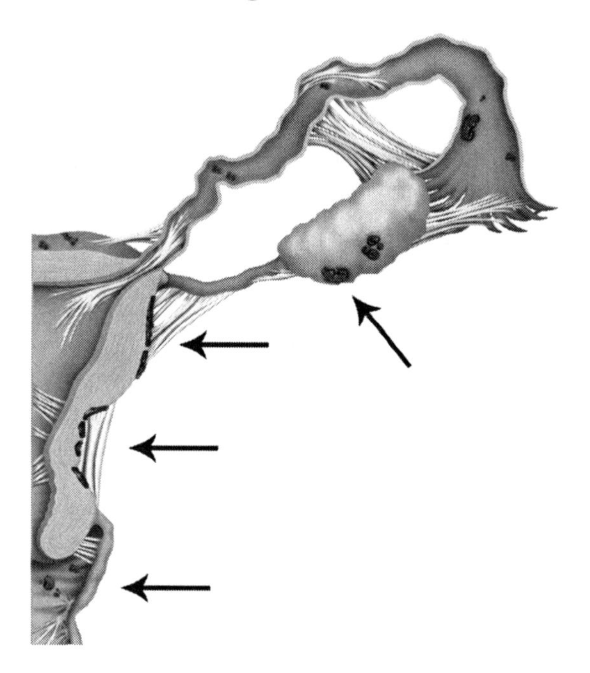

Adhesions are intimately associated with endometriosis forming at sites of endometrial implants.

Endometriosis may also appear at the cervix, within the vagina, and at sites of surgical incision. Because endometriosis may spread via the interstitial spaces of the body (between structures), it has been found in remote areas including the hips, shoulders, and even in the eye.

Understanding the Pain: Endometriosis and Menstruation

During a normal menstrual cycle, hormones signal the lining of the uterus to thicken in preparation for a possible pregnancy. If pregnancy does not occur, hormone levels decrease and the thickened lining sheds. This produces bleeding that normally exits through the vagina during menstruation.

When endometrial tissue is located in other parts of the body, it responds to hormone levels in the same way. It thickens, breaks down, and bleeds each month. But trapped as it is between and within the structures of the body, there is no way for the blood and tissue to exit, as it does from the vagina during menstruation. The trapped blood and tissue can irritate surrounding tissue, cause swelling, and trigger inflammatory responses that lead to scarring and adhesions. In fact, adhesions are frequently found in and near sites of endometrial implants.

Women with endometrial implants often report a great deal of pain, which may occur

- before and during menstruation (dysmenorrhea),
- with ovulation (mittelschmerz),
- with sex (dyspareunia),
- with urination, bowel movements, diarrhea, or constipation.

There is also a strong relationship between endometriosis and infertility, which is discussed in Chapter Seven.

While physicians do not know the exact cause of endometriosis pain, they recognize that an intimate relationship often exists between endometriosis and adhesions; when they find endometriosis, they often find adhesions nearby.

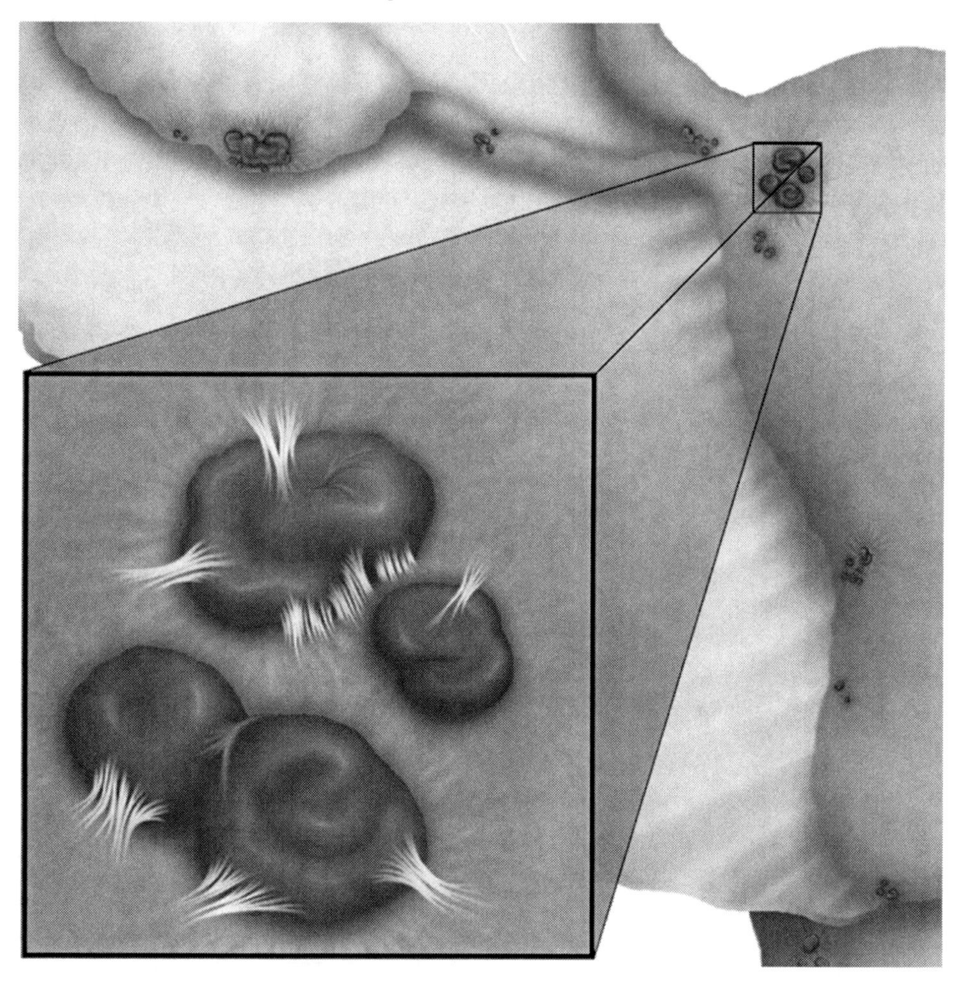

Tiny adhesions bind endometrial tissue to underlying pain-sensitive tissue.

As we have witnessed patient response to our therapy over the years, we have come to believe that the significant pain reported by some women with endometriosis is due to the accompanying adhesions. Here's why:

When endometrial tissue attaches to underlying surfaces, it generally causes irritation and inflammation. The word "endometriosis" literally means a condition (osis) that occurs within (endo) the womb (metra).

The body's response to inflammation is to form adhesions to contain the inflamed area. Over our decades of treating women with endometrial pain, we have come to believe that the adhesions create tiny, but powerful attachments at the sites of endometrial inflammation. As they blanket the inflamed implant, their rope-like fibers attach the endometrial tissue to the underlying organ or structure.

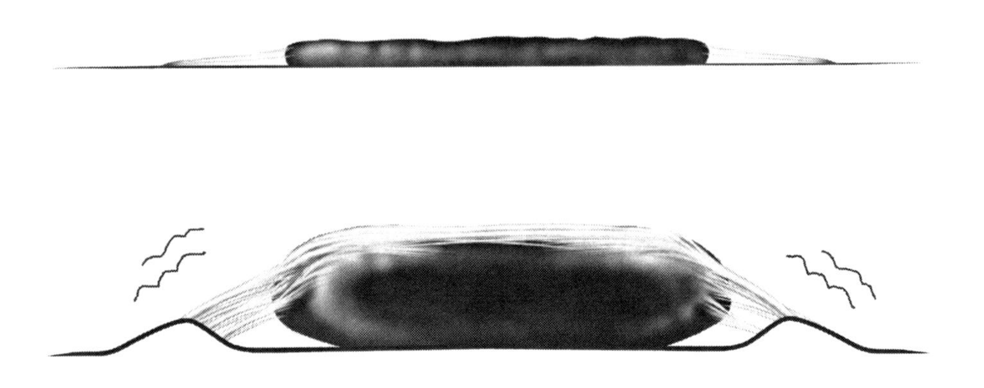

In this conceptual side view, endometrial tissues pull on tiny adhesions when the endometrial tissue swells, with every menstrual period.

Each month when the endometrial tissue swells, we believe that it pulls on those adhesive attachments, causing pain. In severe cases, the adhesions pull on pain-sensitive structures at times other than menstruation — such as when a woman is walking, moving, or even simply breathing.

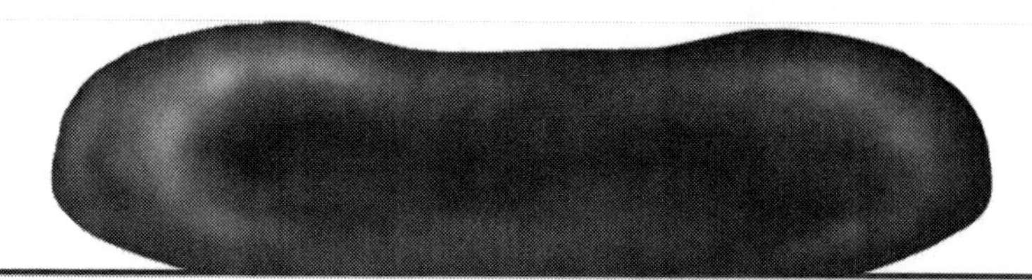

We believe this therapy detaches adhesions, so endometrial tissue can swell without the resulting pull, relieving pain.

Treatment Options

Passing Out from Endometriosis Pain

- Sara's Story

We met our first patient with endometriosis, Sara, when she was just 23. She complained of debilitating pelvic pain during her periods. In fact, her pain was so excruciating that she would regularly pass out from the pain. She marked two days off of her calendar each month when she knew she could not possibly go to school or work. She just hoped she would not have to go to the emergency room for pain treatment — which she did quite often.

She hoped she would not have to go to the ER for pain treatment — which she did quite often.

After hearing Sara talk about her debilitating pain, her poor quality of life two days a month, and the limited treatment options available to her (drugs or surgery), we were determined to help if we could.

Nearly 20 years ago, we had never treated a patient with endometriosis, but we felt our work treating adhesions might help. As we palpated, we could feel adhered tissues deep within Sara's pelvis, beneath our hands. As we did, we could tell that some tissues were moving freely, while others were stuck and virtually immobile. It felt like strong glue had been poured inside of her body.

Slowly and cautiously, we began to unpeel the glue-like adhesions that were tying Sara's organs together. Within the first few hours of treatment, we were able to decrease her pain significantly.

Unfortunately, we were unable to continue Sara's therapy because her insurance provider cut her treatment off, saying, "We have our own physical therapists who can exercise you, if you need physical therapy."

It is frustrating being among the first in the field to make new discoveries. It was doubly frustrating for Sara, because we were making progress with her so quickly. Nevertheless, it opened our eyes to the profound pain some women experience with endometriosis, and to the fact that this non-surgical therapy to address adhesions seems to hold a profound relief for some of them.

Excruciating Endometriosis Pain

- Mary's Story

A few months later, Mary, a PhD researcher, came to see us. She also had days when she could not go to work and was forced to stay home in bed because of pelvic pain due to endometriosis. She told us that on those days she could not even stand upright and had to walk backwards when she wanted to go down stairs. Sex was excruciating no matter what stage of her menstrual cycle, so she and her husband had stopped that activity altogether. Her quality of life was slowly being robbed from her, she told us.

Sex was excruciating no matter what stage of her menstrual cycle.

It was hard to hear Mary's stories of terrible pain, but we were encouraged by our experiences with Sara. We treated Mary in our 20 hour treatment program, the amount we were finding to be most effective for our pelvic pain and infertility patients. Once again, we palpated and found, like Sara, that the soft tissues of Mary's pelvis were stuck and adhered, the organs glued down and unable to glide with normal mobility.

We engaged the tissues with our hands, sinking deep into areas that had become hardened by adhesive glue. Slowly and steadily, pulling out the run in her three-dimensional fascial sweater, we felt the glue-like bonds of the adhesive cross-links began to break, as mobility began to return to her structures.

Mary's next period came without incident, and actually surprised her because she did not have her usual pain and spasm.

She found she was able to return to an active sex life at all times of the month. In fact, intercourse pain decreased to "near zero," accompanied by a noted increase in desire and lubrication.

Mary's next period came without incident, and actually surprised her because she did not have her usual pain and spasm.

These were profound findings. In Chapters Twelve and Thirteen, we discuss more of our findings treating intercourse pain and sexual dysfunction.

Our experiences with Sara and Mary inspired our ongoing investigation into non-surgical treatment of endometriosis pain. Like many healthcare providers, we were initially unaware of the prevalence of endometriosis and the accompanying pelvic pain that plagues women like Mary and Sara.

As therapists, we were beginning to understand the terrible suffering of so many of our patients with endometriosis. However, we had not really grasped the full significance of the relief our patients were experiencing, in comparison to the options that were being offered to them. Then Carol called us.

Carol was a patient at one of our outlying clinics. She experienced such profound relief from endometriosis pain after therapy that she felt compelled to call our home office and urge us to get more involved with national and international experts in endometriosis care. She felt strongly that the world needed to hear about our work, and that we needed to become familiar with experts in the field.

While we were humbled by her suggestion, we did not imagine that we would have much to add to the hundreds of physicians that were already treating endometriosis around the world. Nevertheless, we agreed to attend the Endometriosis Association conference, which is held every five years in Milwaukee, Wisconsin, the home of that organization. Not knowing what to expect, but wanting to share and gather information, we packed our data and headed north.

During the conference, we were struck by three things:

1) The prevalence of the problem. The conference was attended by scientists, physicians, and patients from around the world. Mothers and daughters from England and Eastern Europe were there, searching for answers. Physicians from the US, Mexico, Turkey, and Russia joined colleagues from Japan and South America as they came together to compare notes in their search for a cure — or at least to help women find some relief from the pain and return to a more normal, functional life.

2) The overwhelming need to find answers. These patients knew what they felt, and understood the toll it was taking on their lives monthly, or even daily They knew that there had to be an answer for them and the thousands of new women who are struck every year by the toll that endometriosis takes on their bodies and their quality of life.

3) The limited treatment choices patients faced. It became quickly apparent to us that the choices offered to women who suffered from endometriosis were often inadequate to address the problem. These choices largely fell into several categories, which we will touch on briefly below.

Lifestyle changes

Several lifestyle changes are showing promise in the non-surgical management of endometriosis pain. Among these are changes in environment, diet and exercise regimes. It is not the purpose of this book to list all of the latest science and findings in these areas. We suggest that readers who have interest in learning more of what they can do to help themselves consult their physician or a respected national support or research organization, such as the Endometriosis Association at www.endometriosisassn.org.

Medication

Hormone drug therapy is used to reduce or stop the production of estrogen, a hormone that exacerbates the growth of endometrial tissue. One commonly prescribed drug is Lupron, which slows or stops the production of estrogen, thus preventing menstruation. Some women tolerate Lupron well, while others complain of side effects, such as mood swings. Lupron is often prescribed for a maximum of six months. Other forms of medication include anti-inflammatory drugs, pain-killers, and hormone treatments designed to shrink endometrial tissues such as danazol, gestrinone, GnRH agonist analogs, progesterone derivatives, and progesterone-estrogen combinations.

Surgery

Surgical intervention is generally prescribed as a treatment of last resort to treat the mechanical aspect of endometrial implants. Surgery is typically intended to cut or burn adhesions and to remove endometrial cell clumps. In addition, some surgeons choose to sever the nerves that are transmitting pain.

Surgery to remove endometrial cells appears to have about the same effectiveness as drug treatments, but both are usually temporary measures, as they do not generally eliminate all of the troublesome cells. As a last resort, a hysterectomy to remove the uterus can be performed, sometimes with removal of both ovaries.

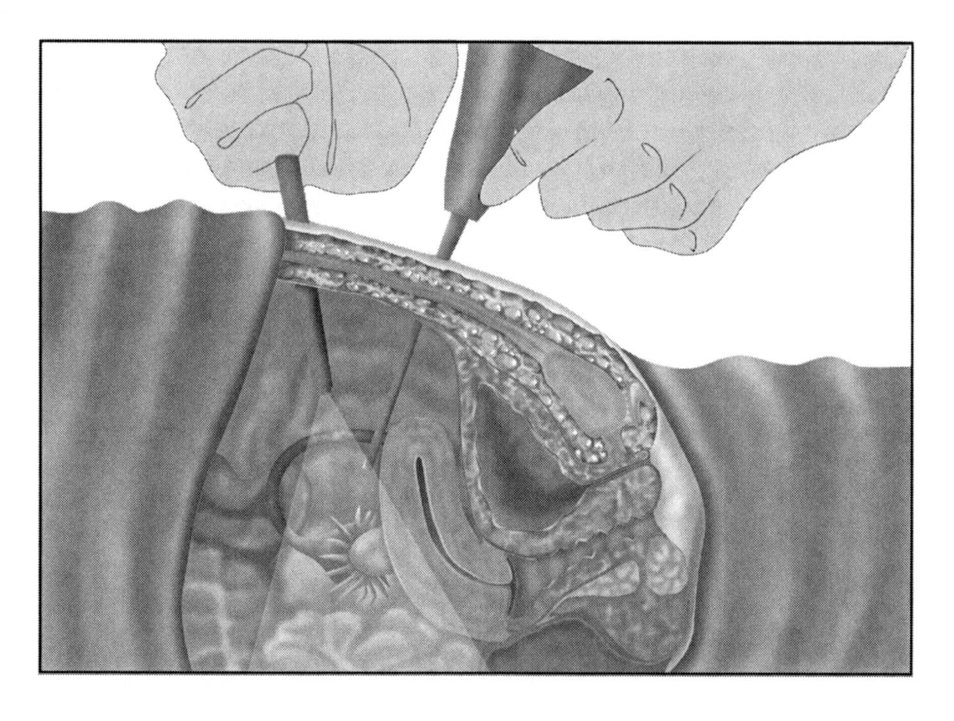

Laparoscopy can cut adhesions and remove endometriosis, but the finest surgeon cannot prevent recurrent adhesion formation.

In essence, medical methods to treat endometrial pain vary considerably. As in most western medicine treatments, the focus has been on medications (to mask pain or to stop periods) and surgery (to destroy endometrial implants, and cut, burn, or remove the adhesions which so often form with this condition). While menstruation-suppressing drugs have been hailed as a great relief for many patients, many women and their physicians (especially those interested in achieving a pregnancy) find that pharmaceuticals are not the answer for them. Many feel that long-term management of a condition using drugs to suppress the body's natural functions may not be the ideal long-term treatment of choice. When pharmaceuticals or changes in diet, environment, and exercise fail to bring lasting relief, many women and their physicians turn to surgery as a last resort.

Most surgeons take the traditional approach of cutting or burning endometrial implants, cauterizing those tissues, and sealing the area. Conscientious surgeons are careful to avoid the delicate areas where they might create further damage to underlying structures, such as the ovaries, bowel, bladder, or fallopian tubes.

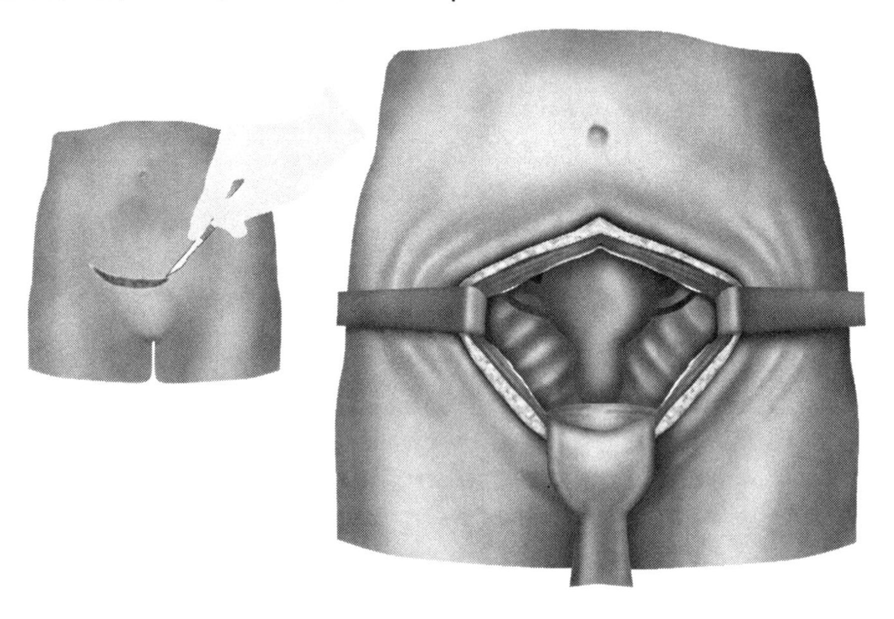

Laparotomy (open surgery) can remove endometriosis and adhesions, but has been implicated as a major cause of adhesion reformation.

Some surgeons choose to dig deeply into the organ from which they are removing the endometriosis. These physicians feel that they can actually find the bottom of the endometrial implantation and cut it out, and that by doing so, they can give a permanent or more lasting effect with their surgical excision. Naturally, the scars they create from the surgeries are much more extensive than less invasive surgeries.

Other surgeons have found success with milder surgical techniques, such as the Helica thermal ablation unit. This device, used in 120 hospitals in the UK, employs helium gas and electricity to cauterize endometrial tissue. Dr. King has had the opportunity to work with this minimally invasive surgical instrument. The designers of this device tell us that the Helica burns only one millimeter deep. They claim, and Dr. King has confirmed in surgery, that if the Helica grazes the tissue with a light cauterization, the surgical damage is mild, but the effects can be profound.

Some women find good resolution of symptoms after surgery, with no recurrence of pain. They go on to lead normal lives like their friends, and may even become pregnant with little or no problem. Other women do not have success with surgery. In fact, despite the best intentions, training, and skills of their doctors, some women are distressed to find that they emerge from surgery with the same or worse pain than before they underwent the procedure.

Part of the problem may be that, being appropriately conservative, the surgeon was unable to access one or more of the areas that caused the pain. For example, the surgeon may feel it is too dangerous to burn or cut endometrial tissue that is found on the intestinal wall, where an errant cut could cause serious damage. Similarly, surgeons may have concerns that they would unduly impair fertility if they were to excise endometrial tissue attached to an ovary or fallopian tube.

In other cases, endometrial tissue may be found deep within the tissues of a muscle or organ, as happens in a condition called adenomyosis (endometrial tissue within the muscle mass of the uterine wall). While the cause of adenomyosis is unknown, the condition has been associated with any sort of uterine trauma or surgery that breaks the barrier between the endometrium (which lines the uterus) and the myometrium (the muscle of the uterine body). Examples of this could include a C-section, D & C, tubal ligation, pregnancy termination or pregnancy itself.

Adenomyosis presents problems for both patients and physicians. While the condition can be very painful to the patient, a surgeon may be reluctant to excise deep endometrial implants for fear of creating greater organ damage than the internal endometrial implants that comprise this condition.

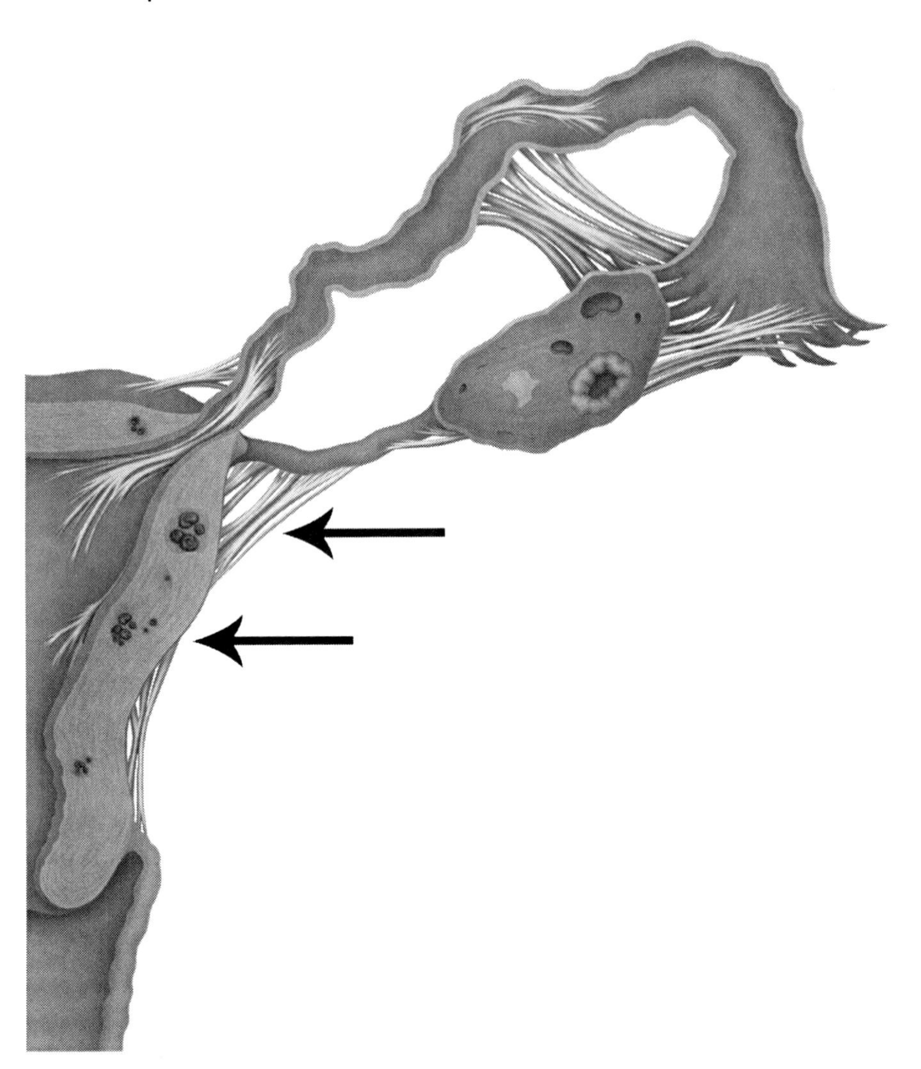

Adenomyosis: endometriosis deep within the muscle of the uterine wall.

Adenomyosis is typically found in women between the ages of 35 and 50, when women often have an excess of estrogen. Near the age of 35, women generally cease to create as much natural progesterone, which counters the effects of estrogen. After the age of 50, women do not create as much estrogen due to menopause.

A final concern is that no matter how gifted the surgeon, adhesions are a nearly inevitable by-product of surgery. Despite the surgeon's best efforts and skills, adhesions form naturally, as the first step in the healing process. This includes surgery to treat endometriosis, and surgery to remove adhesions. In fact, results of an extensive study published in *Digestive Surgery* found that[51]

- adhesions occur in more than 90% of the patients following major abdominal surgery,
- adhesions occur in 55-100% of the women undergoing pelvic surgery, and
- small-bowel obstruction, infertility, chronic abdominal and pelvic pain, and reoperative surgery are the most common consequences of peritoneal adhesions (the peritoneum is the lining of the abdominal cavity).

The article concluded that "despite elaborate efforts to develop effective strategies to reduce or prevent adhesions, their formation remains a frequent occurrence after abdominal surgery."

When living tissue is cut or burned by a scalpel or laser, hundreds of tiny collagen fibers rush in to contain the area that has been traumatized. Like a blanket or the tiny strands of a nylon rope, these fibers lie down next to each other in a random pattern, creating a scar to seal off the area that has been traumatized, much as a scrape on your skin would be healed by scar tissue on the outside of your body.

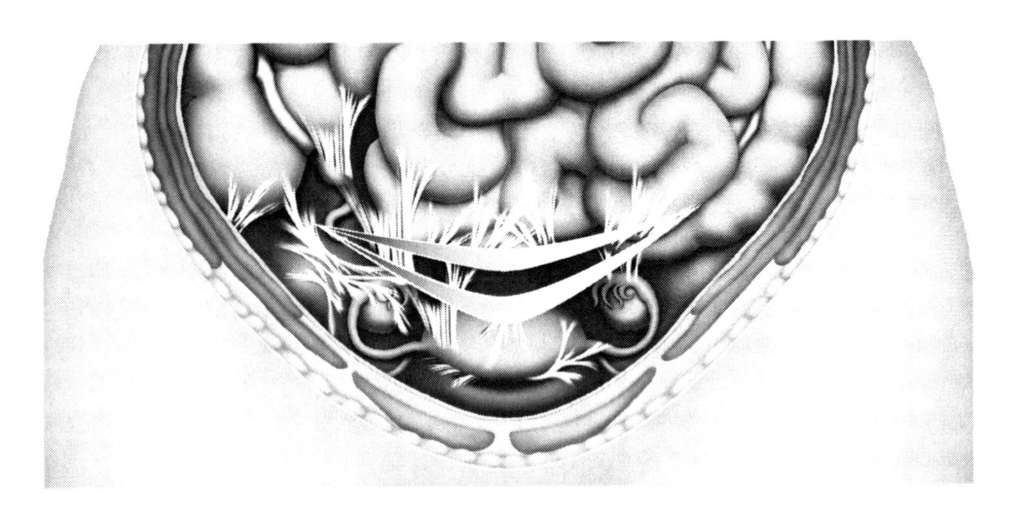

Adhesion formation after surgery

Over time, the scarring tends to bind and pull on the original structure, causing immobility in the area where the healing took place. If the inflammation is more extensive, the adhesions may spread from the surgical site into neighboring structures. Whenever those tiny adhesions attach to any of the extensive network of nerves in the body, they can cause pain. We discuss post-surgical adhesions, pain, and dysfunction extensively in Chapter Sixteen.

My husband and I were elated to find that there was no longer any pain with sex. Another amazing outcome was that I no longer experienced pain from my endometriosis.

– Madison, mother of two after attending CPT for treatment of endometriosis and infertility.

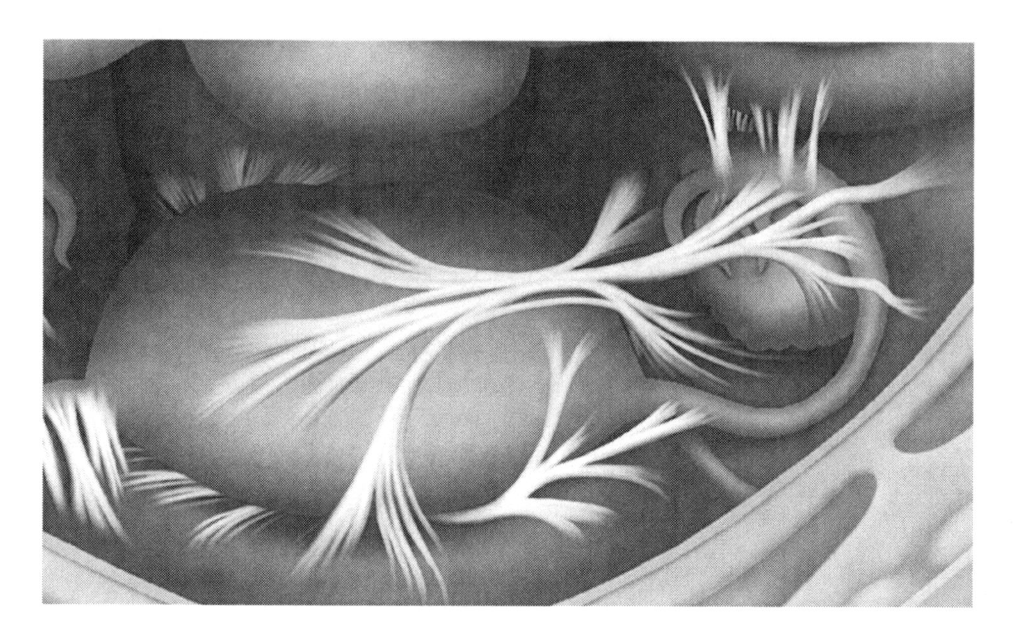

Powerful adhesions can attach to delicate organs within the pelvis.

Driven by pain, the desire to find relief, and frustration with failed surgical results, some women choose to undergo successive invasive surgeries in attempts to address their pain and dysfunction. This can become a vicious circle. Before long, many women eventually find themselves searching for relief from post-surgical adhesions in addition to relief from their endometriosis pain.

From Pain to Pain-Free

When we first began hearing stories from our endometriosis patients of significant pain relief after therapy, we were a bit dumbfounded. Neither we nor anyone else had ever proposed in any scientific setting that a non-invasive manual physical therapy could be used to treat a condition which hitherto had only been treated with surgery or drugs.

But as more and more women with endometriosis pain came to our clinic, we began to take interest in the clinical results. We found that

My pain decreased precipitously during my menstrual cycle. In fact, I didn't even know I started my period until I saw it!

– Danielle, mother of two after attending CPT for treatment of endometriosis and infertility.

when we treated the adhesions that we felt were attaching endometrial tissue to the underlying organs, mobility of those organs would improve. Along with this, we often witnessed a dramatic decrease of pain and an increase in function in these women.

As patients began telling their friends and fellow sufferers, the ranks of our patients with endometriosis grew significantly. We have lost count of the number of patients who came to us saying that they would routinely black out due to severe pain once or twice a month during their period or ovulation. These women scheduled their lives so they would not be debilitated or black out while driving during their cycle.

Some wanted to make sure they were near a hospital, in case they had to be admitted to the emergency room for the pain, or to control spasm.

The first thing that happened following my therapy was that the endometriosis pain I had lived with for over ten years completely disappeared.

– Ava, mother of two after 13 years of infertility and endometriosis pain

Yet after we treated them, many of them called us, very excited. "I had no pain with my period," or "I had little pain with my period," or in some cases, "My period came and I didn't even know it was coming," they told us. A typical first reaction was "I must have stopped ovulating," but the period came, ovulation came, another period came — and still no pain. So many of these women had experienced such severe pain from the time they first began menstruating that they seriously felt something was wrong with them when they had no pain with their periods. Naturally, when we heard these reports we thought they were wonderful, and we were very happy for the women.

Three Prior Laparoscopic Surgeries for Endometriosis

- Kimberly's Story

I have struggled with painful periods since the age of twelve. I would have terrible cramps and have to miss school. At the age of 16 I got on a birth control pill to help with the severe cramps. But I still suffered with painful periods all through college. Over the years the pain increased and became more and more debilitating.

I married at age 23 and knew that my pain was getting worse. I went to my family doctor, my gynecologist, and a nurse practitioner about experiencing painful sex and my worsening period pain. Each medical professional would examine me and then act like I was just crazy and that nothing was wrong. I suggested I might have endometriosis, but they did an abdominal ultrasound and couldn't find anything wrong.

All at once, I would have this stabbing pain like someone was jabbing a knife into my pelvis, and I would fall down.

When I turned 28, my cramps became more severe and felt like intense stabbing pain. I would be standing and all at once, I would have this stabbing pain like someone was jabbing a knife into my pelvis and I would fall down. I turned to my family doctor for help. He sent me for an ultrasound and found that I had ovarian cysts.

From there it seemed to go downhill. I continued to get worse and worse. Instead of having pain one week a month, I was experiencing it all the time. I decided I would go to a male Ob/Gyn a friend recommended. I told him of my experiences and he gave me some pain medication and sent me on my way.

I (got) worse and worse. Instead of having pain one week a month, I was experiencing it all the time.

I continued to see him almost weekly with debilitating pain. By Christmas I was getting where I couldn't function. I went to his office and he said, "I don't know if you have endometriosis, but I can do a laparoscopy and find out." The day after Christmas he did the laparoscopy and found that I had severe endometriosis. In the recovery room, he apologized for the pain I had been living with and said other women he had treated had nothing as severe as I had. He put me on birth control to decrease the pain and told me I could later go off the medication for a while to try and become pregnant.

Later, when my husband and I tried to get pregnant, we were unsuccessful and sought the help of a specialist. With the endocrinologist, we tried fertility medications and intrauterine inseminations, but the medication aggravated my endometriosis and pretty soon the pain was just too much to continue with that.

I continued to see my endocrinologist and had surgery for endometriosis again in 2004. Afterwards she told me she couldn't get it all because it was just too invasive.

My pain only worsened after surgery. I went on Lupron and had worsening pain still. I told the physician it felt like hot pokers were being stabbed into my ovaries and that I felt like my ovaries were on the outside of my body. She finally switched me to Danazol, but I bled during treatment. My specialist said she didn't know why Lupron and Danazol had not provided relief. She said she only knew of one person it had not worked for in the past. I went back on the old standby — birth control.

During this time my doctor recommended acupuncture. I went to an acupuncturist and got some pain relief. I also tried herbs like Red Clover and Evening Primrose, but nothing helped.

I continued to experience terrible pain; none of my doctors knew what to do.

I spent the next three years in pain without any further recommendations from doctors that provided me relief. My husband and I felt at a loss of what to do. We still wanted to become pregnant and my specialist said our best option was to proceed with IVF.

She referred us to her counterpart. Nine months later, we completed an IVF cycle. During the cycle the pain was horrible and I almost couldn't stand it. Unfortunately, the IVF was also unsuccessful.

I continued to experience terrible pain, but none of my doctors knew what to do. They knew a hysterectomy might help, but I still wanted to have a child.

I became isolated because friends didn't understand the pain I was experiencing. I went on medical leave from my job because I couldn't work. I went from having a social life to doing nothing besides sleeping on my heating pad and sitting in our hot tub or the bathtub to help the pain.

I finally convinced my doctor to perform a third laparoscopy. My doctor said my endometriosis was severe and everything was glued together — my ovaries, uterus, and bladder. I had two endometriomas (endometriosis tumors) on each ovary. He had to take 30% of one ovary and 40% of the other to get all of the endometriomas. I had a balloon catheter placed in my uterus so the sides wouldn't grow together from all the scraping out of the endometriosis.

I told (my doctor) I was tired of covering the pain; I wanted to find the source.

Following surgery I went on several medications, but nothing seemed to help my pain. I continued to call the doctor and finally I had a meltdown on the phone with him. I told him I was tired of covering the pain and I wanted to find the source.

When he offered no solutions, I went to a pelvic pain clinic. They helped me identify some of my problems and helped decrease some of my pain, but then I became worse. I was seeing a physical therapist through the clinic, and she recommended I try Clear Passage Therapies (CPT). Ironically, my sister-in-law had read about CPT and told me about it before.

I read about CPT on their website and called them to send me some info. After getting the info and reading the medical info they wanted, I knew they understood my pain from the questions they asked on the forms. My husband and I booked our appointment and headed to Florida for treatment with hope that this would work.

After getting there I got the most thorough medical evaluation I have ever experienced. They could tell that I was guarding and compensating from the way I walked and stood, due to years of pain. They listened to me about my body, my pain, and what wasn't working properly. I felt like I had finally found the people that could help me and it didn't involve trying some kind of medicine! They knew so much about endometriosis, adhesions, and the pain I was experiencing. They could feel tightness in areas that I felt it. It's amazing, all the techniques they have learned and developed to help heal the body.

After treatment my body was more mobile than it had been before because the therapists were able to break up the cross-links of the adhesions. It didn't hurt anymore to go to the bathroom after therapy and sex was less painful. They were able to break up adhesions in my navel area that prevented me from tasks as simple as cutting a piece of meat. The therapy I experienced was finally starting to free up my frozen pelvis!

I can't say enough about CPT. If I had not found them I would not have found the right treatment. Without them I would not have found pain relief or be able to move around. I would recommend this treatment to anyone with endometriosis, experiencing pain, or adhesions.

With the clinical results we were seeing, we knew that we needed scientific review before we could ethically state that our work was helping patients with endometriosis, and quantify success rates, so people might judge the extent to which our therapy might or might not help them.

Our physician and scientific advisors suggested we conduct one or more controlled studies to help in this regard.

At the time, we were working with a highly respected reproductive endocrinologist near our southern California clinic who had become interested in our results. He felt our theories about adhesions made sense, and he had seen positive results from our treatment in patients we shared. He kindly offered to help us quantify our results scientifically, in a publishable format.

My first ovulation after treatment was pain-free. I usually experienced one day of sharp pain because of endometriosis, but this time I didn't feel anything.

– Andie, mother of one after struggling with endometriosis pain and infertility

At his urging, we joined the American Society for Reproductive Medicine (ASRM), a group of several thousand physicians and scientists, with a large base of gynecologists and reproductive endocrinologists. He suggested we conduct a scientific study on our results treating women who came to our clinics with endometriosis-based pain or sexual dysfunction, and submit our data to ASRM.

As it happened, we had already begun two separate studies on treating patients with endometriosis pain. The results of those studies (shown below) revealed that by addressing adhesions with our therapy, we were able to decrease endometriosis pain at all times during the cycle, with the greatest reduction during menstruation.

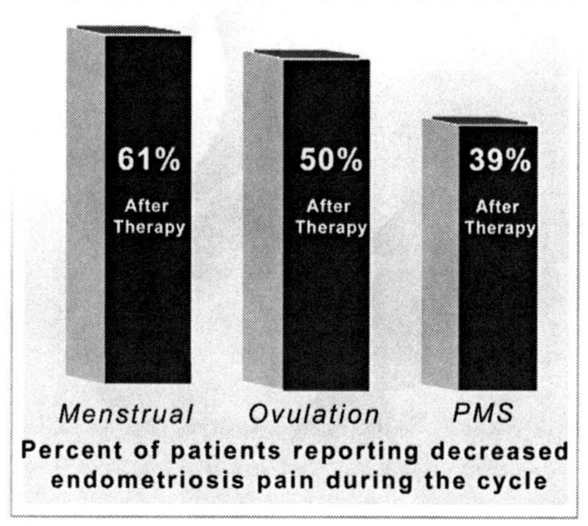

Results reported in "Fertility and Sterility" *in 2006*

In addition, intercourse pain was reduced or eliminated in nearly every subject that we treated who came to us with that condition. These were very encouraging statistics.

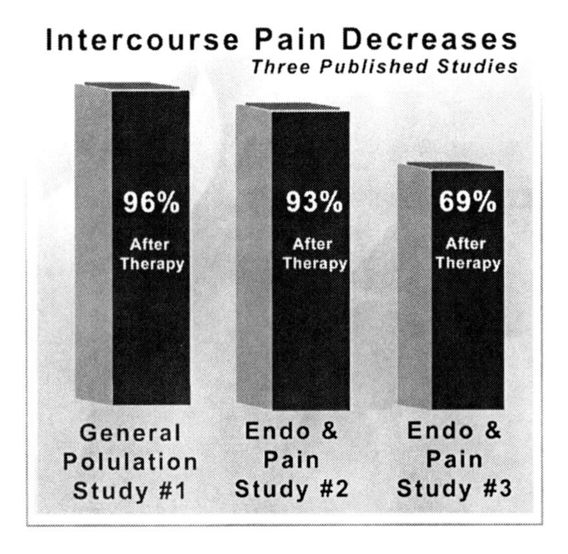

Results reported in "Medscape General Medicine" *(2004)*
and "Fertility & Sterility" *(2006)*

Put into scientific framework by mid-2006, two of our endometriosis investigations (intercourse pain and period pain) were accepted for presentation at the national conference of ASRM. By September of that year, the abstracts of those two studies (along with one on opening and returning function to severely blocked fallopian tubes) had been published in *Fertility and Sterility*,[52] one of the most prestigious medical journals in gynecologic and reproductive medicine.

> ***My primary goal was to become pregnant and one week after treatment – I was! My pregnancy went very well and I was also blessed to no longer experience painful intercourse or lower abdominal pain.***
>
> *– Jasmine, mother of one who struggled with endometriosis pain and infertility*

With data and published citations behind us, we can now confidently offer treatment and relief of period and intercourse pain to women with endometriosis.

Breaking free from endometriosis pain

By the time patients with endometriosis arrive at our door, they have generally been searching for relief for years. In essence, patients who have been shuffled from their family physicians to gynecologists, internal medicine, reproductive specialists, and even mental health counselors report relief of symptoms after just a few hours of our manual physical therapy.

> ***The last day of therapy was the first day of my period. Immediately, I felt a difference. All my abdominal pain was gone without a trace!***
>
> *– Neveah, now pregnant after struggling with endometriosis pain and 10 years of infertility*

The experiences we undergo with our patients and their reactions to our various treatments have placed us and our patients on the forefront of discovery in treating the pain and dysfunction of endometriosis. Spurred by the reliability of scientific testing, we feel we are on the cutting edge for treating this debilitating condition. Having developed and tested our work, we now confidently provide a non-surgical treatment to decrease pain and return quality of life for women and girls who suffer from endometriosis pain.

Chapter Eighteen

Menstrual Pain

Menstrual pain (dysmenorrhea) affects about half of all women of childbearing age. For 30% of this population, it is a nagging inconvenience, easily relieved with medications. If you are among the 20% of women who are significantly affected or incapacitated by menstrual pain, this chapter will likely be of great interest to you.[53]

Menstrual pain symptoms may include cramping in the lower abdomen and pelvis, low back or leg pain, nausea, vomiting, diarrhea, fatigue, or headaches. The combination of menstrual and premenstrual pain can last longer than a week. Some women also experience pain during ovulation, which can last from a few minutes to a couple of days.

Primary dysmenorrhea:
Onset occurs 6-12 months after menarche (beginning of menstruation). Symptoms may include lower abdominal or pelvic pain that lasts 8-72 hours, low back pain, medial/anterior thigh pain, headache, diarrhea, nausea, or vomiting.

Secondary dysmenorrhea:
Onset occurs in the 20s or 30s, after relatively painless menstrual cycles in the past, and is due to some medical cause. Symptoms may include heavy menstrual flow, irregular bleeding, dyspareunia (painful sex), vaginal discharge, or infertility

While we do not regard pain as normal, many women note pain as a consequence of menstruation. Some women experience more pain with their periods than others with no apparent etiology (cause).

Physicians diagnose primary dysmenorrhea when the patient exhibits symptoms from the onset of her first menstrual cycle. Primary dysmenorrhea may be due to medical, hormonal, or mechanical problems, such as adhesions.

In cases of secondary dysmenorrhea, pain is generally the result of a medical condition which occurred in the body after the first menstrual cycle, such as an infection, pelvic inflammatory disease (PID), or endometriosis. These conditions are known precursors of adhesions, which form as the body attempts to isolate and contain the conditions, preventing their spread to neighboring structures.

Women are susceptible to any of a number of inflammatory conditions in the warm, moist tissues of their pelvic cavities. In some cases, inflammation can become extensive, and lead to adhesion formation. As the adhesions bind structures in the pelvis, they can act like strong glue, severely restricting the movement and function of the previously supple and delicate organs in the pelvis. In severe cases, adhesions may bind the internal areas of organs or may attach organs to other structures, causing pain and decreasing mobility or function. The pull of the newly formed adhesions may then cause more inflammation, perpetuating the process.

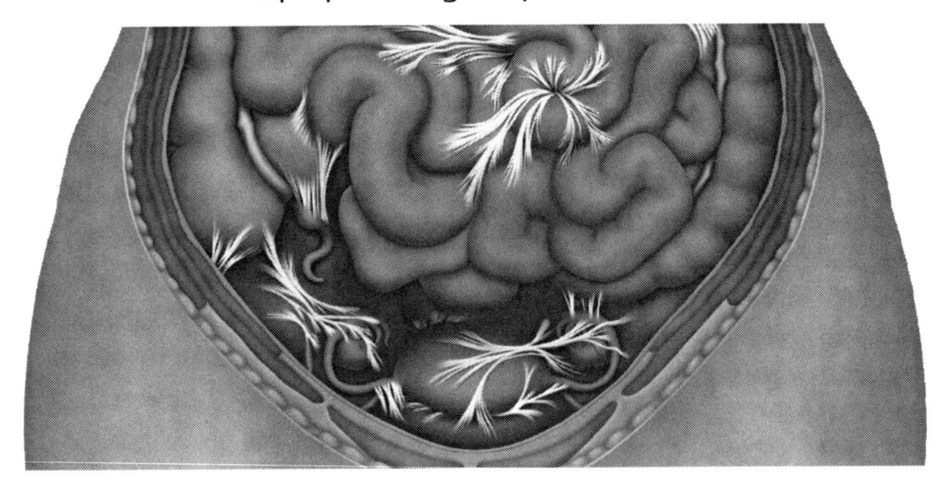

Adhesions bind delicate tissues within the pelvis.

Clinical evidence has shown us that even mild cases of early infection, trauma, endometriosis, or PID can cause strong, filmy adhesions to attach at the sites of inflamed tissues.

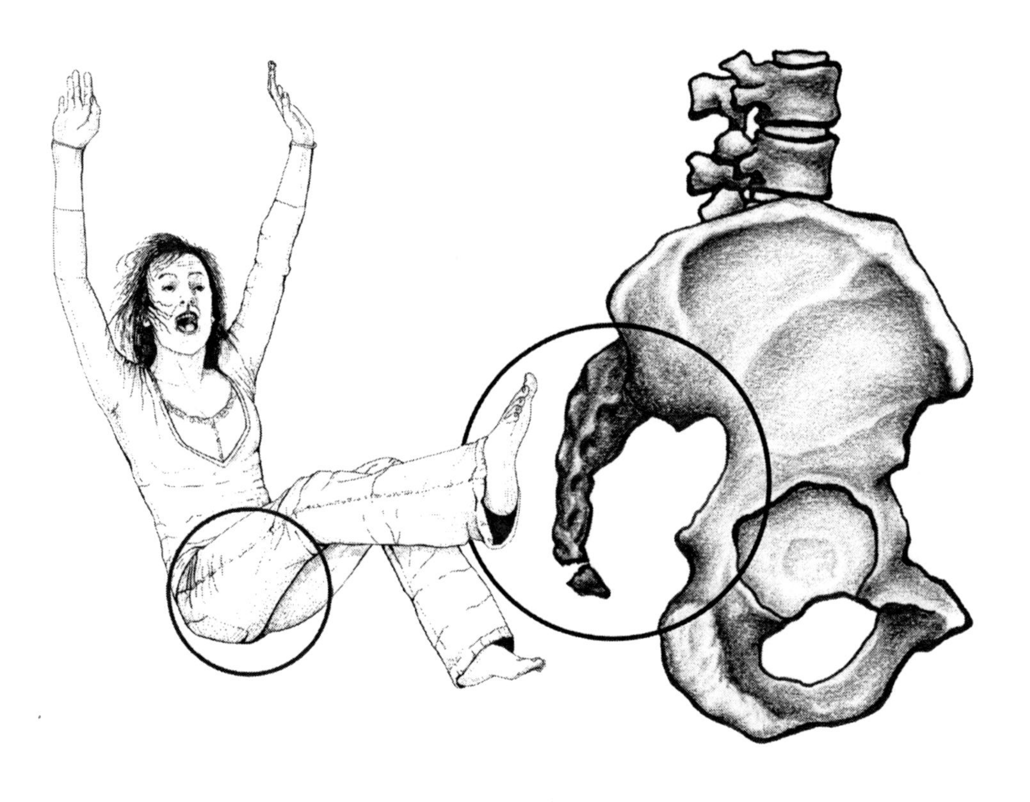

A fall or trauma can cause adhesions that affect the body later in life.

Healing events may also occur at a young age, such as from a fall onto the tailbone or pubic bone. Because of the location of the female urogenital organs (vulva, vagina, bladder, and reproductive organs) at the bottom of the trunk and top of the legs, they are subject to traumas from running, falling, and similar athletic activities The body responds by laying down adhesive cross-links to isolate the injured area. Having recovered from the initial tissue insult, the delicate tissues of these organs undergo a second, more permanent trauma from the adhesions that formed to help the body heal.

Understanding the Menstrual Cycle

The menstrual cycle is divided into three parts: the follicular phase, ovulation phase, and luteal phase.

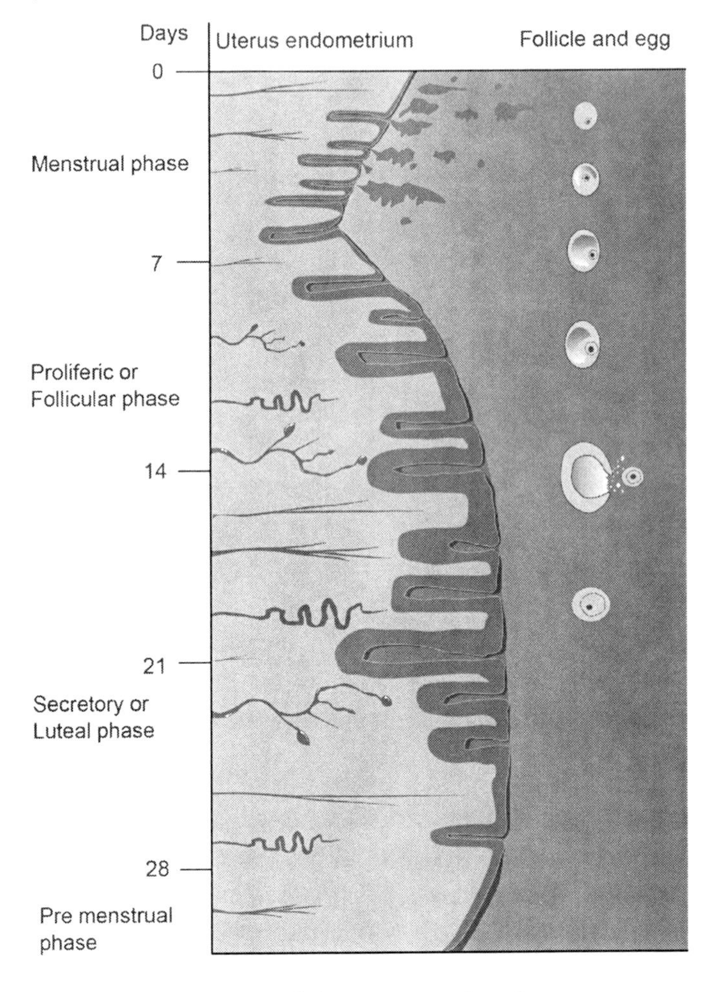

Phases of the menstrual cycle

Follicular phase

Day one of the menstrual cycle is the day menses (a period) starts, and all counting of days begins with day one. When flow begins after mid-afternoon, the next day would be considered day one. The growth of egg follicles appears to start with menses. It is unknown what causes follicles to begin to grow, other than the drop in hormones prior to and with menstruation.

Between days one and ten, there is usually a spike in FSH (follicle stimulating hormone) and LH (luteinizing hormone) as well as an increase in estrogen and progesterone. Generally, several follicles develop; the one follicle that is destined to ovulate puts out the most estrogen.

Ovulatory phase

Ovulation usually occurs within a short 12-24 hour period after the LH surge and rise in estradiol.

Luteal phase

The luteal phase begins after ovulation. The follicle continues to grow and if it is fertilized by a sperm, pregnancy occurs. If it is not fertilized, then the egg will burst from the follicle, leaving its outer casing, the corpus luteum, which precedes the start of the next menstrual cycle. This occurs approximately day 28, in most pre-menopausal women.

> ***After treatment ended, I felt better with less pain in my uterus. I also noticed my cycles were stronger and healthier.***
>
> *- Paulina, mother of one after struggling with pain and infertility*

How Adhesions Can Cause Menstrual Cycle Pain

All of the movement, hormonal changes, and activity that occur during the menstrual cycle are accompanied by swelling and shrinking of the uterus. When adhesions form anywhere on or within the walls of the uterus or its support structures, they tend to decrease that structure's mobility. Bound by these adhesions, the uterus resists the normal swelling and shrinking of the menstrual cycle causing pain. We have come to believe that this same process may be at work at the ovaries, accounting for much of the ovulation pain that we treat.

In primary dysmenorrhea, we sometimes find that the healing bonds that formed from earlier falls or traumatic events have been unnoticed in the system for many years, until the onset of menstruation. When the menstrual cycle first starts, the swelling of the uterus or changes in the ovaries can pull on adhesions which are unnoticed at other times of the cycle. When this happens, the unwelcome side effect can be pain with ovulation or menstruation.

Treatment Options

Many physicians feel that the best treatment for mild to moderate dysmenorrhea is to administer medications such as birth control pills to stop the menstrual cycle. These medications contain estrogen, which decreases hormonal stimulation to the uterus, thus decreasing the amount of blood. We believe that without the normal swelling of menstruation, there is no pull on the tiny adhesions, so pain is decreased.

Because products of menstruation called prostaglandins can also irritate the muscle, birth control pills prevent this irritation as well. Therefore, doctors sometimes prescribe medications such as Aleve® or Motrin® (ibuprofen) to decrease irritation and inflammation within the muscle of the uterus.

For some women, menstrual pain becomes so severe that they opt for surgery to cut or burn adhesions, burn nerves that transmit menstrual pain, or to remove some or all of their reproductive organs. While surgery has returned a quality of life to many of these women, others find that surgical procedures have not helped. In fact in some cases, pain actually increases after surgery. We believe this may occur due to the adhesions that often form as a result of surgery, post-surgical infection, ongoing inflammation, adhesions, or a combination of these factors.

When menstrual pain is so severe that it disrupts a woman's life due to cramping or pain, its imposition on her lifestyle can become a major factor in her life. We have lost count of the number of women who have told us that they have to mark certain days on their calendar when they know they will not be able to go to work due to the pain. The loss of two days in the 28-day cycle means that a woman is sacrificing 7% of her waking life to significant pain and dysfunction. Thus, every year she spends nearly a month of her life in pain, unable to participate in normal activities. During these times, she routinely misses work, avoids sex, and may have pain with the most basic activities, such as standing, walking, exercising, or using the bathroom.

Breaking Free from Birth Control Pills

Manual physical therapy, which addresses the adhesions that seem to cause so much menstrual pain, appears to offer a more permanent solution for many women. It has been gratifying to witness significant pain decreases in women who had undergone years or decades of menstrual pain. Hearing that a woman can add an additional pain-free month to her life each year is very special.

> ***I definitely attribute my treatment at CPT to return of my ovulation.***
>
> *-Sophia, mother of two after struggling with infertility*

In addition to pain relief, some of our patients report that menstrual flows become more normal and length of periods become more regular after we decrease the adhesions that were causing unusual pulls on their reproductive structures. We feel that part of this phenomenon may be due to work we developed to treat the hormone-secreting glands, the pituitary, hypothalamus, and ovaries.

> ***I know (CPT) helped improve my hormones. After just a few days of therapy, my period has returned.***
>
> *- Chloe, whose period had stopped*

In other cases women we were treating for period pain began to report significant increases in desire, lubrication and orgasms when they returned home after therapy. After several such reports, we began to investigate this phenomenon scientifically, and we have now published two studies on the rather remarkable results we were finding. The only explanation we could find was obvious: the same adhesive processes that were binding down uterine or ovarian tissues and causing menstrual pain were also interfering with sensitivity and function of the nearby sites which elicit sexual response. You may read more about this phenomenon in Chapter Thirteen.

Menstrual Pain

- LaRue's Story

(Full Story Featured in Chapter Eleven)

I decided to attend treatment for an intensive week of therapy. The first day of treatment, I knew right away this wasn't typical physical therapy. The therapists evaluated my entire body and they soon found a spot that, when stretched, elicited exactly the kind of pain I experienced during my menstrual cycle. If I had not been a physical therapist, I would not have understood that this was a good sign. Even though this aspect of treatment was somewhat painful, I knew if they could find the area that caused my pain, they would then be able to resolve that pain.

After my first day of treatment, I must have gone to the bathroom at least ten times. It was like their treatment helped clear my bowels and bladder.

I never had menstrual cramps again after that one week of therapy.

By the time treatment was over, the majority of my aches and pains were gone. In fact, I never had menstrual cramps again after that one week of therapy.

Establishing a Pain-free Life

Menstrual pain has plagued womankind for most of reported history. Over the centuries, it has been treated with herbs, poultices, and spells. In modern medicine, the most effective treatments for menstrual pain have been

- drugs to reduce pain or spasm, or to stop the menstrual cycle totally, or
- surgery to remove adhesions and adhered tissue, to block nerves that transmit pain, or to remove the organs.

In the last few years, the manual physical therapy we developed at our clinics has been shown to be effective for treating menstrual pain, without drugs or surgery. Recent studies published in respected peer-reviewed medical journals have shown that the therapy significantly decreased pelvic pain in most women with moderate to severe endometriosis and menstrual pain. Negative side effects of this treatment are rare and may include temporary soreness. Positive side effects include increased desire, arousal, lubrication and orgasm.

Chapter Nineteen

Unfolding the Future

It's been a long and remarkable journey since Belinda's physician first found abnormal cells in her pelvis. During our adventure, we have grown from a myopic view of treating one condition, Belinda's pelvic pain and dysfunction, to developing a system that has been shown to help many conditions that were previously unexplained, or considered untreatable, or were only thought to be treatable with drugs or surgeries.

Along the way, we have been very thankful to patients, physicians, scientists, and healthcare professionals who encouraged and inspired our further inquiry into treating these conditions non-surgically. The doors they have opened for us to investigate further are at once exciting and overwhelming. It has been like starting a new field of healthcare for many of these conditions.

While our clinics are presently small and our patient care is highly individualized, we know that we will grow. However, we plan to grow with respect for our primary goal, success for each patient. When we close the door after entering a patient's room, nothing else exists for us except success for that patient. Patient care and individual success are our primary focus. Without that, nothing else works.

As we look to our growth, we realize that we are at the forefront of several important milestones in conditions that we previously thought were impossible to treat with manual physical therapy. We hope we will be joined, not just by physical therapists, but by physicians and other healthcare providers with a desire to provide effective care for some of their most challenging cases, apparently with little or no risk. In short, we would like to create a national network of physicians and physical therapists who can provide this work. We have already begun that effort.

As we continue, we would also like to follow neurosurgeons suggestions to treat the *substantia nigra* and other areas of the brain and body related to that structure in order to determine if we can assist people in the early stages of Parkinson's Disease by delaying its onset, or decreasing its adverse effects.

We also wonder if the colloidal plaques and tangles that for in the brains of Alzheimer patients have any relationship to the collagenous cross links that we treat every day. How wonderful to think that we might delay onset of that debilitating condition.

We feel that a study of treating partial bowel obstructions may save quality of life, and indeed save the lives of the thousands of women and men who suffer from recurrent abdominal adhesions, or who feel trapped in a cycle of surgery – adhesions – surgery. Indeed, we have already witnessed how gratifying it is to save lives, or to extend the quality of lives in these patients, and to delay or prevent additional surgeries. We have already had this happen in several (often dramatic) cases, and we look forward to expanding that effort.

We would also like to conduct a similar study for women who undergo recurrent surgeries for endometriosis and adhesions, another area in which we see excellent results, and even greater potential.

Oncologists tell us that chemotherapy is often less effective because medications cannot reach their intended sites, due to adhesions. While we have felt that cancer is a contraindication to therapy, we wonder if a therapy that frees adhesions non-surgically might assist in some of these cases.

Belinda and I are but two people. We have certified a few extraordinary therapists from a pool of over 2,000 physical therapists and health care professionals who have asked to be trained. We want to keep our quality and results high, so we tend to be very scrutinous in deciding who has the skills to learn our work and carry the title of "Clear Passage certified." Simply put, we are committed to a very high level of positive results.

In all of our endeavors, patient care comes first and foremost— it always has and it always will. Even though our patients may find that "life is what happens while you are making other plans," we find we can often open the door for patients to create a much greater quality for the rest of their lives, by decreasing their adhesions.

In all of this, we encourage each of our patients to do as we do: "create the vision of where your are taking your life – and then simply step into it, step by step by step."

Appendix

Scientific Studies and Clinical Treatment

Early on, we recognized a responsibility to conduct clinical research to answer questions that physicians, patients and scientists would ask. Does the therapy actually help any conditions? To what extent? Are there any adverse effects? How much treatment is required to yield results?

Most of these questions have been answered in this book, especially in the chapters that deal with specific conditions. Additionally, we have used the following parameters for research, or found the following to be true:

Virtually all of our published research to date (1/2009) was based on a 20-hour therapy treatment protocol, with a one-hour initial evaluation followed by 19 hours of therapy (including about 10 minutes per hour for chart review, consulting other CPT therapists about the progress of therapy, and for any needed room preparation).

Most patients receive their 20 hours over the course of five days: two hours each morning and afternoon starting Monday morning and ending Friday afternoon.

There appears to be no statistical difference in results whether therapy is received in an (intensive) five-day period, or spread over several months.

Very adhered patients sometimes require more than the 20 hours of therapy we used in our published studies; we advise those few who might benefit from additional therapy at the end of their 20-hour protocol.

The positive effects of therapy seem to last for many years. We rarely see a need to treat a condition again, after the initial 20 hours of therapy. In a few cases, patients have chosen on their own to return for more therapy because they felt they still had more issues they wanted cleared.

Roughly 25% of our patients are healthcare professionals (physicians, dentists, nurses, physical therapists, pharmacists, etc.)

Patients come to our clinics from throughout North American and all over the globe, including Africa, Europe, Asia and the Far East. Nearly all patients find us on their own, and contact us as self-referred.

A physician's referral is not required in most of our locations, but it can help with insurance reimbursement. Most patients do not have a problem getting a referral from their physician. A referral is required for patients who are treated in some states (e.g., California).

We request each patient to allow us to use her/his medical data for research or educational purposes, so long as we keep their name in strict confidence. Any patient may refuse to grant this permission, but no one ever has done so.

While we may suggest treatment anywhere on (or in) the body, we recognize that every person comes to therapy with a different history. We do not push anyone to undergo any therapy that they do not want.

We invite, but do not require, all patients to become active members of the team that is addressing their problem.

We suggest that on the first day of therapy (or before) every patient visualize leaving therapy the last day. We suggest: "See the date in your mind's eye. See what you are wearing, and note how the air feels. Now visualize that you are leaving here on that date with exactly the body you want at the end of therapy. This includes leaving behind here anything you have been carrying around that perhaps served you once, but which no longer servers you: adhesions, memories, tightness, and emotions that have become more of a burden than a help. Now own that goal. Share your goal with us along and along during therapy. We are going there together."

Work with Us

Professional requirements

Since our work is a manual soft-tissue therapy program, all of our clinics, whether owned by us or by affiliated therapists or groups, are under the direction of a licensed physical therapist. To be successful with this patient population, our therapists need a significant background (in continuing education and experience) in manual soft tissue skills.

At this time we are accepting resumes from PT's and PTA's. If you are a massage therapist, we encourage you to apply, but please know that we can only train MTs that will be working under the direction of a PT.

If you qualify and are interested, please start the application process by emailing your resume (including continuing education courses taken) to workwithus@clearpassage.com. Please also download and complete the provider questionnaire available at our website and return to us by mail: Clear Passage Therapies, Inc., 4421 NW 39th Avenue , 2-2, Gainesville, FL 32606 .

Background course requirements

We are looking for therapists with extensive manual soft tissue therapy skills. Let us know your background and experience and we'll tell you what additional courses or experience we feel that you need. At our certification training, we will teach you the additional skills you will need in order to succeed with these patients.

On-site training

We are currently only able to offer training to our own staff and affiliated therapists. In order to keep quality of care at its highest standard for our patients, we must find the best manual therapists available. We accept only those who can demonstrate exceptional manual skills.

All training is done in our Gainesville, Florida office. After reading and testing on information contained in a 600-page *Therapist Training Manual* (with over 200 techniques) we provide an intensive 2-week training program. This consists of closely supervised one-on-one training with the Wurns and their certified instructors. Therapists trainees are tested on their understanding of theory, anatomy, body functions and dysfunctions, and on over 200 specific required techniques before they can be certified to practice as a Clear Passage therapist.

Index

Glossary

A

Abortion: Therapeutic: A procedure used to terminate a pregnancy before the fetus can survive on its own.

Adenomyosis: Similar to endometriosis, except that endometrial cells are found within the muscle of the uterus, rather than on the surface of structures.

Adhesions: Scar tissue resulting from infection, inflammation, trauma, or prior surgery occurring in the abdominal cavity, pelvis, or elsewhere in the body. When adhesions occur around the uterus, ovaries, fallopian tubes, or the delicate fimbriae at the end of the uterine tubes, pain or infertility may result. Adhesions can interfere with transport of the egg and implantation of the embryo in the uterus. They can join any structure in the body to its neighbor, or to distant structures. In doing so, they can cause confusing symptoms of pain or dysfunction. Adhesions can become life-threatening when they totally close an organ (such as the bowel or intestine).

Adrenal Corticotropic Hormone (ACTH): Excessive levels of ACTH may lead to decreased fertility. ACTH is secreted from the anterior pituitary in response to corticotrophin-releasing hormone from the hypothalamus. Corticotrophin-releasing hormone is secreted in response to stress. Corticotrophin-releasing hormone is inhibited by glucocorticoids, making it part of a classical negative feedback loop.

Amenorrhea: The absence of menstruation. Primary amenorrhea (no menstruation from the start of puberty) may be caused by developmental problems such as the congenital absence of the uterus, or failure of the ovary to receive or maintain egg cells. Delay in pubertal development can also lead to primary amenorrhea. Secondary amenorrhea (menstruation cycles ceasing) is often caused by hormonal disturbances from the hypothalamus and the pituitary gland, or from premature menopause, or from intrauterine scar formation. Secondary amenorrhea refers to menstruation which has ceased for three months in a woman with a history of regular cyclic bleeding, or for six months in a woman with a history of irregular periods. This usually happens to women aged 40-45. Female athletes or women who perform considerable amounts of exercise on a regular basis are at risk of developing "athletic" amenorrhea. It was thought for many years that low body fat levels and exercise-related chemicals (such as beta endorphins and catecholamines) disrupt the interplay of the sex hormones estrogen and progesterone. Recent studies have shown that there are no differences in the body composition or hormonal levels in amenorrheic athletes. Instead, amenorrhea has been shown to be directly attributable to low energy availability. Many women who exercise at a high level do not take in enough calories to expend on their exercise as well as to maintain their normal menstrual cycles.

Ampullary: This refers to the middle section of the fallopian tube. The ampullary portion is tortuous and gradually widens toward the infundibulum, the outer part of the tube.

Anovulation: The absence of ovulation when it would be normally expected.

Anteverted Uterus: The uterus tips forward toward the bladder with the anterior end slightly concave. This is the normal position of the uterus.

Anterior Deviation of the Uterus: This describes a uterus which tips more forward than normal. This malposition is less frequently seen than lateral deviation. It is often congenital, and occurs frequently following childbirth. This condition commonly leads to dysmenorrhea (it is difficult for the blood to flow through), infertility, bladder irritability, and may lead to prolapse of the uterus.

Antiovarian Antibodies (AOA, AVA): Antibodies which form to attack the ovaries. These antibodies can bind to important functional sites in the ovary and granulosa cells and impair the normal ovarian response. The complete function of the antiovarian antibodies is not well known. It is believed that they cause disturbances that contribute to ovarian failure, non-ovulation or poor ovulation. They are also believed to be a cause of poor response to various medications to stimulate proper ovarian function, and may impair formation of normal eggs.

The treatment of this condition is more or less experimental. Frequently this condition can be helped through in vitro fertilization, and if everything else fails, donation from a fertile donor. When such a pregnancy is properly supported by administration of exogenous hormones — progesterone and sometimes estrogen — it can lead to normal delivery.

Antiphospholipid Antibodies (APA): This syndrome occurs due to the autoimmune production of antibodies against phospholipid (aPL), a cell membrane substance. Phospholipids work to hold dividing cells together. They are necessary for growth of the placenta into the wall of the uterus. They also filter nourishment from the mother's blood to the baby, and filter the baby's waste back through the placenta. The presence of antiphospholipid antibodies may indicate there is an underlying process that results in recurrent pregnancy loss. Antiphospholipid antibody syndrome is a disorder of coagulation, which causes blood clots (thrombosis) in arteries and veins, as well as pregnancy-related complications such as miscarriage, pre-term delivery, or severe preeclampsia.

Antithyroid Antibodies (ATA): Antibodies are proteins produced by the immune system that help fight infections. They are usually produced in response to the introduction of foreign substances into the body. In some situations, the immune system may produce antibodies that act against integral parts of the body, causing inflammation and damage. When antithyroid antibodies are present, the body may generate antibodies that act against the tissue in the thyroid gland that can result in inflammation. This can eventually cause enough damage to lead to underactivity of the thyroid gland. This can interfere with normal thyroid function, thus with normal metabolism. These antibodies are also indicators for a predisposition of the patient to autoimmunity, which may interfere with the reproductive process.

Arcuate Uterus: An arcuate uterus has a single uterine cavity with a convex or flat uterine fundus, and an endometrial cavity with a small fundal cleft or impression. This form is often considered a normal uterine variant because it is not significantly associated with the increased risks of pregnancy loss and the complications found in other uterine malformations.

ART: See Assisted Reproduction Technology.

Artificial Insemination (AI): A procedure which includes placing sperm into the vagina, cervix, uterus or fallopian tubes through artificial means instead of by sexual intercourse — usually injected through a catheter or cannula after being washed. This technique is used to overcome sexual performance problems, to circumvent sperm-mucus interaction problems, to maximize the potential for poor semen, and for using donor sperm. See Intrauterine Insemination.

Asherman's Syndrome: This is a condition characterized by the presence of scars within the uterine cavity, and when uterine walls adhere to one another. The cavity of the uterus is lined by the endometrium. This lining is composed of two layers, the functional layer, which is shed during menstruation, and an underlying basal layer, which is necessary for regenerating the functional layer. Trauma to the basal layer can occur, typically after a dilation and curettage (D&C) performed after a missed or incomplete miscarriage, birth, or elective termination (abortion) to remove retained products of conception or placental remains. Asherman's Syndrome can result after any of the above, and can lead to the development of intrauterine scars or adhesions which obliterate the cavity to varying degrees. In the extreme, the whole cavity can become scarred and occluded. Menstrual anomalies are often but not always correlated with severity of the condition. Adhesions restricted to the cervix or lower uterus may block menstruation.

Asherman's Syndrome can result from other pelvic surgeries including Cesarean sections, or removal of fibroid tumors (myomectomy) and from causes such as IUDs, pelvic irradiation, schistosomiasis and genital tuberculosis. Chronic endometritis from genital tuberculosis is a significant cause of severe intrauterine adhesions in the developing world, often resulting in total obliteration of the uterine cavity.

Asherman's Syndrome affects women of all races and ages as there is no underlying predisposition or genetic basis to its development. It is estimated that 1% to 5% of D&Cs result in Asherman's. Asherman's results from 25% of D&Cs performed 1-4 weeks post-partum, 30.9% of D&Cs performed for missed miscarriages and 6.4% of D&Cs performed for incomplete miscarriages. In the case of missed miscarriages, the time period between fetal demise and curettage increases the likelihood of adhesion formation to over 30.9%. The risk of Asherman's also increases with the number of procedures: one study estimated the risk to be 16% after one D&C and 32% after three or more D&Cs.

Depending on the degree of severity, Asherman's Syndrome may result in infertility, repeated miscarriage, pain during menstruation and ovulation from trapped blood, and high risk pregnancies. There is evidence that if left untreated, the obstruction of menstrual flow resulting from scarring can lead to endometriosis.

Assisted Reproductive Technology (ART): Several procedures employed to bring about conception without sexual intercourse, including IUI, IVF, GIFT and ZIFT.

Asymptomatic: Having no symptoms.

Autoimmune dysfunction: An overactive immune response of the body against substances and tissues normally present in the body. In other words, the body attacks its own cells.

B

Bacterial Vaginosis (BV): Not generally considered to be a sexually transmitted infection, bacterial vaginosis is the most common cause of vaginal infection. The most common symptom of BV is an abnormal vaginal discharge (especially after sex) with an unpleasant fishy smell. Discharge, if present, is usually white or gray and can be thin.

Some women with BV report no signs or symptoms until they get severe cramps caused by the infection. Many women with BV may also experience burning during urination, or itching, swelling and irritation around the outside of the vagina. BV is associated with infertility, miscarriage, pre-term birth, and low-birth-weight babies.

Basal Body Temperature (BBT): This is a woman's body temperature when taken at its lowest point, usually in the morning before getting out of bed. Charting BBT by recording daily on a graph is used to predict ovulation.

Beta hCG Test: A blood test used to detect very early pregnancies and to evaluate embryonic development. A beta test usually refers to a quantitative hCG test (in which the units of hCG are counted), but it sometimes refers to a qualitative (yes/no) test that reads positive or negative with an hCG level under 50.

Bicornuate Uterus: (uterus with two horns) A bicornuate uterus is a congenital malformation of the uterus as the result of abnormal development of the Mullerian duct during embryogenesis. Symptoms (when present) range from amenorrhea, infertility, and/or recurrent pregnancy loss and pain, depending on the nature of the defect. The upper part of the Mullerian system that forms the uterus fails to fuse. The lower part of the uterus is normal and the upper part is bifurcated (divided in half), so the uterus is "heart-shaped."

Biphasic: Having two phases. This term is used to describe BBT charts that show a clear shift from the follicular phase (before ovulation) to the luteal phase (after ovulation).

Blastocyst: An embryo that has developed for five days after fertilization. At this point the embryo has two different cell types and a central cavity. The surface cells will become the placenta and the inner cell mass will become the fetus. A healthy blastocyst should hatch from the zona pellucida by the end of the sixth day. Within about 24 hours after hatching, it should begin to implant into the lining of the uterus, unless obstructed by adhesions, spasm or other causes.

Blighted Ovum: This is a pregnancy that stops developing at an early stage. The amniotic sac may only contain fluid (no fetal tissue) at miscarriage.

Blocking Antibodies: These are antibodies in the mother's immune system that protect her embryo during implantation.

C

Cannula: A hollow flexible tube which can be inserted into the body for the delivery or removal of fluid (i.e. during artificial insemination).

Catheter: A hollow flexible tube that can be inserted into a body cavity, duct or vessel. Catheters allow drainage or injection of fluids or access by surgical instruments. The process of inserting a catheter is catheterization. In most uses a catheter is a thin tube, or a "soft" catheter. In some uses, it is a larger, solid tube, or a "hard" catheter that is used to aspirate or inject fluids.

Cervical Cerclage: When a woman's cervix is weak (called an incompetent cervix) she is more likely to have a baby born prematurely because the cervix shortens or opens too early. In order to prevent premature labor, a gynecologist may recommend a cervical cerclage, a surgical procedure in which stitches (sutures) are put in the cervix to keep it tightly closed in an attempt to prevent miscarriage or early delivery. A cerclage used to prevent these early changes in a woman's cervix helps prevent premature labor. A closed cervix is generally intended to help a developing baby stay inside the uterus until the mother reaches at least 37-38 weeks of pregnancy.

Cervical Mucus: After a menstrual period ends, the external os (opening of the cervix) is blocked by mucus that is thick and acidic. This "infertile" mucus blocks spermatozoa from entering the uterus. For several days around the time of ovulation, "fertile" types of mucus are produced. They have higher water content, are less acidic, and have a "ferning" pattern that helps guide spermatozoa through the cervix. Ferning is a branching pattern seen in the mucus when observed with low magnification under a microscope.

Cervical mucus is one of the body's signals that ovulation is approaching. Women can learn to tell the difference between the different types of mucus their body produces each month and interpret these signals. Mucus production begins a few days before ovulation. The status of the mucus can be determined by observing the cervix with a speculum, or by reaching inside with two fingers, scooping some of the mucus off the face of the cervix and examining it. Secretions can be watery, gel-like, stretchy, sticky or dry. Fertile mucus resembles raw egg whites (watery and stretchy).

Cervical Smear: A sample of the cervical mucus examined microscopically to assess the presence of estrogen (ferning) or white blood cells (which would indicate a possible infection).

Cervical Stenosis: Tightening or closing of the internal cervical os. Cervical stenosis may be congenital or acquired. The most common acquired causes are menopause, surgery (e.g., conization, cautery), infection, cervical or uterine cancer, and radiation therapy. Cervical stenosis may be complete or partial. It may result in a hematometra (accumulation of blood in the uterus) or, (in pre-menopausal women), retrograde flow of menstrual blood into the pelvis, possibly causing endometriosis. Clinically, we have noted that cervical stenosis is often associated with adhesive cross-links which form between the muscle cells of the cervix. When we treat this condition with the Wurn Technique®, stenosis decreases and normal cervical mobility and texture generally return.

Cervicitis: An inflammation of the cervix.

Cervix: The cervix is the opening to the uterus within the vagina. The lower portion is made up of tough fibrocollagenenous fibers which become more porous and muscular toward the uterus. The cervix remains closed during pregnancy and dilates during labor and delivery to allow the baby to be born.

Chemical Pregnancy: A pregnancy that occurs when a fertilized egg does not implant into the uterine wall. If a pregnancy test is taken at just the right time it will be positive, and hCG levels are detected. However, when a repeat test is taken several days later it will be negative. The pregnancy is lost before a heartbeat is seen on an ultrasound. This is a very early miscarriage often before the woman misses a period. The majority of women who have a chemical pregnancy never know they are pregnant before they miscarry, and begin what they think is their normal menstrual cycle.

Chlamydia: Chlamydia is a common sexually transmitted disease (STD) caused by the bacterium, Chlamydia trachomatis, which can damage a woman's reproductive organs. Even though symptoms of chlamydia are usually mild or absent, serious complications that cause irreversible damage including infertility can occur "silently," before a woman ever recognizes a problem. Chlamydia can lead to Pelvic Inflammatory Disease (PID); it can also cause discharge from the penis of an infected man

Chocolate Cyst: These are cysts that form when endometrial tissue (the tissue that lines the inside of the uterus each menstrual cycle) is found in an ovary. It is responsive to monthly hormonal changes, which causes the cyst to fill with blood. It's called a "chocolate cyst" (or endometrioma) because the blood is a dark, reddish-brown color. Although often asymptomatic, chocolate cysts can be painful, especially during the menstrual period or during intercourse. Frequently, patients with large endometriomas do not have any symptoms. If the cyst ruptures or the ovary containing the cyst twists, emergency surgery may be necessary to remove the cyst, usually laparoscopically. See endometrioma.

Chronic: A disease, condition or injury that is long-lasting or recurrent. The term chronic describes the course of the disease, condition or injury or its rate of onset and development. A chronic course is distinguished from a recurrent course; recurrent diseases, conditions or injuries relapse repeatedly, with periods of remission in between. As an adjective, chronic can refer to a persistent and lasting medical condition. Chronicity is usually applied to a condition that lasts more than three months.

Chromotubation/Chromopertubation: These terms each refer to a dye test performed to help determine the condition of the fallopian tubes, and to confirm that they are patent (open). This test is usually done in combination with a diagnostic laparoscopy. Similar to an HSG, methylene blue dye is injected into the uterus. While looking inside the uterus with the laparoscope or by x-ray, physicians can see if the dye fills the fallopian tubes and spills out the tubes into the abdominal cavity. Free spillage of dye indicates totally patent (open) tubes.

Cilia: Millions of tiny hair-like fibers which line the fimbriae and interior surface of the fallopian tubes. The cilia beat in waves hundreds of times a second. It is theorized that they help catch the egg at ovulation and move it through the tube toward the uterus.

Clomid®: A commonly prescribed fertility medication (also known as Serophene® and clomiphene citrate). Clomid is taken orally to stimulate ovulation through the release of gonadotropins from the pituitary gland. Studies have found a weak association between prolonged use and ovarian cancer.

Clomiphene Citrate Challenge Test (CCCT, CCT): This test consists of the oral daily administration of 100 milligrams of clomiphene citrate on menstrual cycle days 5-9. Blood levels of FSH are measured on cycle day 3 and again on cycle day 10. Elevated blood levels of FSH on cycle day 3 or cycle day 10 are associated with very low pregnancy rates.

Collagen: Collagen is the main protein of connective tissue in animals and the most abundant protein in mammals, making up about 25% of the protein content of the entire body. Collagen fibers have a mechanical support role; they provide strength and stiffness to the tissues. Collagen is one of the long, fibrous structural proteins whose functions are quite different from those of globular proteins such as enzymes. Tough bundles of collagen called collagen fibers are a major component of the extracellular matrix that supports most tissues and gives cells structure from the outside, but collagen is also found inside certain cells. Collagen has great tensile strength, and is the main component of fascia, cartilage, ligaments, tendons, bone and teeth. Along with soft keratin, it is responsible for skin strength and elasticity, and its degradation leads to wrinkles that accompany aging.

It strengthens blood vessels and plays a role in tissue development.

Collagenous Cross-Links: Cross-links are the tiny fibrous building-blocks of adhesions. They form as a normal part of the healing process. Cross-links form in response to infection, inflammation, surgery and trauma.

The fascia reorganizes itself along the lines of tension imposed upon it in order to support and protect the structure. Where there is excess stress, cross-links can form, thickening the fascia to add strength and support. Adhesion cross-links can equally reinforce poor posture and motion. With stress or trauma, in addition to the development of elastocollagenous cross-links, the lubricating fluid (ground substance) of the fascia tends to solidify. Over time, cross-links can bind tissues and structures together that should be able to move freely. These bonds can decrease function of organs, or cause pain.

Colposcopy: This is a medical diagnostic procedure to examine an illuminated view of the cervix and the tissues of the vagina and vulva.

Conception: Conception is the fusion of gametes, or the union of sperm fusing with an ovum which eventually leads to the development of an embryo to produce a new organism.

Cone Biopsy: A cone biopsy is a surgical procedure in which a cone-shaped tissue sample from the cervix is removed for examination. Also called cervical conization, a cone biopsy is done to diagnose cervical cancer or to remove cancerous or precancerous tissue. The procedure may occasionally damage the cervix and thus disrupt normal mucus production or cause an incompetent cervix. See Incompetent Cervix.

Congenital Adrenal Hyperplasia (CAH): Congenital adrenal hyperplasia refers to a condition which can affect both fetal and infant boys and girls. People with congenital adrenal hyperplasia lack an enzyme needed by the adrenal gland to make the hormones cortisol and aldosterone. Without these hormones, the body produces more androgen, a male sex hormone. This causes male characteristics to appear early, or inappropriately.

Elevated androgens suppress the pituitary gland and interfere with spermatogenesis or ovulation. Women may have ambiguous genitalia from the excess production of male hormone, making their genitalia appear more like a male. Parents of children with CAH often elect early surgery to correct the visual anomaly. About 1 in 10,000 to 18,000 children are born with congenital adrenal hyperplasia.

Controlled Ovarian Hyperstimulation (COH): Several drugs can be used to induce ovulation in a process called controlled ovarian hyperstimulation. These drugs are prescribed for women who do not ovulate or ovulate infrequently, and also for couples with other infertility problems. The fertility medications stimulate the growth of multiple follicles for ovulation. COH is also called Superovulation.

Corpus: This refers to the body of the uterus.

Corpus Luteum: The corpus luteum, which means "yellow body" in Latin, is what is left of the follicle after ovulation. When a woman ovulates, the egg will burst from the follicle. Then what is left of the follicle will become the corpus luteum. The corpus luteum produces progesterone until the placenta begins to take over progesterone production at around ten weeks' gestation. **Progesterone** thickens the lining of the uterus to assist implantation and to sustain a healthy pregnancy.

Cul-de-sac: The space between the rectum and the uterus is called the cul-de-sac. It is defined as the area which encompasses the uterosacral ligaments (which help support the uterus in the pelvic cavity), the cervix, the top of the vagina and the rectum.

Cushing's Syndrome: A condition characterized by an overproduction of adrenal gland secretions. The person will suffer from high blood pressure, water retention, and several other symptoms. A concurrent elevation of adrenal androgens will suppress pituitary output of LH and FSH and result in ovulatory failure or in low sperm production. A woman may also develop some male sex characteristics, including abnormal hair growth. Cushing's Disease is another condition in which these same symptoms occur, but as the result of a pituitary tumor.

Cycle Day: The day of a woman's menstrual cycle. The first day (day 1) is when full flow starts before mid-afternoon.

Cyst: A fluid-filled sac.

D

D&C: See Dilation and Curettage.

D&E: See Dilation & Evacuation.

Danazol (Danocrine®): A synthetic androgen frequently prescribed to treat endometriosis. Danazol suppresses LH and FSH production by the pituitary and causes a state of amenorrhea during which the endometrial implants waste away. Side effects may include oily skin, acne, weight gain, abnormal hair growth, deepening of the voice and muscle cramps.

Day 1: The first day of a woman's cycle with menses in full flow (not just spotting). Flow should begin before mid-afternoon; otherwise the next day would be considered Day 1.

Days Post-Ovulation (DPO): The number of days a woman is past ovulation. Counting begins the day after ovulation, so if ovulation is on Wednesday, Saturday would be 3 DPO.

Days Post-Transfer (DPT): The number of days a woman is past embryo transfer. Counting begins the day after transfer, so if it is on Monday, Friday would be 4 DPT.

Dilation and Curettage (D & C): A procedure used to dilate the cervical canal and scrape out the lining and contents of the uterus. The procedure can be used to diagnose or treat the cause of abnormal bleeding and to terminate an unwanted pregnancy. We believe that D & C may cause adhesion formation on the inner uterine walls.

Dilation and Evacuation (D & E): A procedure in which the cervix is dilated and the baby and placenta are removed. D&E is used to describe two different procedures. One is similar to a D & C and uses more suction than scraping, and is performed on first-trimester pregnancies. A D & E can also be used to describe a surgical removal of a fetus between 14-20 weeks gestation as an alternative to induced labor. We believe that D & E may cause adhesion formation on the inner uterine walls.

DNA: Deoxyribonucleic Acid. The primary material of chromosomes, DNA carries the genetic code.

Donor Egg: Eggs donated by one woman to another.

Donor Insemination: Artificial insemination with donor sperm. See Artificial Insemination, Intrauterine Insemination.

Dysfunction: Abnormal function.

Dysmenorrhea: Painful menstruation.

Dyspareunia: Difficult or painful intercourse for either the man or the woman. Female dyspareunia may occur at the vaginal opening, with deep penetration, or both.

E

Ectopic Pregnancy: A pregnancy located outside of the uterus, usually in a fallopian tube. Such a pregnancy can rarely be sustained. Early treatment involves use of the chemotherapy drug methotrexate that attacks fast growing cells and may dissolve the pregnancy without causing major damage to the tube. If not treated early enough, surgery may be required to remove the trapped embryo from the tube.

Egg: The female reproductive cell is the egg; it is also called an oocyte or ovum.

Egg Donation: The donation of eggs from one woman to another for use in attempting pregnancy through IVF.

Egg Donor: A woman who donates eggs to an infertile woman for in vitro fertilization.

Egg Retrieval: A surgical procedure used to obtain eggs from ovarian follicles for use in assisted reproductive techniques such as in vitro fertilization, GIFT, and ZIFT. The procedure may be performed during laparoscopy or by using a long needle and ultrasound to locate the follicle in the ovary.

Elective Abortion: The voluntary termination of a pregnancy for non-medical reasons.

Embryo Toxic Factor (ETF): An immune response a woman may have against her own fetus in a pregnancy that may result in the loss of the pregnancy. Treatment consists of high doses of progesterone until the 16th week of pregnancy.

Embryo Transfer (ET): Placing an egg which has been fertilized outside the womb into a woman's uterus or fallopian tube.

Embryologist: A scientist who specializes in embryo development.

Empty Sella Syndrome: A condition that occurs when spinal fluid leaks into the bony chamber housing the pituitary gland (sella turcica). The sella turcica (literally "Turkish saddle") is a saddle-shaped depression in the sphenoid bone deep within the human skull. The leaking spinal fluid causes pressure which may compress the pituitary gland and adversely affect its ability to secrete LH and FSH, or elevate prolactin levels.

Endocrine Gland: Any of a number of glands that secrete hormones directly into the blood rather than through a duct. These glands include the pituitary, thyroid, parathyroid, pineal, pancreas, adrenals, ovaries and testicles.

Endocrine System: An integrated system of small glands that involve the release of signaling molecules known as hormones. The endocrine system is instrumental in regulating metabolism, tissue function, growth, development and puberty. It also plays a part in determining mood.

Endometrial Biopsy (EB, Ebx, EMB): A procedure during which a sample of the uterine lining is collected for microscopic analysis. The biopsy results confirm or deny ovulation and the proper preparation of the endometrium by estrogen and progesterone stimulation. It is usually done to check for Luteal Phase Defect or Hyperplasia.

Endometrioma: A solitary, non-cancerous pelvic mass containing endometrial tissue and blood. See Chocolate Cyst.

Endometriosis: A condition in which there is growth of endometrial tissue (the tissue that normally lines the uterus) outside the uterus. The cause of endometriosis is still uncertain. Endometriosis is most commonly found in the lower region of the female pelvis, such as on the ovary (approximately half of the cases). The broad ligaments (beneath the ovaries), uterosacral ligaments (supporting structures of the cervix) and Douglas' pouch (peritoneum between the rectum and the cervix) are frequently-involved areas and can produce intense to no pain felt in the pelvis, low back, and during pre-menstruation.

Less commonly, endometrial lesions can be found on the bladder, intestines, ureters, and diaphragm. Bowel endometriosis affects approximately 10% of women with endometriosis, and can cause severe pain with bowel movements. Each month the endometrial tissue bleeds with the onset of the menses. The resultant bleeding and irritation causes adhesions in the abdominal cavity and in the fallopian tubes. Endometriosis may also interfere with ovulation and with the implantation of the embryo. Symptoms may be painful menstruation, painful bowel movements and/or painful intercourse. It may be asymptomatic in some cases. Infertility is a common result of endometriosis.

Endometritis: Inflammation of the endometrium.

Endometrium: The inner tissue lining of the uterus which grows and sheds in response to estrogen and progesterone stimulation; the bed of tissue designed to nourish the implanted embryo.

Estradiol (E2): The principal estrogen hormone produced by the ovary, estradiol is responsible for formation of the secondary female sex characteristics such as breasts and pubic hair. It supports the growth of the follicle and the development of the uterine lining. At mid-cycle, the peak estrogen level triggers the release of the LH spike from the pituitary gland. The LH spike is necessary for the release of the ovum from the follicle. Fat cells in both obese men and women can also manufacture estrogen from androgens, and can interfere with fertility. The blood test to monitor estradiol is E2 - Rapid Assay. Women on injectable fertility drugs have routine E2 monitoring.

Estrogen: The primary female sex hormone, estrogen was first recognized around 1915. Estrogen is responsible for the development of the secondary feminine sex characteristics, which include breasts, rounded hips, and pubic hair. Together with progesterone (another female hormone made by the ovaries) estrogen regulates the changes that occur with each monthly period and prepares the uterus for pregnancy. See Estradiol.

F

Fallopian Tubes: These tiny cylindrical transport organs stretch from the uterus to the ovaries and measure about 4 to 6 inches in length. The egg travels through the tubes toward the uterus once it is released from the follicle. Sperm normally meet the egg within the fallopian tube, the site where fertilization usually occurs. The fallopian tube is divided anatomically into a few regions: closest to the uterus and within the uterine wall is the "interstitium" (where interstitial pregnancies develop), next is the "isthmus" (immediately outside the uterine wall), then the "ampulla" (midsection of the tube) and then the "infundibular or fimbrial portion " (adjacent to the ovary at the end of the tube). The ends of the fallopian tubes lying next to the ovaries feather into ends called fimbriae (Latin for "fringes" or "fingers").

Fascia: The body's primary shock absorber, fascia is a continuous three-dimensional weave of collagen and elastin fibers that divides the body's tissues and organs into different compartments (like the divisions of an orange). It unifies them into complex systems, and into a single integrated organism. The fascia transforms the pulls of gravity and muscular contractions into the controlled and harmonious movement of all our body parts. It acts to stabilize and maintain upright posture through its attachments at the lumbodorsal (thoracic and lumbar) fascia, the iliotibial band (along the outer thigh), the gluteal (buttocks) fascia, and superiorly through the thoracic and cervical fascia and into the head.

The fascia may be loose or dense, depending on its location and structure. The loose fascia wraps and protects the organs. It provides the immediate environment for exchanges between blood and cells, inflammatory reactions to trauma, immunological phenomena, and scarring. The fascia has important functions in protection, cellular respiration, elimination, metabolism, and in fluid and lymphatic flow. It can have a profound effect on the health of the cells and ultimately on the immune system. Trauma, injury or malfunction of the fascia can set up the environment for poor cellular efficiency, necrosis (tissue death), disease, pain and dysfunction throughout the body.

The dense fascia is made up of collagen and elastin fibers surrounded by a gel-like ground substance. Collagen fibers have a mechanical support role; they provide strength and stiffness to the tissues. The elastic fibers allow flexibility and extensibility to the body. The ground substance allows the fibers to glide over each other, and it absorbs the shock from any trauma and disperses it through the body. When there are restrictions in the fascial system, the forces or energy of any trauma are not able to discharge from the body, so the ground substance thickens and hardens, as collagenous cross-links form.

Due to the interconnectedness of the fascial system with all of the other body structures, any alterations in tension due to postural imbalance, gravitational pull, surgery, trauma or inflammatory processes can result in variations in connective tissue tensions and mobility throughout the body. Areas of hypertonicity (increased tone) can impose functional restrictions on the natural longitudinal glide of the fascial sheets. One area of restriction can influence and affect tissue tone in body areas both near and far.

Fertile Mucus: Mucus that allows sperm to thrive and make its way into the cervical canal, into the uterus and tubes. It resembles raw egg whites and is both stretchy and watery. Non-fertile mucus blocks sperm from entering the cervix.

Fertility Specialist: A physician specializing in the practice of fertility. Included are both gynecologists and reproductive endocrinologists. The American Board of Obstetrics and Gynecology certifies a subspecialty for Ob/Gyns who receive extra training in endocrinology (the study of hormones) and infertility. Those who acquire certification are reproductive endocrinologists (REs).

Fertility Treatment: Any method or procedure used to enhance fertility or increase the likelihood of pregnancy, such as ovulation induction treatment, varicocoele repair, microsurgery to repair damaged fallopian tubes, or various alternative/complementary therapies. The goal of fertility treatment is to assist couples in having a baby.

Fertilization: The combining of the genetic material carried by sperm and egg to create an embryo. Fertilization normally occurs inside the fallopian tube (in vivo) but may also occur in a petri dish (in vitro). See also In vitro Fertilization.

Fetus: The developing baby from the second month of pregnancy until its birth.

Fibroid (Myoma or Leiomyoma): Benign tumors of the uterine muscle and connective tissue.

Fibromyalgia: Fibromyalgia (FM) is a disorder classified by the presence of chronic widespread pain and tactile allodynia, which is a painful response to a usually non-painful stimulus such as light touch, pressure or brushing. Allodynia can occur in areas other than the one stimulated.

While the criteria for such an entity have not yet been thoroughly developed, the recognition that fibromyalgia involves more than just pain has led to the frequent use of the term "fibromyalgia syndrome. It is not contagious, and recent studies suggest that people with fibromyalgia may be genetically predisposed. The disorder is not directly life-threatening. The degree of symptoms may vary greatly from day to day with periods of flare-up (severe worsening of symptoms) or remission, however, the disorder is generally perceived as non-progressive.

Fimbriae: Finger-like projections at the end of the fallopian tube nearest the ovary. An ovary is not directly connected to its adjacent fallopian tube. When ovulation is about to occur, the sex hormones activate the fimbriae, causing them to hit the ovary in a gentle, sweeping motion. An oocyte is released from the ovary into the peritoneal cavity and the cilia of the fimbriae sweep or draw the ovum into the fallopian tube.

Follicle: A woman's eggs develop in the ovaries inside fluid-filled cysts (sacs), called follicles. During a natural menstrual cycle, several follicles begin to enlarge Over the next few weeks, only one of these follicles develops to maturity. It ruptures, and releases its egg during the process of ovulation. This follicle grows to about one inch in size when it is ready to ovulate. The other follicles that had begun to develop stop growing, degenerate and dissolve, therefore, only a small percentage of eggs present in the ovaries are ever ovulated during the woman's reproductive life span

Follicle Stimulating Hormone (FSH): A pituitary hormone that stimulates growth of the ovarian follicle in women. FSH also stimulates the Sertoli cells in the testicles and supports male sperm production. Elevated FSH levels are indicative of gonadal failure in both men and women, and of decreasing fertility in women as they age.

Frozen Embryo Transfer (FET): A procedure in which frozen embryos are thawed and then placed into the uterus.

FSH: See Follicle Stimulating Hormone.

Fundus: the upper portion of the uterus.

G

Galactorrhea: A clear or milky discharge from the breasts associated with elevated prolactin, and unassociated with childbirth or nursing.

Gamete Intrafallopian Transfer (GIFT): A technique that may be used in lieu of in vitro fertilization for women with patent (clear and open) tubes. After egg retrieval, the eggs are mixed with sperm and then immediately injected through the fimbriae into the woman's fallopian tubes for in-vivo fertilization. This procedure is done through laparoscopy.

Gestation: The period of fetal development in the uterus (womb) from implantation to birth.

GnRH: See Gonadotropin Releasing Hormone.

Gonadotropin Releasing Hormone (GnRH): The hormone produced and released by the hypothalamus which controls the pituitary gland's production and release of gonadotropins, which stimulate the gonads. See FSH, LH.

Gonadotropins: Two primary hormones control reproductive function: Follicle Stimulating Hormone (FSH) and Luteinizing Hormone (LH). In women, they stimulate the ovaries; in men, they stimulate the testicular function.

Gonads: The glands that make reproductive cells and sex hormones: the ovaries, which make eggs (ova) and estrogen, and the testicles, which make sperm and testosterone.

Gonal-F: Recombinant FSH injectable fertility medication that is used for superovulation.

Gonorrhea: A sexually transmitted disease that may lead to infertility, gonorrhea is caused by the bacteria Neisseria Gonococcus.

Gynecologist: A doctor who specializes in the diseases and the routine physical care of the reproductive system in women.

H

Habitual Abortion: A condition defined by a woman experiencing repetitive miscarriages, usually marked by two or more consecutive pregnancy losses.

Hemorrhage: Profuse, life-threatening bleeding.

Home Pregnancy Test (HPT): A test a woman can use at home to test urine for pregnancy by detecting the presence of hCG.

Hormone: Produced by an endocrine gland, a hormone is a substance that travels through the bloodstream to a specific organ, where it creates a stimulatory effect.

Hormone Replacement Therapy (HRT): Medically prescribed or administered estrogen and progesterone replacement in menopausal women.

HPT: See Home Pregnancy Test.

HRT: See Hormone Replacement Therapy.

HSC: See Hysteroscopy.

HSG: See Hysterosalpingogram.

Human Chorionic Gonadotropin (HCG): A naturally produced hormone released in early pregnancy, hCG keeps the corpus luteum producing progesterone. HCG is also administered via injection (Profasi) to trigger ovulation after some fertility treatments, and used in men to stimulate testosterone production.

Hyperplasia: The growth and proliferation of cells within an organ or tissue beyond that which is ordinarily seen. Hyperplasia may result in the gross enlargement of an organ, the formation of a benign tumor, or may be visible only under a microscope. Hyperplasia is considered to be a physiological response to a specific stimulus, and the cells of a hyperplastic growth remain subject to normal regulatory control mechanisms.

Hyperthyroidism: Overproduction of thyroid hormone by the thyroid gland. The resulting increased metabolism "burns up" estrogen too rapidly and interferes with ovulation.

Hypothalamus: A part of the brain, the hormonal regulation center, located adjacent to and above the pituitary gland. In both the man and the woman, this tissue secretes GnRH every 90 minutes or so. The pulsatile GnRH stimulates the pituitary gland to secrete LH and FSH, which stimulate the gonads. See also FSH; LH; Ovary; Pituitary Gland; Testicle.

Hypothyroidism: A condition in which the thyroid gland produces an insufficient amount of thyroid hormone. The resulting lowered metabolism interferes with the normal breakdown of "old" hormones and causes lethargy. Women with hypothyroidism will suffer from elevated prolactin and estrogen, both of which will interfere with fertility, and men will suffer from a lower sex drive and elevated prolactin (see Hyperprolactinemia).

Hysterectomy: A hysterectomy (from Greek hystera "womb") is the surgical removal of the uterus, usually performed by a gynecologist. Hysterectomy may be total (removing the body, fundus, and cervix of the uterus; often called "complete") or partial (removal of the uterine body but leaving the cervical stump, also called "supracervical").

Hysterosalpingogram (HSG): A radiological procedure to investigate the ovaries and shape of the uterine cavity, and the shape and patency (unobstructed condition) of the fallopian tubes. It entails the injection of a water-based or oil-based radio-opaque material into the cervical canal and usually fluoroscopy with image intensification. A normal result shows the filling of the uterine cavity and the bilateral filling of the fallopian tubes with the injection material. If the fallopian tubes are open (patent), the contrast medium will fill the tubes and spill out into the abdominal cavity. It can be determined whether the fallopian tubes are open or blocked and whether the blockage is located at the junction of the tube and the uterus (proximal), in the middle of the tube (mid-tubal) or at the end of the fallopian tube (distal).

Hysteroscopy (HSC): A procedure which uses a hysteroscope, (a thin telescope that is inserted through the cervix into the uterus) to visualize the interior of the uterus. Modern hysteroscopes are so thin that they can fit through the cervix with minimal or no dilation. Because the inside of the uterus is a potential cavity, like a collapsed air dome, it is necessary to fill (distend) it with either a liquid or a gas (carbon dioxide) in order to see it. Diagnostic hysteroscopy and simple operative hysteroscopy can usually be done in an office setting. Minor surgical repairs can be executed during the procedure.

I

ICSI: See Intracytoplasmic Sperm Injection.

Idiopathic Infertility: Unexplained inability to conceive, with no known cause or pathology. Idiopathic Infertility is the diagnosis given when a comprehensive array of screening tests and investigations fails to identify a cause for the infertility.

Implantation: An event that occurs early in pregnancy in which the embryo adheres to the wall of uterus. At this stage of prenatal development, the embryo is a blastocyst. By this attachment to the uterine wall, the fetus receives the oxygen and nutrients from the mother to help it grow. Implantation usually occurs in the lining of the uterus 5-10 days after ovulation; however, in an ectopic pregnancy it may occur in the fallopian tube.

Implantation Failure: Inability of the fertilized egg to properly implant in the uterine lining.

Implantation Spotting: Bleeding associated with an embryo implanting into the endometrium inside the uterus around 5-10 days after ovulation. It is not uncommon, but it is not the norm. Implantation spotting does not look like a regular menstrual period. Implantation bleeding is scanty and usually is a pink or brownish discharge.

Incompetent Cervix: A weakened cervix which opens prematurely during pregnancy, an incompetent cervix is a cause of premature birth and miscarriage. As the baby gets heavier during pregnancy, it presses down on the cervix. This pressure may cause the cervix to start to open before the baby is ready to be born. An incompetent cervix happens in only about 1 out of 100 pregnancies. A cervical cerclage is a procedure in which a stitch or two is put around the cervix to prevent its opening until removed when the pregnancy is at term.

Incomplete Abortion: A miscarriage where some fetal tissue has passed, but some remains in the uterus.

Infection: The state or condition in which the body or a part of it is invaded by a pathogenic agent (microorganism or virus) that can multiply or produce injurious effects, such as adhesions.

Infertility (IF): The inability to conceive after a year of unprotected intercourse in women under 35, or after six months in women over 35; also the inability to carry a pregnancy to term. Diagnosed problems such as anovulation, tubal blockage, and low sperm count are also included in the definition of this term. Conditions that end in the suffix "-itis" refer to infection.

Inflammation: Swelling, redness, heat and pain caused by injury such as infection. Conditions that end in the suffix "-osis" refer to inflammation.

Inhibin-F (Folliculostatin): A female feedback hormone made in the ovary to regulate FSH production by the pituitary gland.

Injectables, Injectable Fertility Medications: Medications given by injection. On some infertility forums, the word injectables is commonly used to refer to ovulation induction medications such as hMG (brands: Pergonal®, Humegon® and Repronex®), urofollitropins (brands: Fertinex® and Metrodin®), and recombinant FSH follitropins alpha and beta (brands: Follistim® and Gonal-F®).

Intracervical Insemination (ICI): One of the more commonly used types of artificial insemination, ICI is a painless and quick procedure that helps to deposit the sperm samples directly into the uterus via the cervix. This can help increase the chances that sperm will swim through the uterus and into the fallopian tubes, where they will fertilize an egg. Couples often opt for ICI because it is associated with good success rates and is less expensive than IUI procedures. ICI is typically performed by a reproductive specialist at a fertility clinic. See Artificial Insemination.

Intracytoplasmic Sperm Injection (ICSI): An in vitro fertilization procedure in which a single sperm is injected directly into an egg. This procedure is most commonly used to overcome male infertility problems, although it may also be used where eggs cannot easily be penetrated by sperm, and occasionally as a method of in vitro fertilization associated with sperm donation.

Intratubal insemination (ITI): The least commonly performed type of artificial insemination due to the fact that it is more invasive than other types of artificial insemination. ITI is associated with much higher costs. ITI consists of placing washed sperm directly into the fallopian tubes, where sperm has a better chance of fertilizing an egg and producing a viable pregnancy.

ITI is not recommended for everyone facing fertility difficulties. It is best suited for couples that are experiencing difficulty in conceiving by other types of artificial insemination, such as IUI. Women who have cervical mucus that is impeding conception may choose this procedure, and ITI is sometimes used in some cases of unexplained fertility, ejaculation dysfunction and ovulation problems. See Artificial Insemination.

Intrauterine Insemination (IUI): The process of placing sperm into the female reproductive tract to impregnate the female by using means other than sexual intercourse.

During this procedure, freshly ejaculated sperm or sperm which has been frozen and thawed is placed in the female's uterus by artificial means.

IUI is a relatively "low-tech" ART which bypasses cervical mucus and deposits the sperm closer to the fallopian tubes, where fertilization occurs. It is used to bypass hostile cervical mucus, and to overcome sperm count and motility problems. See Artificial Insemination.

Intravaginal Culture: A fertilization and culture container (e.g., for intravaginal use) with an orifice for introducing a culture medium, one or more oocytes and sperm, and a microchamber for collecting and retrieving one or more embryos.

The container body has elements for restricting access of a retrieval catheter or pipette relative to the microchamber. At least a portion of a sidewall of the container body defining the microchamber is transparent and of optical quality for microscopic inspection of embryos prior to and/or during retrieval with a catheter or a pipette.

In Vitro Fertilization (IVF): In vitro fertilization (IVF) is a process, by which egg cells are fertilized by sperm outside the woman's uterus (in vitro). IVF is a major treatment in infertility when other methods of assisted reproductive technology have failed. The process involves hormonally controlling the ovulatory process, removing ova (eggs) from the woman's ovaries, and allowing or assisting sperm to fertilize them in a fluid medium. The fertilized egg (zygote) is then transferred to the patient's uterus with the intent of creating a successful pregnancy. For IVF to be successful, it requires healthy ova, sperm that can fertilize, and a uterus that can maintain a pregnancy. Cost considerations generally place IVF as a treatment when other less expensive options have failed.

Isthmus: The portion of the fallopian tube which begins at the point where the tube emerges from the uterus.

ITI: See Intratubal Insemination.

IUI: See Intrauterine Insemination.

IVC: See Intra-vaginal Culture.

IVF: See In Vitro Fertilization.

J

K

L

Laparoscope: The instrument used to perform a laparoscopy, a laparoscope is a small telescope that can be inserted into a hole in the abdominal wall for viewing the internal organs. It is used to diagnose and treat a number of fertility problems including endometriosis, abdominal adhesions, and polycystic ovaries; it is also used in egg retrieval for in vitro fertilization. Examination of the pelvic region by using a laparoscope is called a laparoscopy.

Laparoscopy (LAP): A surgical procedure where small incisions are made in the abdomen and in the navel, where a fiberoptic scope is inserted to examine and repair any of the pelvic organs.

Laparotomy: Major open abdominal surgery where abdominal and pelvic abnormalities can be corrected, such as tubal repair and the removal of adhesions.

Lateral deviation of the uterus: This position occurs frequently and can cause infertility and genital pain. It can be caused by inflammatory lesions of the peritoneum, shortness or restriction of the round ligament on one side, restrictions along the broad ligament on one side, and/or rotated or flared ilia (the major bones of the pelvis).

LH: See Luteinizing Hormone.

LH Surge: See Luteinizing Hormone Surge.

Low Responder: A woman who does not produce many follicles after using injectable fertility medications.

LPD: See Luteal Phase Defect.

Lupron: An injectable medication used to treat endometriosis pain by down-regulating the pituitary gland and preventing the release of substances such as luteinizing hormone (LH) and follicle stimulating hormone (FSH). Without LH or FSH, the ovary will not produce follicles that will in turn decrease the production of estrogen and progesterone.

Luteal Phase: The post-ovulatory and pre-menstrual phase of a woman's cycle lasting approximately ten to sixteen days. During this phase the corpus luteum produces progesterone, which causes the uterine lining to thicken to support the implantation and growth of an embryo.

Luteal Phase Defect (or Deficiency) (LPD): A condition that occurs when the uterine lining does not develop properly due to inadequate progesterone stimulation, or because of the inability of the uterine lining to respond to progesterone stimulation. LPD may prevent embryonic implantation or cause an early miscarriage.

Luteinizing Hormone (LH): A pituitary hormone that stimulates the gonads. In the woman, LH is necessary for the production of estrogen. In the man, LH is necessary for spermatogenesis and for the production of testosterone. When estrogen reaches a critical peak in a woman, the pituitary releases a surge of LH (the LH spike or LH surge), which releases the egg from the follicle.

Luteinizing Hormone Surge (LH Surge): The spiking release of luteinizing hormone (LH) that causes release of a mature egg from the follicle. Ovulation test kits detect the sudden increase of LH, signaling that ovulation is about to occur (usually within 24-36 hours).

M

Magnetic Resonance Imaging (MRI): A procedure that uses a large magnet linked to a computer to create pictures of areas inside the body.

Meiosis: The cellular process, characteristic of reproductive cells, which allows genetic material to divide in half. Each new cell will contain twenty-three chromosomes. The spermatids (immature sperm) and ova (eggs) each contain twenty-three chromosomes, so when they combine (fertilize), the baby will have a normal complement of forty-six chromosomes.

Menarche: The time when a woman first menstruates.

Menopause: The time in her life when a woman stops menstruating.

Menorrhagia: Heavy or prolonged menstrual flow.

Metrodin (Pure FSH): An injectable form of follicle stimulating hormone used to stimulate ovulation.

Metrorrhagia: Menstrual spotting during the middle of the cycle.

Miscarriage (MC, m/c): Spontaneous loss of an embryo or fetus from the womb. See Abortion.

Missed Abortion, Missed Miscarriage: The fetus dies in the uterus but there is no bleeding or cramping. A D&C will be needed to remove the fetal remains and prevent complications. See Abortion.

Mittelschmerz: The discomfort felt on one or both sides of the lower abdomen at the time of ovulation.

Morphology: Term meaning shape. When sperm is diagnosed as having poor morphology, it means the sperm is misshapen and often incapable of fertilization.

Motility: The measurement of motion and forward progression of sperm, e.g., during a semen analysis.

Mucus: See cervical mucus.

Myofascial Pain Syndrome (MPS): A term used to describe one of the conditions characterized by chronic pain, MPS is associated with and caused by "trigger points" which are sensitive and painful areas between the muscle and fascia. These contractile knots have been documented and identified through electromyographic imaging, ultrasound, and biopsy. The symptoms can range from referred pain through myofascial trigger points to specific pains in other areas of the body.

MPS may be related to a closer-studied complex condition known as fibromyalgia (FM). By accepted definition, the pain of fibromyalgia is generalized, occurring above and below the waist and on both sides of the body. Myofascial pain is more often described as occurring in a more limited area of the body, for example, only around the shoulder and neck, and on only one side of the body.

Neither MPS nor FM is thought to be an inflammatory or degenerative condition, and the best evidence suggests that the problem is one of an altered pain threshold, with pain reported for a given amount of painful stimuli. This altered pain threshold can manifest as increased muscle tenderness, especially in the certain areas, e.g., the trapezius muscle. Both of these syndromes tend to occur more often in women than in men, and the pain may be associated with fatigue and sleep disturbances.

Myofascial Release (MFR): A form of manual soft tissue therapy, t**he primary goal of MFR** is to increase mobility and decrease pain in muscles (myo) and fascia (fascial) by using specific techniques to break down the excess collagenous cross-links which are at the core of adhesion formation. These excess cross-links may cause pain and limited movement.

Myoma (Fibroid or Leiomyoma): A non-cancerous, benign tumor of the uterine muscle and connective tissue of the uterus.

Myomectomy: A surgical procedure used to remove a fibroid tumor from the uterus, and leave the uterus intact.

N

Natural Killer Cells (NK, CD56+): Large granular lymphocytes that bond to cells and lyse to them (causing dissolution) by releasing cytotoxins. NK cells are known to be effective against cells infected with viruses and some types of tumor cells. When activated, NK cells function to fight, kill and destroy their targets. Their excessive number in the blood is correlated with pregnancy loss and reduced success in IVF cycle outcome.

Necrospermia: Condition in which sperm are produced but are found dead in the semen, thus unable to fertilize eggs.

NEST: See Non-surgical Embryonic Selective Thinning.

Non-obstructive Azoospermia: Severely impaired or non-existent sperm production. See Azoospermia.

Non-stimulated Oocyte Retrieval In (office) Fertilization (NORIF): A procedure in which the egg is removed by ultrasound aspiration from the ovaries. Unlike SCORIF, no ovulation induction hormones are used for this process. This procedure is done in the doctor's office. The egg is mixed with sperm and placed in a small plastic dish and left in the incubator for two days. The fertilized egg is then transferred to the uterus through a small plastic catheter.

Non-surgical Embryonic Selective Thinning (NEST): A form of assisted hatching using a chemical to thin the outer membrane of the zona pellucida of the egg.

NORIF: See Non-stimulated Oocyte Retrieval In (office) Fertilization.

NSA: See Non-surgical Sperm Aspiration.

O

Obstetrician-Gynecologist (Ob/Gyn): A doctor who specializes in the diseases and the routine physical care of the reproductive system of women, including treating women through pregnancy and childbirth.

Obstructive Azoospermia: The result of a blockage in the male reproductive tract. Sperm production may be normal but the sperm are trapped inside the epididymis. See Azoospermia.

Occlusion: Blockage. If fallopian tubes are occluded, it means they are blocked.

OHSS: See Hyperstimulation.

Oligomenorrhea: Infrequent menstrual periods.

Oligo-ovulation: Infrequent ovulation, usually less than six per year.

Oligospermia: Having few sperm.

Oocyte (Egg): The female reproductive cell.

Oophorectomy: Surgical removal of the ovaries.

OPK/OPT: See Ovulation Predictor Kit/Test.

Ostium: The opening of the cervix to the uterus, also called the os.

Ovarian Cyst: A fluid-filled sac inside the ovary. An ovarian cyst may be found in conjunction with ovulation disorders, tumors of the ovary, and endometriosis. See also Chocolate Cyst.

Ovarian Drilling: During a laparoscopy, an electro surgery needle is used to burn 10-12 small holes into each ovary. This procedure may help reduce androgen levels and restore cycles in women with polycystic ovaries.

Ovarian Failure: The failure of the ovary to respond to FSH stimulation from the pituitary. It is diagnosed by elevated FSH levels in the blood.

Ovarian Hyperstimulation Syndrome (OHSS): See Hyperstimulation.

Ovary: The female gonad which produces eggs and female hormones.

Ovulation: The release of the mature egg (ovum) from the ovarian follicle.

Ovulation Induction: Medical treatment performed to initiate ovulation. See also clomiphene citrate, Humegon®, Pergonal®, Repronex®, Follistim®, Gonal-f®, Fertinex® and Metrodin®.

Ovulation Predictor Kit/Test: A test kit a woman can use at home to predict forthcoming ovulation based on a surge of luteinizing hormone.

Ovulatory Dysfunction: A problem existing in the ovary where either something is abnormal in the process of developing the follicle, or the egg is not released from the follicle.

Ovulatory Failure (Anovulation): The failure to ovulate.

Ovum: The egg; the reproductive cell from the ovary; the female gamete; the sex cell that contains the woman's genetic information.

P

P4: See Progesterone.

Palpation: In manual therapy, palpation is the act of physically touching a patient's skin over his/her soft tissues, muscles, organs and bony structures in order to evaluate the structures below. A physical therapist or osteopathic physician is trained and licensed to evaluate the texture, temperature, range of motion, mobility, motility, asymmetry, spasm, tone, tenderness and resistance to deep touch. As such, palpation is used as part of their professional evaluation and treatment.

Panbypopituitarism: Complete pituitary gland failure.

Pap Smear: The removal of cells from the surface of the cervix to study microscopically to check for the presence of abnormal or cancerous cells.

Parametrium: The connective tissue of the female pelvic floor that extends from above the cervix of the uterus laterally (to the sides) between the layers of the broad ligaments.

Parlodel®: See Bromocriptine.

Partial Zona Dissection (PZD): A predecessor to ICSI in which the zona pellucida, or shell, surrounding a woman's egg is opened using either chemical dissolution or a sharp instrument to file through the shell. This is performed in order to allow easier access for the sperm to reach the egg. One concern is that PZD may result in too many sperm entering the egg.

Patent: The condition of being open, as with the fallopian tubes of the female reproductive system. For tests of patency, see chromotubation or hysterosalpingogram.

Paternal Leukocyte Immunization (PLI): Injecting a woman with her husband's (or male partner's) white blood cells to increase her fetal blocking antibodies and lower the amount of her natural killer cells.

PCO, PCOD, PCOS: See **Polycystic Ovarian Syndrome.**

PCT: See Post Coital Test.

Pelvic Inflammatory Disease (PID): An infection of the pelvic organs that can cause severe illness, high fever, and extreme pain. PID has been implicated as a frequent cause of fallopian tube blockage and pelvic adhesions.

Penis: The male organ of sexual intercourse.

Percutaneous Epididymal Sperm Aspiration (PESA): A small needle is passed directly into the head of the epididymis and fluid is aspirated. Sperm found via PESA are often used in conjunction with **Intracytoplasmic Sperm Injection** (ICSI).

Perinatologist: A doctor specializing in treating the fetus/baby and mother during pregnancy, labor, and delivery, particularly when the mother and/or baby are at a high risk for complications.

Pergonal (hMG): A medication used to replace the pituitary hormones LH and FSH. It is similar to Humegon and Repronex. It may be used to induce ovulation in women who do not respond to clomiphene citrate. It is most frequently used with women who do not normally produce estrogen because of a pituitary gland or hypothalamic malfunction. It may also be used with men to stimulate sperm production.

PESA: See Percutaneous Epididymal Sperm Aspiration.

PI: See Primary Infertility.

PID: See Pelvic Inflammatory Disease.

Pituitary Gland: The pituitary is considered to be the master gland of the body and of female reproduction. It determines when and in what quantity hormones are released. The gland is stimulated by the hypothalamus and controls virtually all hormonal functions. The pituitary gland, or hypophysis, is an endocrine gland about the size of a pea. It is a protrusion off the bottom of the hypothalamus at the base of the brain, and is well-protected in a small, bony cavity (sella turcica) covered by a dural fold. The pituitary fossa, in which the pituitary gland sits, is situated within the sphenoid bone, deep inside the skull. The pituitary controls hormonal secretions of several glands in other parts of the body, including the gonads, the adrenal and the thyroid glands.

Placenta: The embryonic tissue that implants in the uterine wall and provides a mechanism for exchanging the baby's carbon dioxide and waste products for the mother's nutrients and oxygen. The baby is connected to the placenta by the umbilical cord.

PLI: See Paternal Leukocyte Immunization.

PMS: See Premenstrual Syndrome.

POC: See Products of Conception.

POF: See Premature Ovarian Failure.

Polar Body: The discarded genetic material resulting from female germ cell division. See Meiosis.

Polycystic Ovarian Syndrome (PCOS, PCOD, or "Stein-Leventhal Syndrome"): An endocrine disorder that affects approximately 5% of all women, PCOS occurs among all races and nationalities, is the most common hormonal disorder in reproductive age women, and is a leading cause of infertility. The principal symptoms include lack of regular ovulation and/or menstruation, multiple ovarian cysts, and excessive amounts or effects of androgenic (masculine) hormones. Symptoms may also include acne and male pattern hair growth (hirsutism). Insulin resistance, diabetes, and obesity are all strongly correlated with PCOS. Symptoms and their severity vary greatly among women, and PCOS may occur without outward symptoms.

In some cases of PCOS, adhesions will partially or totally envelop the ovary like a thick sock, preventing the ovum from escaping. Surgical treatment can involve drilling several holes in the adhesive envelope to allow the egg to escape. The Wurn Technique® has shown good results clinically in some women who presented for therapy with PCOS.

Polyp: A polyp is an abnormal growth of tissue projecting from a mucous membrane. If it is attached to the surface by a narrow elongated stalk it is said to be pedunculated. If no stalk is present it is said to be sessile. Polyps are commonly found in the colon, stomach, nose, sinuses, urinary bladder and uterus. They may also occur in other mucous membranes of the body, such as the cervix and small intestine

Post Coital Test (PCT): A microscopic examination of the cervical mucus performed several hours after intercourse to determine compatibility between the woman's mucus and the man's semen, sperm-mucus interaction problems, the presence of sperm antibodies and the quality of the cervical mucus.

Post-Traumatic Stress Disorder (PTSD): A psychological disorder that develops in some individuals after a major traumatic experience such as war, rape, domestic violence or accident. There are some articles written about PTSD as a complication of infertility or as a result of pregnancy loss. Some symptoms include avoidance, guilt, depression, flashbacks, nightmares and excessive irritability.

Posterior deviation of the uterus: This common malposition of the uterus can cause infertility. Hypotonia of the round ligament or laxity in the uterovesical ligament can cause this condition, as can post-operative adhesions which attach the uterus to the broad ligament. Lumbar or sacral restrictions can also cause this deviation.

Preclinical Pregnancy: Synonym: chemical pregnancy. An early pregnancy loss that ends before the next period is due. There are usually no pregnancy symptoms, but a blood test can reveal small amounts of the pregnancy hormone hCG.

Pre-embryo: A fertilized egg before cell division begins.

Pregnyl®: Injectable hCG.

Premature Ovarian Failure, Ovarian insufficiency, POF, Primary Ovarian Insufficiency: This refers to a condition in which a woman's ovaries stop functioning and she stops having periods earlier than might normally be expected. It is associated with high levels of gonadotropins and low levels of estrogen before a woman is 40 years old. This can be natural or caused by surgery, chemotherapy or radiation. Some women with POF still have occasional periods, and the ovary may intermittently produce mature follicles. POF is sometimes called premature menopause. Many physicians believe that women with POF cannot become pregnant naturally. Fertility treatments help some women, while others use donor eggs to have children.

Premature Rupture of Membranes (PROM): Spontaneous rupture of fetal membranes at least one hour before the onset of labor. This is characterized by a trickle or gush of fluid from the vagina.

Pre-menstrual Syndrome (PMS): Emotional and physical symptoms that occur after ovulation and usually end with menstruation. In some women, the symptoms may vanish after the menstrual flow begins, but in others, it may continue even after the flow has begun.

Primary Infertility (PI): Refers to women experiencing infertility without ever having conceived. Popular usage has been extended to include those who have conceived but not had a live birth.

Products of Conception (POC): Tissues resulting from a pregnancy, such as the embryo/fetus and placenta. The term is often found on pathology reports where miscarriages are analyzed.

Profasi®: Injectable hCG.

Progesterone (P4): The hormone produced by the corpus luteum during the second half (luteal phase) of a woman's cycle. It helps to thicken the lining of the uterus in preparation for implantation of a fertilized egg. It is released in pulses, so the amount in the bloodstream is not constant.

Progesterone Withdrawal: A diagnostic procedure used to analyze menstrual irregularity and amenorrhea; a procedure used to demonstrate the presence or absence of estrogen and to demonstrate the ability of the uterus and reproductive tract to "bleed." Also, uterine "bleeding" that occurs within two weeks after taking progesterone. Prior to ovulation induction therapy, the progesterone withdrawal procedure may be used to induce a menstrual period.

Progestin: Progestin is a synthetic progesterone (Provera®).

PROM: See Premature Rupture of Membranes. It also stands for passive range of motion exercises in the physical therapy field.

Prostaglandins: Prostaglandins are hormone-like substances found in men and women. It is hypothesized that prostaglandins secreted by active, young endometrial implants may interfere with the reproductive organs by causing muscular contractions or spasms. Prostaglandins not "washed" from sperm can cause severe cramping during IUI procedures.

Prostate Gland: A gland encircling the male urethra that produces a third of the fluid in semen, including a chemical that liquefies the coagulated semen 20 minutes to one hour after entering the vagina.

Provera®: See Progestin.

PTSD: See Post-Traumatic Stress Disorder.

Pyospermia: The presence of white cells in the semen indicates possible infection and/or inflammation.

PZD: See Partial Zona Dissection.

Q

Qualitative hCG Test: A pregnancy test that gives a yes or no answer. Home pregnancy tests are qualitative.

Quantitative hCG Test: A pregnancy test in which the units of hCG are measured.

R

Radiation: A general term for any form of radiant (emitting beams of light) energy emission. Ionizing radiation has the ability to penetrate cells and deposit energy and can cause radiation injury to the cells. Radiation therapy, used as a treatment for a localized cancerous tumor, may cause massive adhesion formation.

RE: See Reproductive Endocrinologist.

Reactive Oxygen Species (ROS): Oxygen free radicals. High levels of ROS generation are linked to a reduced ability of sperm to bind to the zona pellucida. Vitamin E may significantly improve this aspect of sperm function.

Recombinant (Human) Follicle Stimulating Hormone (R-FSH, R-hFSH): Genetically engineered follicle stimulating hormone as opposed to FSH extracted from the urine of post-menopausal women. It is synthesized in vitro by cells into which genes encoding for FSH subunits have been inserted. Brand names are Gonal-f and Follistim.

Recurrent Pregnancy Loss (RPL), Recurrent Miscarriage, Recurrent Spontaneous Abortion (RSA): Repeated miscarriages. Testing can be done to try to determine the cause of such losses. If an underlying condition is found, the woman may need to be treated for the problem before a pregnancy can be carried to term.

Reproductive Endocrinologist (RE): A medical specialty combining obstetrics and gynecology with endocrinology to treat reproductive disorders that are related to endocrine problems.

Reproductive Immunologist (RI): A medical specialty combining obstetrics and gynecology with immunology to treat reproductive disorders that are related to immune problems.

Reproductive Immunophenotype (RIP): A test which looks for cells that have the CD56+ marker in order to determine the portion of natural killer cells. An NK (CD56+) cell range above 12 percent is abnormal.

Reproductive Surgeon: An Ob/Gyn or urologist who specializes in the surgical correction of anatomical disorders that affect reproductive function.

Repronex® (hMG): A medication used to replace the pituitary hormones LH and FSH. It is similar to Humegon and Pergonal and may be used to induce ovulation in women who do not respond to clomiphene citrate. Most frequently, it is used with women who do not normally produce estrogen because of a pituitary gland or hypothalamic malfunction. It may also be used with men to stimulate sperm production.

Retrograde Ejaculation: A male fertility problem in which the sperm travels backwards into the bladder instead of forward out the opening of the penis due to a failure in the sphincter muscle at the base of the bladder.

Retroverted Uterus: The uterus is tilted back toward the rectum. In most cases a retroverted uterus is congenital, but some cases are caused by pelvic surgery, pelvic adhesions, endometriosis, fibroids, pelvic inflammatory disease or the labor of childbirth. It usually does not pose any medical problems, though it can be associated with dyspareunia (pain during sexual intercourse) and dysmenorrhea (pain during menstruation).

Reversal: Term used in infertility for undoing a sterilization procedure such as a tubal ligation (tubes surgically closed), or vasectomy.

R-FSH, R-hFSH: See Recombinant (Human) Follicle Stimulating Hormone.

RIP: See Reproductive Immunophenotype.

ROS: See Reactive Oxygen Species.

RPL: See Recurrent Pregnancy Loss.

RSA: See Recurrent Spontaneous Abortion.

S

Sacroiliac joint (S-I Joint): The joint between the sacrum (at the base of the spine) and the ilia which is joined by ligaments. It is a strong, weight-bearing synovial joint The sacroiliac joint has irregular elevations and depressions that produce interlocking of the bones.

Inflammation of this joint, or sacroiliitis, may cause pain in the low back, buttocks or thighs. Another condition of the sacroiliac joint is called sacroiliac joint dysfunction (also termed SIJD). While S-I joint dysfunction also causes low back and leg pain and results from inflammation of the sacroiliac joint, it differs from sacroiliitis in that its origin is a disruption in the normal movement of the joint (too much or too little movement within the joint).

Salpingectomy: Surgical removal of the fallopian tubes.

Salpingitis: An inflammation or infection of one or both fallopian tubes.

Salpingitis Isthmica Nodosa (SIN): The term for nodular scarring of the fallopian tubes. Salpingitis refers to inflammation of the salpinx (fallopian tube); isthmica refers to the isthmus area of the fallopian tube, near the uterus. Nodosa describes the nodular appearance of the fallopian tube. In very early stages, the tubes may appear almost normal. As scarring and nodularity progress, the changes become more apparent.

Salpingolysis: Surgical removal of adhesions that restrict the movement and function of reproductive organs.

Salpingo-oophorectomy: Surgical removal of the fallopian tubes and ovaries.

Salpingostomy: A surgical incision made in a fallopian tube. This may be done to remove an ectopic pregnancy or to recreate an opening in an obstructed tube. Also: Salpingotomy.

Salpingotomy: See Salpingostomy.

SCORIF: See Stimulated Cycle Oocyte Retrieval In (office) Fertilization.

Scrotum: The sac of skin and thin muscle surrounding the man's testicles, epididymis, and vas deferens.

Secondary Infertility (SI): The inability to conceive or carry a pregnancy to term after successfully conceiving one or more children naturally. This strict medical definition describes couples for whom the pregnancy did not go to term.

Secondary Sex Characteristics: The physical qualities that distinguish man and woman, such as beard, large breasts, and deep voice. Formed under the stimulation of the sex hormones (testosterone or estrogen), these characteristics also identify those people who have gone through puberty (sexual maturity).

Semen (Seminal Fluid): The fluid that is secreted from the testicles, seminal vesicles, prostate gland, and several other glands in the male reproductive tract during ejaculation. The semen provides nourishment and protection for the sperm and a medium in which the sperm can travel to the woman's vagina. Semen may also refer to the entire ejaculate, including the sperm.

Semen Analysis (SA): A laboratory test used to assess semen quality: sperm quantity, concentration, morphology (form), and motility. In addition, it measures semen (fluid) volume and whether or not white blood cells are present, which would indicate an infection.

Semen Viscosity: The liquid flow or consistency of the semen.

Seminal Vesicles: Pair of pouch-like glands at the base of the bladder that produce much of the semen volume, including fructose (sugar) for nourishing the sperm and a chemical that causes the semen to coagulate on entering the vagina.

Seminiferous Tubules: The network of tubes in the testicles in which the sperm are formed, mature and move toward the epididymis.

Septate Uterus: A uterine abnormality in which the uterus is divided into two halves by a wall of tissue (septum).

Septum: A dividing wall within a body cavity, such as a wall dividing the uterus in half.

Serophene®: Brand name for clomiphene citrate. (See Clomid.)

Sexually Transmitted Disease (STD): An infectious disease transmitted during sex.

Sheehan's Syndrome: A condition caused by profuse hemorrhage at the time of delivery. The severe blood loss shocks the pituitary gland, which becomes nonfunctional and dies.

Short Luteal Phase: See Luteal Phase Defect.

SI: See Secondary Infertility.

SLE: See Systemic Lupus Erythematosus.

Slow Responder: A woman who takes longer than average (10 days) to produce mature follicles after receiving injectable fertility medications.

Soft tissues: In medicine, the term soft tissue refers to tissues that connect, support, or surround other structures and organs of the body. Soft tissue includes muscles, tendons, ligaments, fascia, nerves, fibrous tissues, fat, blood vessels, and synovial membranes.

Sonogram (Ultrasound): The use of high-frequency sound waves in order to visualize the female pelvic organs, specifically the uterus, ovaries, fallopian tubes, bladder, and Douglas' pouch.

The examination can be performed transabdominally, generally with a full bladder, which acts as an acoustic window to achieve better visualization of pelvic organs, or transvaginally with a specifically designed vaginal transducer head.

Larger lesions reaching into the abdomen are better seen transabdominally. The procedure is regarded as painless, noninvasive, and relatively safe, as no radiation is used. Scans are performed by healthcare professionals call sonographers, or gynecologists trained in performing ultrasounds.

Gynecologic sonography is used extensively:

to assess pelvic organs,

to diagnose and manage gynecologic problems including endometriosis, leiomyoma, adenomyosis, ovarian cysts and lesions,

to identify adnexal masses, including ectopic pregnancy,

to diagnose gynecologic cancer, and

to track the response of ovarian follicles to fertility medication (i.e. Pergonal).

Ovarian cysts can be aspirated through transvaginal sonography. This technique is used to obtain human eggs (oocytes) through sonographic directed transvaginal puncture of ovarian follicles in certain IVF procedures.

Sonohystogram: An ultrasound/sonogram in which sterile saline is injected into the uterine cavity to check for abnormalities. The procedure delineates intrauterine pathology such as polyps, Asherman's syndrome, or submucous leiomyoma. The procedure is similar to a hysterosalpingogram, but does not require iodine dye injection or radiation.

SPA: See Sperm Penetration Assay.

Sperm: The microscopic cell that carries the male's genetic information to the female's egg; the male reproductive cell; the male gamete.

Sperm Agglutination: Sperm clumping caused by antibody reactions or by infection.

Sperm Bank: A place where sperm is collected and frozen to be used at a later time by a couple or to be donated for use in an Assisted Reproductive Technique (ART).

Sperm Penetration Assay: Also called a Hamster Test, the SPA is a test used to measure the ability of sperm to penetrate a hamster egg that has been stripped of the Zona Pellucida (outer membrane).

Sperm Count: The number of sperm present in ejaculate. Also called sperm concentration or sperm density and given as the number of sperm per milliliter.

Sperm Density: The number of sperm per milliliter or cc. Sperm may be measured by its motility, morphology, count (density) and viability.

Sperm Maturation: A process during which the sperm grow and gain their ability to swim. Sperm take about ninety days to reach maturity.

Sperm Morphology: The size and shape of the sperm. This is routinely evaluated as part of a standard semen analysis. The results of a sperm morphology exam indicate the percentage of sperm that appear normal when semen is viewed under a microscope. Abnormal sperm morphology may be a contributing factor in infertility.

Normal sperm have an oval head with a long tail. Abnormal sperm may have head or tail defects — such as a large or misshapen head or a crooked or double tail. These defects may impair the ability of the sperm to reach and fertilize an egg.

Causes of abnormal morphology include:

- Testicular abnormalities that are present at birth (congenital)
- Enlargement of veins within the scrotum (varicocoele)
- High fever
- Illicit drug use
- Infections

The semen analysis may be repeated in four to six weeks to determine if the changes in morphology are temporary or permanent. Pregnancy may be possible even with poor morphology. Intrauterine insemination or in vitro fertilization methods are sometimes needed.

Sperm Motility: The ability of sperm to swim. Poor motility means the sperm have a difficult time swimming toward their goal — the egg.

Sperm Penetration: The ability of the sperm to penetrate the egg so it can deposit the genetic material during fertilization.

Sperm Viability: Refers to whether or not the sperm is alive.

Sperm Washing: A laboratory technique in which sperm are separated from semen, and motile sperm are separated from non-motile sperm. Used in assisted reproduction techniques.

Spermatic Cord: The cord suspending the testes. It is composed of veins, arteries, lymphatics, nerves and the vas deferens.

Spermatocyte: An immature sperm cell.

Spermatogenesis: Production of sperm within the seminiferous tubules.

Spermatozoa: The male reproductive cell or gamete that is also called the sperm.

Split Ejaculate: The method of collecting a semen specimen so that the first half of the ejaculate, which is rich in sperm, is caught in one container and the rest, which is mostly seminal fluid, in a second container.

Spontaneous Miscarriage, Spontaneous Abortion: An unplanned end to a pregnancy during the first 20 weeks.

STD: See Sexually Transmitted Disease.

Stein-Leventhal Syndrome: Also called Polycystic Ovarian Syndrome (PCOS). In 1935, Stein and Leventhal reported the classic symptomatology of PCOS in a group of women who had irregular menstrual cycles, amenorrhea, infertility, obesity or weight gain, acne, excessive or male pattern hair growth (hirsutism) and an accumulation of incompletely developed and enlarged follicles in the ovaries, or polycystic ovaries. The authors found that, after ovarian biopsy, the women began to menstruate regularly. As was discovered over time, women may have polycystic ovaries, yet their cases may not conform to all of the original criteria for this condition. Therefore, Stein-Leventhal syndrome became a subgroup of a more encompassing syndrome called PCOS.

Sterility: The quality or state of being unable to reproduce, of being infertile. An irreversible condition that prevents conception.

Sterilization: A surgical procedure designed to cause infertility, such as a tubal ligation or vasectomy.

Stillbirth: The death of a fetus between the twentieth week of gestation and birth.

Stimulated Cycle Oocyte Retrieval In (office) Fertilization (SCORIF): A procedure performed in the doctor's office in which the woman's ovaries are stimulated with medications such as hMG or pure FSH. The eggs are removed by ultrasound aspiration from the ovaries. The eggs are mixed with sperm and placed in a small plastic dish and left in the incubator for two days. The fertilized eggs are then transferred to the uterus through a small plastic catheter.

Subzonal Insertion (SUZI): A predecessor to ICSI, where the zona pellucida is punctured and sperm inserted into the area between the zona and the egg. Having more than one sperm enter the egg is a potential problem with this procedure.

Superovulation: Using fertility medications to stimulate the growth of multiple follicles for ovulation. This is also known as Controlled Ovarian Hyperstimulation (COH).

Surrogate Mother: A woman who agrees to become impregnated and carry a baby for another couple. She agrees to give the baby to the couple shortly after birth. This can be done using the sperm of the male and the egg of the female or with the egg of the surrogate. It may also be performed using both donor sperm and eggs from another party.

Synarel®: A synthetic hormone used for the hormonal management of endometriosis including pain relief and reduction of endometrial lesions. Synarel is also indicated for use in controlled ovarian stimulation programs prior to in vitro fertilization.

Synthetic: Made through artificial means

T

T4: See Thyroxin.

Terratogen: Any substance capable of causing malformations in a developing embryo.

Termination: The ending of a pregnancy by choice by induced labor (resulting in a live birth or stillbirth) or abortion. See Abortion.

Testes: The two male sexual glands contained in the scrotum. They produce the male hormone testosterone and the male reproductive cells (sperm).

Testicle: The male gonad. It produces sperm and male sex hormones.

Testicular Biopsy: A minor surgical procedure used to take a small sample of testicular tissue for microscopic examination; a test used to diagnose male fertility problems when no other means is available (because the biopsy procedure itself may cause testicular damage).

Testicular Enzyme Defect: A congenital enzyme defect that prevents the testes from responding to hormonal stimulation. This can result in oligospermia or azoospermia.

Testicular Failure: Occurs when the testes do not produce a normal number of mature sperm and when the hormones needed for normal sperm are abnormally elevated.

Testicular Feminization: An enzymatic defect that prevents a man from responding to the male hormone testosterone. The man will look like a woman, but karyotyping will reveal a normal XY male chromosome pattern, and testosterone levels will be in the normal male range.

Testicular Sperm Aspiration (TESA): A needle biopsy of the testicle used to obtain small amounts of sperm. A small incision is made in the scrotal skin and a spring loaded needle is fired through the testicle. Usually does not result in enough sperm to freeze for later use.

Testicular Sperm Extraction (TESE): An open biopsy where a small piece of testicular tissue is removed through a skin incision. The tissue is placed in culture media and separated into tiny pieces. Sperm are released from within the seminiferous tubules where they are produced and are then extracted from the surrounding testicular tissue. This procedure can be done using local anesthetic or IV sedation. It is possible to get enough sperm to freeze for future use.

Testicular Stress Pattern: A semen analysis result showing depressed sperm production, poor sperm motility, and poor sperm morphology. The pattern is consistent with secondary testicular failure or illness.

Testicular Torsion: A condition in which the testicle twists on itself, cutting off its own blood supply, testicular torsion causes extreme pain, and requires immediate surgical repair to reduce damage to the testicle

Testosterone: The male hormone responsible for the formation of secondary sex characteristics and for supporting the sex drive, testosterone is also necessary for spermatogenesis.

Teratospermia: Abnormally shaped sperm.

Therapeutic Abortion: Termination of a pregnancy due to severe abnormalities in the fetus, or where the mother's health is at risk. See Abortion.

Threatened Miscarriage: A threatened miscarriage occurs when certain symptoms such as vaginal bleeding or severe cramping occur during the first half of pregnancy. The symptoms may stop, or may progress to a complete miscarriage.

Thyroid Gland: The endocrine gland in the front of the neck that produces thyroid hormones to regulate the body's metabolism.

Thyroid Releasing Hormone (TRH): A peptide hormone synthesized in the hypothalamus and passed through the hypophyseal portal venous system. In the anterior pituitary, TRH stimulates synthesis and release of thyrotropin (TSH).

Thyroid Stimulating Hormone (TSH): Also called thyrotropin, TSH is a hormone produced by the pituitary gland (at the base of the brain) that promotes the growth of the thyroid gland (in the neck) and stimulates it to function.

Thyroxin (T4): Thyroxin (T4), one of the most important thyroid hormones made by the thyroid gland, has four iodine molecules attached to its molecular structure. Thyroid hormones are essential for the function of every cell in the body. They help regulate growth and the rate of chemical reactions (metabolism) in the body.

Tinnitus: Derived from the Latin word for "ringing," tinnitus is the perception of sound in the human ear in the absence of corresponding external sound. Tinnitus can be perceived in one or both ears or in the head. It is usually described as a ringing noise, but in some patients it takes the form of a high-pitched whining, buzzing, hissing, humming, whistling, or a "whooshing" sound, as of wind or waves. People have also described ticking, clicking, roaring, crickets, tree frogs, locusts or beeping. Tinnitus can be intermittent or it can be continuous, which can create great distress in the sufferer.

TMJ: Temporomandibular Joint disorder (TMJ or TMJD) refers to a complex set of conditions that can cause pain in the area of the jaw joint and associated muscles and/or problems using the jaw. Both or just one of the TM joints may be affected. TMJDs can affect a person's ability to speak, eat, chew, swallow, make facial expressions, and even breathe. Because the disorder transcends the boundaries between several health-care disciplines — in particular, dentistry, neurology, physical therapy, and psychology — there are a variety of quite different treatment approaches, and a multi-disciplinary approach is often indicated.

TORCH Organisms: TORCH organisms include toxoplasmosis, syphilis, rubella, cytomegalovirus, herpes simplex, and other diseases which may harm the embryo/fetus.

Torsion: Twisting, such as the twisting of the testes inside the scrotum. Besides causing extreme pain and swelling, the rotation twists off the blood supply and causes severe damage to the testicle. Torsion of the ovary may also occur in a woman suffering from hyperstimulation, a complication of ovulation induction treatment.

Total Effective Sperm Count: An estimate of the number of sperm in an ejaculate capable of fertilizing an egg represented by the formula: total sperm count X percent motility X percent of forward progressive motility X percent normal morphology.

Toxin: A poison produced by a living organism (plant or animal).

Transuterine Fallopian Transfer (TUFT): The placement of an embryo inside the fallopian tube after in vitro fertilization. The transfer is made by threading a tube through the cervical canal and uterus and depositing the embryo into the fallopian tube. The process is meant to mimic the natural process of a fertilized embryo traveling down the tube and implanting in the uterus.

Transvaginal: Through the vagina or across its wall, as in a surgical procedure

Transvaginal Ultrasound: An ultrasound examination performed by means of inserting a probe into the vagina. This type of ultrasound is common for viewing follicle growth This can produce better images in early pregnancy than could be obtained with conventional abdominal sonograms.

Transvaginal Ultrasound Aspiration: A technique used in in vitro fertilization to retrieve or aspirate the eggs.

TRH: See Thyroid-releasing Hormone.

Triphasic: Having three phases. This term is used to describe a basal body temperature chart that shows three levels of temperatures: low temperatures before ovulation, a shift up of at least .4 degrees Fahrenheit after ovulation, and then another shift upward that may coincide with the implantation of an embryo.

Trophoblastic Disease: See Molar Pregnancy.

TSH: See Thyroid Releasing Hormone.

Tubal Embryo Transfer (TET): The placement of an embryo inside the fallopian tube after in vitro fertilization. The process is meant to mimic the natural process of a fertilized embryo traveling down the tube and implanting in the uterus.

Tubal Ligation: A procedure to surgically tie or obstruct the fallopian tubes in order to sterilize a woman.

Tubal Patency: Open and unobstructed fallopian tubes.

Tubal Pregnancy: See Ectopic Pregnancy.

Tubocornual Anastomosis: Surgery performed to remove a blocked portion of the fallopian tube and to reconnect the tube to the uterus. Tubouterine implantation may also be performed to remove fallopian tube blockage near the uterus and reconnect the tube to the uterus.

Tuboplasty: Reconstructive surgery to correct abnormality of the fallopian tubes that is causing infertility.

Tubotubal Reanastomosis: Surgery performed to remove a diseased portion of the fallopian tube and reconnect the two ends; sterilization reversal.

TUFT: See Transuterine Fallopian Transfer.

Tumor: An abnormal growth of tissue that can be either benign (non-cancerous) or malignant (cancerous).

Tumor Necrosis Factor (TNF): a monokine produced in various parts of the body, important in attacking a tumor by stimulating leukocytosis, fever and necrosis (death of some tissues surrounded by healthy tissue). This might be described as the body's natural form of chemotherapy.

Turner's Syndrome: The most common defect contributing to genetic female fertility problems. The ovaries fail to form and appear as slender threads of atrophic ovarian tissue, referred to as streak ovaries. Karyotyping will reveal that this woman has only one female (X) chromosome instead of two or a mosaic (46XX and 45X).

U

Ultrasound (Sonogram): Used to reveal images of internal organs without the use of an x-ray. In fertility treatment, it helps to monitor follicular growth and to detect abnormalities such as cysts. The sonogram uses high-frequency sound waves. This procedure is also known as a sonogram.

Umbilical Cord: Two arteries and one vein encased in a gelatinous tube leading from the baby, in the womb to the placenta. The cord is used to exchange nutrients and oxygen from the mother, and for waste products from the baby.

Undescended Testicles (Cryptorchidism): The failure of the testicles to descend from the abdominal cavity into the scrotum by one year of age. If not repaired by age six, this may result in permanent fertility loss in a male.

Unexplained Infertility: The reasons for infertility are unable to be determined. Approximately 10 to 15 percent of couples will receive the diagnosis of unexplained infertility. Unexplained infertility is a diagnosis of exclusion, once both members of a couple have been evaluated and all tests have been negative.

Unicornuate Uterus: Uterine abnormality where the uterus is one-sided and smaller than normal. Only one side of the Mullerian duct forms. The uterus has a typical "penis shape" on imaging systems.

Ureaplasma (similar to Mycoplasma): An infection that may cause the formation of sperm antibodies and an inflammation of the uterine lining, either of which may interfere with implantation of the embryo.

Urethra: The tube-like structure through which urine passes between the bladder and the outside of the body. In the man this tube also carries semen from the area of the prostate to the outside.

Urinary Tract Infection (UTI): Infection of the kidney, ureter, bladder, or urethra. Common symptoms include a frequent urge to urinate and a painful burning when urinating, but symptoms are not always present.

Urologist: A physician/surgeon specializing in the urinary tract and male reproductive tract.

Uterus: The hollow, muscular female reproductive organ that houses, protects, and nourishes the fetus until birth. The uterus is primarily supported by the pelvic diaphragm and the urogenital diaphragm. It is also supported by several pairs of ligaments, anteriorly, posteriorly and laterally.

UTI: See Urinary Tract Infection.

V

Vagina: The female organ of sexual intercourse; the birth canal that connects the external and internal sex organs.

Vaginismus: A spasm of the muscles around the opening of the vagina, making penetration during sexual intercourse either impossible or very painful. It can be caused by physical or psychological conditions.

Vaginitis: Vaginitis is inflammation due to yeast, bacterial vaginosis, or trichomonas infections of the vagina. Frequent vaginitis may indicate the presence of pelvic adhesions and tubal blockage from other infections, such as chlamydia. Vaginitis may interfere with sperm penetration of the cervical mucus, and the symptoms may interfere with desire and the ability to have intercourse.

Venereal Disease: Any infection that can be sexually transmitted, such as chlamydia, gonorrhea, ureaplasma, and syphilis. Many of these diseases will interfere with fertility and some will cause severe illness. See also PID.

Viable: Capable of sustaining life. Often used to describe an early pregnancy in which a heartbeat has been seen.

Virus: A microscopic infectious organism that reproduces inside living cells.

Viscosity: The thickness of semen.

Vulva: The female's external genitalia.

W

X

X Chromosome: The congenital, developmental, or genetic information in the cell that transmits the information necessary to create a female. All eggs contain one X chromosome, and half of all sperm carry an X chromosome. When two X chromosomes combine, the baby will be a girl.

Y

Y Chromosome: The genetic material that transmits the information necessary to make a male. The Y chromosome can be found in one-half of the man's sperm cells. When an X and a Y chromosome combine, the baby will be a boy.

Z

ZIFT: See Zygote Intrafallopian Transfer.

Zona Pellucida: The protective outer membrane surrounding the egg.

Zygote: A fertilized egg which has not yet divided.

Zygote Intrafallopian Transfer (ZIFT): An ART in which eggs are removed from a woman's ovaries, fertilized with the man's sperm in a lab dish, and the resulting zygotes are transferred into the woman's fallopian tubes during a minor surgical procedure.

About the Authors

Larry Wurn

Larry Wurn, the third child of Lonnie and Emily Wurn, was born in 1948 in Jacksonville, Florida. His late father, Lonnie, was an immigrant from Poland at the age of nine who became a respected attorney, developer, and beloved philanthropist. His mother Emily, a Florida native, is a strong woman with a gentle heart and love of art whom Lonnie frequently called "B.W." for beautiful wife.

Inspired by his parents at an early age with the unique combination of hard work, compassion for others, a love of art and travel, Larry learned he was most happy when he explored the infinite possibilities for making the world a better place.

After graduating from the Creative Writing Department of San Francisco State University in 1972, Larry immersed himself in the Arts. He was Guest Curator for the Fine Arts Museum of San Francisco where he developed a large exhibition called "The Rainbow Show" – a celebration of art and music which took place simultaneously at all art museums throughout San Francisco and neighboring cities. Larry wrote for, and was Associate Editor of The "Rainbow Book", dedicated to color symbolism in art, science, and history.

In the mid-1980s his wife, Belinda, was diagnosed with cancer, which took him down a more humble path. For the last 20 years he has devoted himself to the profession of manual bodywork to treat adhesions, pain, and infertility which he describes as "the best art I have been involved in."

Encouraged by physician friends and associates, he graduated from the Florida Institute of National Health in 1990, and became a licensed massage therapist. He and Belinda co-developed the Wurn Technique® and co-founded Clear Passage Therapies. Together they have co-authored seven scientific studies published in peer-reviewed medical journals, and continue to conduct research and treat patients from the US and abroad.

Maintaining his love of travel, Larry has visited more than a hundred countries. He and Belinda live with their two golden retrievers in a log cabin built circa 1930 on a lake outside of Gainesville, Florida.

Belinda Wurn

Belinda Wurn was born in Cuba in 1951, the daughter of Leon and Sara Felhandler. Her grandparents all fled to Cuba from Poland, where most of their siblings were killed in concentration camps. Leon worked as a diamond cutter in Cuba, and then moved to the USA with Sara and their newborn daughter. Leon built homes with Lonnie Wurn, Belinda's future father-in-law.

Raised in Jacksonville, Florida, Belinda and Larry played together as children, not knowing that their paths would one day cross again as adults who would fall in love, and marry. But first, Belinda would earn her physical therapist degree from the University of Florida and graduate summa cum laude at the top of her class in 1975.

In 1984, while working as a physical therapist and teaching at the University of Florida as an adjunct instructor of physical therapy, she learned she had cancer of the cervix. She survived the cancer but the surgery and radiation therapy treatments left her pelvic organs totally adhered to each other. Her cure left her infertile, in debilitating pain and unable to work. Unfortunately, conventional medicine provided no relief for her.

Searching for alternatives to ease her pain, Belinda and Larry began their journey across the US and abroad. After years of travel, study and treatment by many experts in the osteopathic and physical therapy fields, Larry and Belinda began conducting their own trial and error treatments on Belinda's adhered organs. Together, they developed the techniques that relieved Belinda's pain, and gave her back her quality of life.

Together, Belinda and Larry opened several physical therapy clinics in North Florida to treat patients with chronic pain and dysfunction. When they discovered that their work could also open blocked fallopian tubes and restore reproductive function for infertile women, they co-founded Clear Passage Therapies.

Belinda has co-authored seven scientific studies published in peer-reviewed medical journals and is the author of the 600+ page Therapist Training Manual used to train and certify Clear Passage therapists.

Belinda shares Larry's passion for travel and seeing as much of the world as possible. Together, they have visited over a hundred countries. Belinda and Larry live in a log cabin built circa 1930 on a lake outside of Gainesville, Florida with their two beautiful golden retrievers.

C. Richard King

Dr. King was born in April, 1946 to Richard King, M.D., a thoracic surgeon in Atlanta, Georgia, and Barbara Nelson King. Following in his father's footsteps, he became a doctor and surgeon.

Dr. King graduated from Vanderbilt University then received his M.D. from the Medical College of Georgia and completed his residency at the University of Florida College of Medicine in 1976. He served as lieutenant commander for two years in the Navy stationed in Guam. After practicing Ob/Gynin Moultrie, Georgia for six years, he established a gynecologic practice in Gainesville, Florida in 1984. He is a Board-certified gynecologist with the American College of Obstetrics and Gynecology and a practicing clinician, surgeon and researcher.

His relationship with Larry and Belinda Wurn began in the early 1990s while serving as Chief of Staff at North Florida Regional

Hospital in Gainesville, Florida. Fascinated by the Wurns' work, Dr. King has provided medical advice and research guidance gratis to Clear Passage Therapies® since that time.

Dr. King is presently Vice-Chairman of the Board of Trustees of North Florida Regional Medical Center in Gainesville, Florida and Co-Medical Director of Florida Medical and Research Institute, a division of Southeastern Integrated Medical, PA. This is a clinical and research facility conducting research in multiple areas of medicine, including gynecology and research in women's health.

Dr. King lives in Gainesville, Florida with Susan, his wife of 37 years. Together, they have two sons and three grandchildren.

(Endnotes)

1 Wurn BF, Wurn LJ, King CR, Heuer MA, Roscow AS, Scharf ES, Shuster JJ. Treating female infertility and improving IVF pregnancy rates with a manual physical therapy technique. Med Gen Med. 2004; Jun 18; 6(2): 51. PMID 15266276.

2 Can noninvasive pelvic physical therapy open occluded fallopian tubes? Contemporary Ob/Gyn Technology. April 15, 2008; 53:12.
Wurn BF, Wurn LJ, King CR, Heuer MA, Roscow AS, Hornberger K, Scharf ES. Treating fallopian tube occlusion with a manual pelvic physical therapy. Altern Ther Health Med. Jan.-Feb. 2008; 14(1):18-23. PMID 18251317.

3 Keye et al. Infertility Evaluation and Treatment, W.B. Sanders Co.; 1995: p.

4 Domar AD, Clapp D, Slwasby EA, Dusek J, Kessel B, & Freizinger M. Impact of group psychological interventions on pregnancy rates in infertile women. Fertility and Sterility. 2000; 73 (4):805-11.

5 Paulus WE, Zhang M, Strehler E, El-Danasouri I, & Sterzik K. Influence of acupuncture on the pregnancy rate in patients who undergo assisted reproduction therapy. Fertility and Sterility. 2002; 77(4),(4): 721

6 Smith C, Coyle M, & Norman RJ. Influence of acupuncture stimulation on pregnancy rates for women undergoing embryo transfer. Fertility and Sterility. 2006: 85 (5):1352-8.

7 Wurn BF, Wurn LJ, King CR, Heuer MA, Roscow AS, Hornberger K, Scharf ES. Treating fallopian tube occlusion with a manual pelvic physical therapy. Alternative Therapies Health Medicine. 2008; 14(1): 18-23.

8 Wurn BF, Wurn LJ, King CR, Heuer MA, Roscow As, Scharf ES, Shuster JJ. Treating female infertility and improving IVF pregnancy rates with a manual physical therapy technique. Medscape General Medicine. 2004; 6(2):51

9 Glelcher N, Confino E, Cofrman R, et.al. The multicentre transcervical balloon tuboplasty study: conclusions and comparison to alternative technologies. Hum Reprod. 1993; 8(8): 1264-1271.

10 Wurn BF, Wurn LJ, King CR, Heuer MA, Roscow AS, Hornberger K, Scharf ES. Treating fallopian tube occlusion with a manual pelvic physical therapy. Altern Ther Health Med. Jan-Feb,2008; 14(1):18-23. PMID 18251317.

11 Can noninvasive pelvic physical therapy open occluded fallopian tubes? Contemporary Ob/Gyn Technology, April 15, 2008; 53:12.

12 Wurn BF, Wurn LJ, King CR, Heuer MA, Roscow AS, Hornberger K, Scharf ES. Treating fallopian tube occlusion with a manual pelvic physical therapy. Altern Ther Health Med. Jan-Feb,2008; 14(1):18-23. PMID 18251317.

13 Sato M, Yamada R, Kimura M, Maeda H, Shioyama Y, Sonomura T, et al. Transvaginal fallopian tube catheterization–diagnostic and therapeutic usefulness. Radiat Med 1993;11:49–52.

14 Wurn BF, Wurn LJ, King CR, Heuer MA, Roscow AS, Hornberger K, Scharf

ES. Treating fallopian tube occlusion with a manual pelvic physical therapy. Altern Ther Health Med. Jan-Feb, 2008; 14(1):18-23. PMID 18251317.
15 Gleicher N, Confino E, Corfman R, Coulam C, DeCherney A, Haas G, et al. The multicenter transcervical balloon tuboplasty study: conclusions and comparison to alternative technologies. Hum Reprod. 1993;8:1264–71.
16 Rier SE, Martin DC, Bowman RE, Becker JL. Immunoresponsiveness in endometriosis: implications of estrogenic toxicants. Environmental Health Perspectives. 1995; 103 (Supp 7): 151-156. The National Institute of Environmental Health Sciences (NIEHS).
17 What are the Symptoms of Endometriosis? US Dept. of Health and Human Services. http://www.4woman.gov/faq/endomet.htm#b.
18 Wurn LJ, Wurn BF, King CR, Roscow AS, Scharf ES, Shuster JJ. Treating endometriosis pain with a manual physical therapy. Fertil Steril. 2006; 86 (Supp 2): S262. Abstract.
19 http://www.cdc.gov/ART/ART2005/faq.htm#10
20 http://www.cdc.gov/ART/ART2005/faq.htm#10
21 Stephen EH: Projections of impaired fecundity among women in the United States: 1995 to 2020. Fertility and Sterility 1966;66 (2):205
22 Basson R, Berman J, Burnett A, et al. Report of the international consensus development conference on female sexual dysfunction: definitions and classifications. J Urol. 2000;163:888-893. PMID 10688001.
23 Margaret R. H. Nusbaum, DO, MPHGeorge Gamble, PhDBron Skinner, PhDJulia Heiman, PhD. The high prevalence of sexual concerns among women seeking routine gynecological care. J Fam Pract . 2000; 49:229-232.
24 Laumann EO, Paik A, Rosen RC. Sexual dysfunction in the United States: prevalence and predictors. JAMA 1999;281:537-544. PMID 10022110.
25 Wurn BF, Wurn LJ, King CR, Heuer MA, Roscow AS, Scharf ES, Shuster JJ. Treating female infertility and improving IVF pregnancy rates with a manual physical therapy Technique. Med Gen Med. Jun 18, 2004; 6(2): 51. PMID 15266276. Wurn LJ, Wurn BF, King CR, Roscow AS, Scharf ES, Shuster JJ. Improving sexual function in patients with endometriosis via a pelvic physical therapy. Fertil Steril. 2006; 86 (Supp 2): S29-30. Abstract.
26 The Female Sex ual Function Index (FSFI): A multidimensional self-report instrument for the
assessment of female sexual function. R. Rosen. Journal of Sex & Marital Therapy. 2000; 26:191–208.
27 Wurn LJ, Wurn BF, King CR, Roscow AS, Scharf ES, Shuster JJ. Increasing orgasm and decreasing dyspareunia by a manual physical therapy technique. Med Gen Med. Dec. 14, 2004; 6(4): 47. PMID 15775874
28 Wurn BF, Wurn LJ, King CR, Heuer MA, Roscow AS, Scharf ES, Shuster JJ. Treating female infertility and improving IVF pregnancy rates with a manual physical therapy technique. Med Gen Med. Jun 18, 2004; 6(2): 51. PMID 15266276.

Wurn LJ, Wurn BF, King CR, Roscow AS, Scharf ES, Shuster JJ. Improving sexual function in patients with endometriosis via a pelvic physical therapy. Fertil Steril. 2006; 86 (Supp 2): S29-30. Abstract.
29 http://diss.kib.ki.se/2005/91-7140-236-5/thesis.pdf
30 World Health Organization. Female Genital Mutilation. Fact Sheet N 241. May 2008. http://www.who.int/mediacentre/factsheets/fs241/en/
31 The American Fibromyalgia Syndrome Association. FMS Fact Sheet. http://www.afsafund.org/Fact%20Sheet.pdf.
32 Bennett RM. Beyond fibromyalgia: ideas on etiology and treatment. J Rehumatol. (suppl 19) 16:185, 1989.
33 Smythe H. Fibrositis syndrome: a historical perspective. J Rheumatol (suppl 19) 16:2, 1989.
34 Moldofsky HD et al. Musculoskeletal symptoms and non-REM sleep disturbance in patients with "fibrositis syndrome" and healthy subjects. Psychosom Med. 1975; 37: 341-351.
35 Campbell SM, et al. Clinical characteristics of fibrositis. I. A "blinded" controlled study of symptoms and tender points. Arthritis Rheum. 26:817-24, 1983.
36 McCain GA, et al. A controlled study of the effects of a supervised cardiovascular fitness training program on manifestations of primary fibromyalgia. Arthritis Rheum. 31:1135, 1988.
37 Hobson, JA. Sleep after exercise. Science 162: 1503, 1968.
38 Schneider MJ. Tender points/fibromyalgia vs. trigger points/myofascial pain syndrome: a need for clarity in terminology and differential diagnosis. J Manipulative Physiol Ther. Jul-Aug, 1995;18(6):398-406. PMID: 7595112.
39 Travell JG, Simons DG. Myofascial Pain and Dysfunction, The Trigger Point Manual. 1983. Waverly Press, Baltimore, MD.
40 Ellis H, Moran BJ, Thompson JN, Parker MC, Wilson MS, Menzies D, McGuire A, Lower AM, Hawthorn RJ, O'Brien F, Buchan S, Crowe AM. Adhesion-related hospital readmissions after abdominal and pelvic surgery: a retrospective cohort study. Lancet Br J Med. 1999; 353: 1476-80. PMID 10232313.
41 Liakakos T, Thomakos N, Fine PM, Dervenis C, Young RL. Peritoneal adhesions: etiology, pathophysiology, and clinical significance. Dig Surg. 2001; 18: 260-273. PMID 11528133.
42 Fanucci A, Cerro P, Fraracci L, Ietto F. Small bowel length measured by radiography. Gastrointest Radiol & Abdominal Imaging Journal. 1984;9(4):349-51. PMID 6500246.
43 Eskenazi B and M Warner. 1997. Epidemiology of endometriosis. Obstet Gynecol Clin North America 1997; 24(2):235-258..
44 Impact of endometriosis on women's health: comparative historical data show that the earlier the onset, the more severe the disease," Ballweg ML, Best Practice and Research Clinical Obstetrics and Gynaecology, Vol. 18, No. 2, pp. 201-218, 2004.

45 Cramer D, Missmer S. Epidemiology of endometriosis. Ann NY Acad Sci. 2002; 955:11-22.
46 Laufer MR et al. Prevalence of endometriosis in adolescent girls with chronic pelvic pain not responding to conventional therapy. J Pediatr Adolesc Gynecol. 1997; 10(4):199-202.
47 Human Reproduction 2005 20(1):279-285; doi:10.1093/humrep/deh575
51 Liakakos T, Thomakos N, Fine PM, Dervenis C, Young RL. Peritoneal adhesions: etiology, pathophysiology, and clinical significance. Dig Surg. 2001; 18: 260-273. PMID 11528133.
52 Wurn LJ, Wurn BF, King CR, Roscow AS, Scharf ES, Shuster JJ. Treating endometriosis pain with a manual physical therapy. Fertil Steril. 2006; 86 (Suppl 2): S262. Abstract.
53 Zondervan KT, Yudkin PL, Vessey MP, et al. The prevalence of chronic pelvic pain in the United Kingdom: a systematic review. Br J Obstet Gynaecol 1998;105:93–99. Search date 1996; primary sources Medline, Embase, and Psychlit. PMID 9442169.
54 An Osteopathic Approach to Diagnosis and Treatment, E.L. DiGiovanna and S. Schiowitz, Chapter One, page 4, Essay by David J. Martinke, D.O., © 1991 J. B. Lippincott Company, Philadelphia, PA54
55 National Center for Health Statistics http://www.cdc.gov/nchs/data/series/sr_23/sr23_019.pdf

For more information:

Miracle Moms, Better Sex, Less Pain

Book Orders and Inquiries:	(352) 336-3466
Online Orders:	www.medartpress.com
Fax Requests:	(352) 336-9980
Postal Requests:	Med-Arts Press PO Box 358692 Gainesville, FL 32635 USA

Clear Passage Therapies

Email info@clearpassage.com,
or fax this form to (352) 336-9980 to request:

- ❑ Postal Mail (Brochures/DVD)
- ❑ Email (Information Emails and Newsletters)

Name: ______________________________

Address: ______________________________

City: ____________________ State: ________ Zip: __________

Country: ______________________________

Telephone: ______________________________

Email address: ______________________________

For more information:

Miracle Moms, Better Sex, Less Pain

Book Orders and Inquiries:	(352) 336-3466
Online Orders:	www.medartpress.com
Fax Requests:	(352) 336-9980
Postal Requests:	Med-Arts Press PO Box 358692 Gainesville, FL 32635 USA

Clear Passage Therapies

Email info@clearpassage.com,
or fax this form to (352) 336-9980 to request:

- ❑ Postal Mail (Brochures/DVD)
- ❑ Email (Information Emails and Newsletters)

Name: ______________________________

Address: ______________________________

City: ____________________ State: ______ Zip: ________

Country: ______________________________

Telephone: ______________________________

Email address: ______________________________

LaVergne, TN USA
30 March 2010
177616LV00009B/2/P

9 780981 186801